JOB READINESS
for HEALTH PROFESSIONALS

Soft Skills Strategies for Success

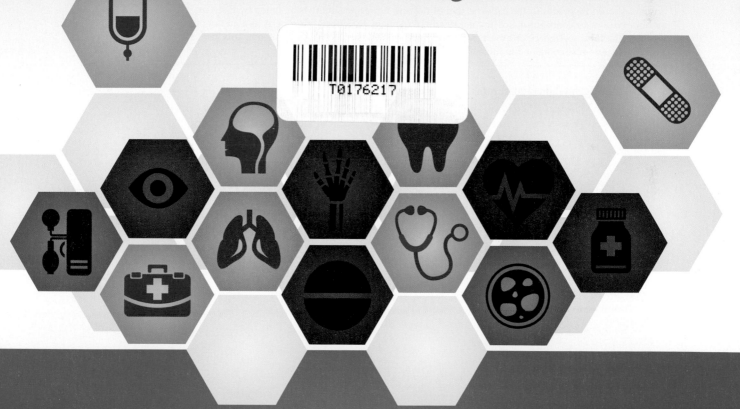

T0176217

FOURTH EDITION

ELSEVIER

Elsevier
3251 Riverport Lane
St. Louis, Missouri 63043

JOB READINESS for HEALTH PROFESSIONALS:
SOFT SKILLS STRATEGIES for SUCCESS, Fourth Edition

ISBN: 978-0-443-11108-2

Notice

Practitioners and researchers must always rely on their own experience and knowledge in evaluating and using any information, methods, compounds, or experiments described herein. Because of rapid advances in the medical sciences, in particular, independent verification of diagnoses and drug dosages should be made. To the fullest extent of the law, no responsibility is assumed by Elsevier, authors, editors, or contributors for any injury and/or damage to persons or property as a matter of products liability, negligence or otherwise, or from any use or operation of any methods, products, instructions, or ideas contained in the material herein.

Senior Content Strategist: Luke E. Held
Senior Content Development Specialist: Priyadarshini Pandey
Publishing Services Manager: Deepthi Unni
Senior Project Manager: Manchu Mohan
Design Direction: Renee Duenow

Printed in India

Last digit is the print number: 9 8 7 6 5 4 3 2 1

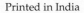

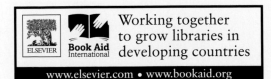

Working together
to grow libraries in
developing countries

www.elsevier.com • www.bookaid.org

CONTRIBUTOR

JAIME NGUYEN, MD, MPH, MS
Director of Healthcare Programs
Penn Foster College
Scranton, Pennsylvania

REVIEWERS

GLENDA ALGAZE, CPHT, CDA, MED
Dental Assisting Instructor, Pharmacy Technician
NAF Health Science Academy Leader
Miami Lakes Educational Center and Technical College
Miami, Florida

DEBRA BLAIS, LPN
Career Services Coordinator, Medical Assistant/Medical
    Office Specialist Instructional Lead
Nevada Career Institute
Las Vegas, Nevada

L. TAYLOR DEATHERAGE, CPC
Medical Coding Instructor
Tulsa Technology Center
Tulsa, Oklahoma

JENNIFER L. DILLARD, RMA (AMT)
Former Medical Program Chair
Everest College
Thornton, Colorado

TAMELA FREEMAN, BS, CMAA, CEHRS, CBCS
Medical Office Support Instructor
Sierra Nevada Job Corps Center
Reno, Nevada

LISA HUEHNS, MA Ed
Allied Health Instructor (AMT)
Lakeshore Technical College
Cleveland, Wisconsin

**BETH M. LAURENZ, MBA, BS Healthcare
Management, AAS, CMA, Health IT certifications**
Clinician Practitioner Consultant, Implementation
    Manager, Project Management
Director of Healthcare Education
National College
Columbus, Ohio

AMY DIANE LAWRENCE, MBA/HR, CPC, CCA
Online Program Chair for Medical Administrative
    Assistant and Medical Office Billing Specialist
Ultimate Medical Academy
Tampa, Florida

BRIGITTE NIEDZWIECKI, RN, MSN, RMA
Medical Assistant Program Director
Chippewa Valley Technical College
Eau Claire, Wisconsin

JUDITH PERELLA-ZIRKLE, MED
Certified and Registered Dental Assistant, Director of
    Dental Assisting
Cumberland County Technical Education Center
Bridgeton, New Jersey

ELIZABETH ANN PETRELLA, MSN, RN
President and CEO
Genesee Health Careers
Flint, Michigan

JULIE POPE, CMA(AAMA), CPMA, CPC, CPC-H, CPC-I
Program Director
ATA College
Louisville, Kentucky

CYNTHIA LEWIS PORTER, CDA, EFDA, PhD
Dental Coordinator
Centura College
Norfolk, Virginia

TRACY TOMKO SCHLIEP, RN
Allied Health Instructor, Healthcare Consultant
Laurel Technical Institute
Sharon, Pennsylvania

JAIME TRACKTENBERG, BS
Program Manager, Assessment and Training
Goodwill of Southwestern Pennsylvania
Pittsburgh, Pennsylvania

**BARBARA A. WILSON, MHA, BSEd, CPC, CCS-P, RHIT,
CRC, CIMC, CPC-P, CPMA**
Director of Coding Operations/Medical Billing and
    Coding Education Consultant
I-Code-For-You
Charlotte, North Carolina

AUDREY A. WOZNIAK, BS, AHI, RMA, EMT
MTTI/Women and Infant's Hospital
Seekonk, Massachusetts

MINDY WRAY, MA, BS, CMA(AAMA), RMA
Program Director, Medical Assisting
ECPI University
Greensboro, North Carolina

Health care professionals get jobs because of their hard skills—their clinical skills and their knowledge of their profession. They *keep* jobs because of their soft skills.

You don't hire for skills; you hire for attitude.
You can always teach skills.

–Herb Kelleher

Regardless of what field you are in, soft skills are essential for professional and personal success. Health care is no different, with professional or soft skills playing a significant role in ensuring high-quality patient care and creating a positive work environment for both the health care team and patients.

In addition to specific clinical and technical skills and training required for the position, the health care field requires exceptional soft skills, which include effective communication, collaborating with co-workers, successful interactions with patients, and critical thinking and time management skills. In fact, more employers are making soft skills core recruitment criteria during the hiring process.

This book will focus on the different types of soft skills you will need to be successful in your health care profession. Additionally, it will discuss and include strategies to develop different soft skills to help you as a new graduate or to advance in your current field.

Background

Oftentimes, the lack of soft skills is what holds people back in their careers and causes them to fall short of their goals and potential. This book is designed to give you the tools necessary to be successful in your chosen profession and to achieve your career goals.

How We Made Sure the Content of This Book Will Help You Succeed

There are thousands of different soft skills. This book identifies the top soft skills that are the most important to be successful as health care professionals. The book's content, format, and method of teaching were also developed from feedback from more than 135 health care professions instructors who were extensively surveyed. These health care professions instructors are from vocational-technical schools, career colleges,

community colleges, and colleges and universities and have decades of experience in the classroom as instructors and out of the classroom as health care professionals. They all work with local employers, place students in externships, and write recommendations for graduates. They all generously contributed ideas and learning strategies that have been effective in their professional experience. We are grateful for the expertise they provided in helping to create a practical guide to help. The format and features they suggested are explained further in *"Distinctive Features of This Textbook."*

Opportunities for Employment

Due to the increasing demand for health care professionals, many new graduates are being employed; however, many are having issues staying employed. Although many health care professionals are well qualified, many lack the experience and skills necessary to know how to act on the job.

Losing a job or being reprimanded for inappropriate conduct can be embarrassing and devastating. The soft skills discussed in this book will help you become a valuable member of the health care team. As a health care professional, you must possess empathy and offer meaningful care to your patients. You have worked hard to learn the skills and knowledge of your profession. It is just as important to have the soft or professional skills for your profession.

The health care field is one of the fastest-growing industries. As a health care professional, you have made a great choice. Your career opportunities are astounding! Make the most out of all the opportunities available to you by thriving in your new job.

Who Will Benefit From This Book?

Whether you are a current student, a recent graduate, or a new employee in the health care field, this book was created for you. Every new employee in any field needs soft skills to be successful. This book focuses on the health care professions because of the specific challenges you will face in this field.

Jobs in the health care professions can be stressful. Patients needing health care services are in pain, scared, and may be anxious. Not only will you have to manage these patients, but you most likely will have to interact with concerned family members and care-givers. In some cases, the patient's anxiety and fear may be inappropriately expressed as anger and even violence and directed toward the health care professionals. Additionally, health care professionals often must endure long hours and unique stressors as they uphold standards of care and follow procedures. Even co-workers and supervisors can present additional challenges. You must be able to master the different soft skills needed to handle stressful situations.

Approach

This book's approach is to make the content useful and practical by using stories, vignettes, and patient scenarios to make the content more applicable and relatable. Every patient has a story, and every shift has a tale of its own. Stories and patient scenarios are presented in features, such as Case Studies and "A Different Path," designed to illustrate what can happen to health care professionals who either possess soft skills or need help in developing them.

Each skill is presented in an easy-to-read format with summaries of the research and reasoning that supports it. The style of this book is intended to be approachable and engaging, as well as authoritative. All the features explained below in *"Distinctive Features of This Textbook"* are designed to make your learning personal and engaging and to help you relate this knowledge to your own life, background, abilities, and profession.

Organization

People learn to relate to the world using an "inside-out" process. Your personal experiences reflect your beliefs about yourself and subsequently govern your behaviors.

This book is organized to reflect this process using four key focus points:

* Self-Management and Interpersonal Skills
* Communication Skills
* Career Building Skills
* Professional Skills and Development

The book is divided into 15 chapters. Within these chapters, there are more than 40 different soft skills presented to promote your interactive learning.

Distinctive Features of This Textbook

Mastering soft skills must be a highly engaged, hands-on process. This book presents the learning process through a series of activities and thought processes designed to help you relate and integrate these skills to your own personal and professional life and circumstances.

Learning Objectives

Learning objectives are provided for each chapter to prepare you for what you will be learning. Being able to mentally prepare yourself will contribute to successful and meaningful behaviors. To affirm your learning, first read the objectives before you begin each chapter and again after you finish the chapter. Assess your understanding and learning by asking yourself if you are able to incorporate these objectives into actions and behaviors.

Quotes

Quotes can be fun and inspiring. Regardless of the quote, a quote may have different interpretations and meanings from one person to another. They can impart wisdom, encourage self-reflection, and offer new perspectives or ideas to your own set of thoughts and beliefs. Further, reading a quote from a famous and prominent individual helps remind you that every person had obstacles to overcome in their success. The iconic actress Marlene Dietrich put it well:

I love quotations because it is a joy to find thoughts one might have, beautifully expressed with much authority by someone recognized wiser than oneself.

—Marlene Dietrich

Journal Boxes

Throughout this book, you will be encouraged to keep a journal. Writing in a journal helps you internalize thoughts and process and personalize this material. We suggest journal topics throughout the book, but we also hope you will add your own topics as you think of them. By the time you have finished this book, your journal will serve as a personalized version of this book. An example of a journal box is shown below.

JOURNALING 2.4

Write about two instances in your life—one when you gave up more easily than you should have, and one when you were resilient in the face of a challenge. Which characteristics did you display in each of these situations? What were the differences and similarities in both situations that resulted in different actions?

What If? Boxes

The health care profession can be challenging and filled with dilemmas. Challenges occur at unexpected times and in unexpected ways. Your success as a health care professional depends on your ability to handle challenges. We include "What If?" boxes throughout the book to challenge your thinking with theoretical scenarios you might encounter. An example of a What If? box appears below.

> **? WHAT IF?**
>
> You live in a small town where there are few medical facilities. How can you increase your chances of finding a job?

Boxed Material

Content in boxes makes information concise and memorable and provides summaries. These boxes may include lists and steps in a process. An example of boxed material is shown below.

> **BOX 11.3**
>
> **Examples of Transferable Skills**
>
> - Work well with people from a variety of backgrounds.
> - Provide good customer service.
> - Resolve customer complaints satisfactorily.
> - Perform accurate word processing.
> - Demonstrate empathy.
> - Apply ethical standards.
> - Apply active listening skills.

Case Studies

Much of the content of this book is presented in the form of Case Studies. These are intended to bring each skill to life in a way that allows you to imagine how you would act if faced with similar circumstances. We offer "Questions for Thought and Reflection" after each case study to promote comprehension and critical thinking.

"A Different Path" Vignettes

As a companion to the Case Studies, the "A Different Path" vignettes provide different scenarios to illustrate what can go wrong when a health care professional fails to master a soft skill or take its importance

seriously. These stories are meant to open your eyes to the real reasons why soft skills are essential to your success in your health care career. We offer "Questions for Thought and Reflection" after each vignette to promote comprehension and critical thinking.

Experiential Exercises

After each skill, we offer several experiential exercises you can practice and apply outside of the classroom or workplace. You might even look at them before you read the skill material to gain advanced insights. These exercises will help you learn more about yourself and how you can use these skills to improve your as well as the skill itself. An example of an Experiential Exercises box is shown below.

> **★ EXPERIENTIAL EXERCISES**
>
> 1. Select an appropriate outfit for interviewing and make sure everything is clean and pressed.
> 2. Review your fingernails, tattoos, accessories, and hair to make sure they are appropriate for interviews.

Cross Currents With Other Soft Skills

One of the most difficult aspects of writing a book about soft skills has been the effort to isolate one skill at a time, as if these skills are not interrelated. Therefore "Cross Currents With Other Soft Skills" identify related skills and describe how they are related throughout the book. An example is shown below.

> **CROSS CURRENTS WITH OTHER SOFT SKILLS**
>
> *DRESSING FOR SUCCESS:* So much of what you wear to work and at work has a direct bearing on your grooming, hygiene, and cleanliness.
> *READING AND SPEAKING BODY LANGUAGE:* Your personal hygiene is part of your body language. Poor personal hygiene screams in body language.

New Features in the Fourth Edition

In the fourth edition, the content has been extensively reorganized to provide a more logical flow for instructors and students. The first section of the book begins with the development of soft skills, such as self-management and interpersonal skills. The next section focuses on developing successful relationships at work and mastering professional communication skills. The third section discusses being a successful student and preparing for a job. The fourth section focuses on being on the job, how to be successful in your profession and personal life, and how to advance in your job.

New Chapter and More Content

A new chapter has been added in the fourth edition, "Preparing for the Externship." With many health care training programs requiring externships, internships, or practicums, this chapter hopes to guide students through the process, be successful, and get the most benefit from this clinical experience. This edition also includes more content to help students navigate current trends and advancing technology, such as managing their social media profiles and preparing for virtual interviews.

With 15 chapters starting from being a student to a professional advancing in your career, the fourth edition of *Job Readiness for Health Professionals* is a comprehensive resource for introductory professional and soft skills and for students preparing for a successful career in the health care field.

The fourth edition will also include revised TEACH handouts, PowerPoint presentations, lesson plans, and test bank questions.

For the Instructor

TEACH for *Job Readiness for the Health Professional* is designed to help health care profession instructors prepare for class by reducing preparation time, providing new and innovative ideas to promote student learning, and helping to make full use of the rich array of resources available. Available on Evolve, TEACH includes:

* Detailed lesson plans
* Chapter-specific PowerPoint presentations
* Examview Test Bank
* Video Case Assessments and Implementation Tools.

If you can't fly then run, if you can't run then walk, if you can't walk then crawl, but whatever you do you have to keep moving forward.

—Rev. Martin Luther King, Jr.

A Note to the Reader

Remind yourself as you move forward that there are a number of people behind you, pushing and supporting you. You have already done the hard part of your profession by learning the technical skills associated with your profession. To complete your preparation and to propel yourself to even greater success, challenge yourself to master these soft skills. If you already possess some of these soft skills, share your skills and serve as a mentor to your co-workers and classmates.

Soft skills are about personal growth. This book will challenge you to step outside of your comfort zone and adopt an open mind. As the Supreme Court Judge Oliver Wendell Holmes explained it, "The imagination, once stretched by a new idea, never regains its original dimensions." Take this opportunity and challenge yourself, not just now but as you move forward in your career.

CONTENTS

SELF-MANAGEMENT AND INTERPERSONAL SKILLS

CHAPTER 1

Beginning Your Career

- Understand Your Current Approach to Work
- Explain the Benefits and Challenges of Working
- Describe How to Create a Positive Work Environment
- Explain the Benefits of Being Organized
- Develop a Plan for Managing Your Time
- Define Adaptability as an Effective Change Strategy
- Identify the Impact of Dependability
- Differentiate Between Honesty and Integrity

Dealing With the Realities of Work

What the mind can conceive and believe, it can achieve.
—Napoleon Hill

**LEARNING OBJECTIVE 1:
DEALING WITH THE REALITIES OF WORK**

- Understand the many benefits of working.
- Identify different challenges that may occur at work and with co-workers.
- List five strategies you can implement to make your approach to work more positive.
- Keep a journal and decide how you are going to use this tool for personal and professional growth and development.

Whether or not you have ever had a job before, your experiences and environment have shaped your attitudes about work. These attitudes, in turn, can affect how you approach the challenges and opportunities you may face in your career, such as finding your first job, advancing in your career, or managing conflict with co-workers. It is likely that there will be aspects of your work that you dislike. You may have to perform tasks you find boring or tedious or that are simply not your favorites. You may not agree with every managerial initiative or everything your supervisor says. You might have co-workers you do not care for.

To be successful in your work, however, you will have to accept some things you do not like. In this chapter, we will examine the realities of work a little more closely and offer strategies to help you manage your approach to work more effectively.

Realities of Work

For most of us, working is a reality and necessity of life. In order to support ourselves and pay for housing, food, and transportation, we must have a paid job. Financial security is an important reason why we work. However, there are many other benefits to working.

Work may give you a sense of identity and accomplishment. This is particularly true if your job aligns with your interests. For example, a person who likes to help people may want to work in health care while a person who likes numbers may become an accountant. It is human nature to want to grow emotionally and intellectually, and work often provides that growth and challenge. Some people enjoy working because they like taking on new challenges and learning new skills. Work also provides a social outlet or a work community. Although you may not become friends with everyone you work with, it is common for people to become friends with some of their co-workers since so much time is spent at work. Additionally, people in the same field or profession often have common interests or outlook on life (Figure 1.1).

There are, however, many challenges with work regardless of the profession and field. Some of the challenges we must overcome are occasional lack of control, the need to adapt to change, and having to manage stress and conflicts at work.

Lack of Control

Life is full of things you cannot control, including many aspects of your job. Although you may be able to exert influence upon some aspects of your work environment, there will likely be many things outside of your control, such as your co-workers, supervisors, and the type of patients you will see. What do you do about the things you have little or no control over?

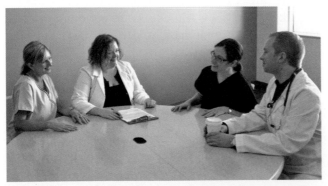

FIGURE 1.1 People in the same profession often have common interests or outlook on life.

First, recognize which elements are out of your control and accept them. Second, seek elements you *can* control and concentrate on them.

So, what can you control? In fact, you can control a lot. You have already chosen your education, and your aspirations and goals. Having options and being able to make decisions in your life can be very empowering. When you recognize you have a choice and can make a choice, you have control.

One choice you always have is how you choose to see and interpret your circumstances and the way you react to a situation. You can be understanding or surrender to your emotions. You can be tolerant or prejudiced. You can be happy, or you can be unhappy. You can forgive or hold a grudge. It is ultimately up to you. As Carlos Castaneda, an author and anthropologist, said, it takes the same effort either way.

We either make ourselves miserable, or we make ourselves happy. The amount of work is the same.
—Carlos Castaneda

Constant Change

The ancient philosopher Heraclitus claimed that change is the only constant in life or, more precisely, "life is flux." Change occurs in all areas of life, including your work. The health care industry is constantly changing with innovation, technology, research, and an ever-changing patient population. For example, electronic medical records, clinical decision software, and the use of robotics for surgical procedures would have seemed foreign just a few years ago.

Change is something you cannot always control, but you can control how you adapt to that change. But how you perceive a change often affects your ability to successfully transition. For example, if you see a change as positive and full of opportunities, you will embrace it and adapt quickly. However, if you think the change is negative and may have a detrimental effect on you, then you are likely to be resistant. Box 1.1 explains the stages people typically go through in the process of accepting change.

To be successful as a health care professional, you will need to continually adapt and be prepared to change. However, whether it is positive or negative, change can be stressful because it involves the unknown, which tends to cause fear. If you are able and open to accepting change as an ongoing and unstoppable facet of your life (and much of it positive), the better able you will be able to deal with change, and the happier you will be. Finding ways to embrace change is the key to personal and professional success.

Six Stages of Change Acceptance

1. Recognize that change can cause anxiety, disruption, and other negative emotions. You may be losing something you liked or were accustomed to.
2. Whenever you experience a loss, you are likely to feel anger. Choose to withhold judgment rather than lash out and say or do something you will regret later.
3. Recognize that the new way will take practice, learning, reinforcement, and habit change. Some people will stall, refuse to cooperate, or try to sabotage the change, but this will only make a difficult process worse.
4. Determine the positive aspects of the change.
5. Do not look back. Experience the benefits of the change, and start to see the change as the "new normal."
6. Integrate the change into your life. Look at how you have changed, perhaps becoming more versatile and resilient, by accepting the change.

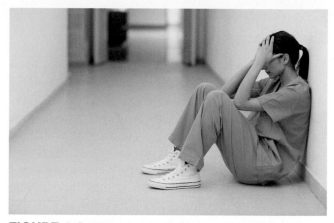

FIGURE 1.2 When in conflict, try to separate personal feelings from professional behavior. (Copyright © istock.com.)

Conflict

Very few of us get to choose our co-workers, supervisors, or patients, and nobody gets along with *everyone*. However, you do have to learn to work effectively and professionally with everyone, regardless of your personal likes or dislikes or how you feel about a person. For example, to deal better with personality clashes with your co-workers, first try to analyze the situation. What is at the root of the conflict? Then ask yourself whether there is anything you can do to improve the situation. Consider whether you might adjust your actions to work more productively with that person. For instance, communication issues are a common source of workplace conflict, whether due to a lack of information, unsuitable or irrelevant information, or misinformation. If a personality clash with one of your co-workers seems to boil down to a problem with communication, there is a lot you can do to improve the situation.

If you are concerned that a co-worker seems to dislike you, or your conflict is based on differing values or clashing personalities, you have the choice of whether to avoid or confront the issue. Although it is wise to pick your battles and avoid conflict for the sake of a cordial working relationship, there may be times when dealing with conflict head-on is the better

option. Once you acknowledge the issue with your co-worker, you can work to understand what the other person's perspective and goals are and, ideally, better understand one another. However, if there is a serious problem with a co-worker that interferes with your ability to work in a productive and positive manner, you have resources at work to help you. For example, if a co-worker acts unethically or tries to humiliate and intimidate you, then you need to present the problem to your supervisor and, if necessary, your company's Human Resources Department.

Whatever the source of the issue or conflict, try to separate your personal feelings from your professional behavior to minimize the impact of workplace conflict (Figure 1.2). Consider that your co-worker's behavior may have little or nothing to do with you. An individual's cultural background, work goals, personal motivations, or management style may all affect how they interact with you. For example, you may feel motivated to be thorough and discuss options in greater detail before making a decision on a project, whereas a co-worker who may be working on multiple projects may be more concerned with accomplishing tasks as quickly as possible. Understanding each other's goals will help you work together more effectively and successfully.

Although you may feel that you are doing your job and have done nothing wrong, remember that part of your responsibility as an employee and a professional is to work effectively with your co-workers. Providing clear, accurate, and timely information to your co-workers in a respectful way will likely go a long way toward avoiding problems. You should also remind yourself that, as co-workers, you are on the same team and share similar goals. As a result, your co-workers' goals are also yours.

Alone we can do so little; together we can do so much.
—Helen Keller

Creating a Positive Work Environment

You will likely find many aspects of your work to be positive and fulfilling. As a health care professional with specialized knowledge and skills, you are likely to find meaning in your everyday duties of helping patients with their health problems. You will most likely build a comradery with your co-workers and look forward to seeing them at work every day. There will be fun events, morale-building activities, celebrations, and team meetings to look forward to.

Your positive approach, your willingness to work hard, be friendly and professional, offer solutions to problems, and support your co-workers in their job will create a positive environment where your co-workers will enjoy working with you and will greatly improve the quality of your day-to-day work experience. The big takeaway here is that you must adapt and *choose* the attitude you adopt to face the world's challenges and your personal problems. Although you may not have total control over your work environment, you are completely in charge of your attitude, your actions, and your reactions to people and situations.

Creating Positive Expectations

One of the most beneficial things you can do is *plan* for positive outcomes. A part of planning is preparing and visualizing how you will get positive results. This process of planning and visualizing future events applies to every aspect of your day, such as scheduling your day, encountering patients, or dealing with a difficult co-worker. Planning and using visualization and having positive expectations will improve many aspects of your life, including your work. Box 1.2

BOX 1.2

Ten Steps to a Positive Attitude at Work

1. Visualize and plan for success.
2. Focus on the fun, positive aspects of your work.
3. Associate with other positive people.
4. Look at the bright side of things.
5. Do not give up easily.
6. Attack problems when they first arise.
7. Engage in positive self-talk.
8. Seek balance in your life.
9. Embrace change, as it is inevitable.
10. Have a support system in place at work and at home.

provides some important tips for creating a positive attitude at work.

Put this into practice by asking yourself what you know about, for example, an upcoming meeting. You may know the topic and the agenda. You may know the people who will attend and the purpose of the meeting. Based on this knowledge, be prepared by doing the following:

* **Plan for the meeting.** Prior to the meeting, get the agenda and review it. Is there any research you can do ahead of time to be better prepared or to contribute to the meeting? Consider who is coming. Ask yourself, who will lead this meeting and who will be influential there? Are there some people who always think alike, or others who usually disagree? Who are the positive people, and who are the negative people?
* **Plan your actions, involvement, comments, and role.** This process is part of visualization (Figure 1.3). Imagine how the meeting will go and how you will behave during it. Imagine entering the meeting room and seeing everyone. Imagine talking to people and where you will sit. Think about your own role and what outcomes you would like to see. Be prepared that the meeting may not go exactly as you visualized it, but you may be surprised at how similar many things will be to your visualization.

The future belongs to those who prepare for it today.
—Malcolm X

Changing Negative Self-Talk Into Positive Self-Talk

Think about the kinds of things you may say to yourself and what effect they have on you. For example, suppose you often say to yourself, "I do not deserve to be treated so nicely." Next, put these words in the mouth of someone who really cares about you—your supervisor, a co-worker, your mother, or your best friend. Imagine one of these people saying to you, "Tasha, you do not deserve to be treated so nicely." How would that sound and make you feel? You would probably be hurt and insulted! So, why is it all right for you to say that to yourself?

Next, think of someone you do not particularly like. Imagine that this person said, "Tasha, you do not deserve to be treated so nicely." If this happened in

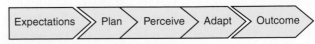

FIGURE 1.3 The process of visualization.

real life, you would likely defend yourself, if not argue with this person. You would tell them you deserve every good thing that happens to you. You would not tolerate this person saying something negative to you. Why do you then tolerate saying it to yourself?

People do not engage in negative self-talk because they think it is a good idea. They do it because it becomes a habit – a bad habit. Most of the time people are not even aware they are doing it. These are old, deeply ingrained messages that we repeat to ourselves almost unconsciously. These messages are likely not even true!

If you sometimes participate in negative self-talk, try to argue with yourself. Whenever you notice negative self-talk, reject it. Tell yourself that you will *not* accept these messages unchallenged anymore. Instead, every time you catch yourself thinking negative thoughts, replace them with affirmations about the best parts of yourself. For example, imagine you make a mistake and start saying to yourself, "You are so stupid!" Reject that statement. Tell yourself instead: "I am not stupid; I just made a mistake. I am still learning, but I have come a long way already." Show yourself the same patience and generosity that you would show a co-worker, friend, or loved one.

Tell yourself that you're not pretty. Look at you, you're beautiful.

—Natalie Merchant

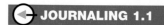 JOURNALING 1.1

Write a list of your 10 most positive qualities.

Finally, tell yourself not to take everything personally. If people cut you off in traffic, were they specifically targeting you? Probably not. It is much more likely that they had something on their mind or got distracted and made a mistake. Or maybe they are just lousy drivers.

Take these opportunities to show them some grace and patience. Even if they were rude to you, ignored you, or made a mean comment, their behavior says more about them than it does about you. You may not be able to control what others do or even your initial emotional response, but you can control your actions. You can decide what you do next. Whatever the cause, if you carry around anger and resentment all day long, then you allow the incident to have more effect on you than it needs to.

Keep a Journal

Another method to be self-motivating and to create positivity personally and professionally is keeping a journal. You may have already noticed throughout this book, there are several journaling activities.

We encourage you to keep a journal and to record your thoughts. By keeping a journal, you write down your thoughts and intentions to help you reflect and reinforce any goals. You can map your journey of change and then revisit significant moments along the way, reminding yourself of your aspirations and your strengths and building on your earlier insights. At the end of this term or course, your journal will serve as a living document of change and self-reflection, which can be used to guide you in your future development.

CASE STUDY 1.1
Shifting Gears

Claudette Wilson was born with a lot of disadvantages in her life. Her father disappeared shortly after her birth, and he was never in her life growing up. She has six half-brothers and half-sisters, all with different fathers, who are also long gone. When she was 15, Claudette dropped out of high school to help her mother take care of her younger brothers and sisters. As Claudette says with a laugh today, "I came from humble beginnings."

A year later, their financial situation worsened. Her mother realized they needed money, so she asked Claudette to get a job. Claudette began working evenings at a nearby nursing home. She had no training or certification, but she did have a natural ability to work with patients, especially the elderly. She liked them and tried to make them laugh. She was concerned about their comfort, and she worked hard to help them bathe, change their clothes and linens, and make sure they got plenty to eat. Claudette had the patience for this kind of work. She loved to talk to her patients and encouraged them to talk about their lives.

Eventually, Claudette and her boyfriend, Bob, moved to Rock Island, Illinois, where Bob got a job as a welder at a John Deere tractor factory. In Rock Island, Claudette found out about a Job Corps Center across the river in Clinton, Iowa, and she completed her high school education there and got more nursing assistant training. Over the next 5 years, she worked at different nursing homes. She and Bob got married and had three children together, two boys and a girl. Congress passed a law that required nursing assistants working in a facility that receive federal funds, such as Medicare and Medicaid, to be certified, so Claudette completed a certification program. Bob had become a foreman at John Deere, and the young family bought a small house in a nice neighborhood with good schools.

One evening at work, Claudette heard some shouting coming from one of the patient's rooms. As she ran to the room, she burst in just as Harry, one of the nurses, threw Mr. Fischer, a patient, onto a commode chair and sent him crashing into a wall. Harry started yelling and swearing at Mr. Fischer, when Claudette shouted, "Harry, stop it!"

"I've just about had it with this stubborn, old coot," said Harry, and pushed past Claudette on his way out of the room. Claudette went over to Mr. Fischer. He was shaking and crying, asking for his glasses. She got him cleaned up and dressed and brought him to the TV room where his friends congregated after dinner. She got him involved with his friends, and she was pretty sure he had forgotten all about the incident with Harry. Nevertheless, Claudette reported Harry to the Nursing Director the next day.

"That's hard to believe that Harry would do that," the Nursing Director told her.

"I couldn't believe it either," Claudette said.

Later that day, Claudette was called back into the Nursing Director's office. "Harry denies your charge," the Director said. "And Mr. Fischer doesn't remember anything about it."

"Mr. Fischer has Alzheimer's disease. Harry is not telling the truth."

"Well, I don't know. It's one person's word against another. I don't doubt your word, Claudette. But it's not easy to get RNs, and I can't go around firing a nurse without being certain. I'll keep a close eye on him." She paused, waiting for an argument from Claudette. Claudette said nothing. "Under the circumstances, it doesn't seem that you and Harry are going to be able to work together."

"No, it doesn't," said Claudette.

"So, I think it would be best for everybody if you just quietly resigned. Give us 2 weeks' notice, but leave today,

and we'll pay you for the 2 weeks and any vacation time you have coming. I'll give you a good recommendation."

"Then, I resign," said Claudette quietly. "I'll take the money, but I don't want your recommendation. It would be meaningless to me."

When Bob got home from work that afternoon, she told him what had happened. "We don't need the money," he told her. "The kids are young. Why don't you just stay home?"

"Yes," she said. "I'm going to take a break from work."

They sat in silence for several minutes. Claudette thought back to her childhood in Lexington, Kentucky, where she had sometimes been a victim of discrimination and where she saw a lot of prejudice and injustice. It had been many years since she felt discriminated against. She felt that the Nursing Director had fired her because that was the easiest thing for her to do, the simplest solution to the problem that Claudette had brought to her attention. She had to tell herself not to let those old feelings intrude into the day she was having today.

Finally, Bob broke the silence. "Today was a bad day," he said. "What did you learn from it?" Claudette sat up ramrod straight. "I'll tell you what I learned, Bobby. I'm going to become a nurse." And she did.

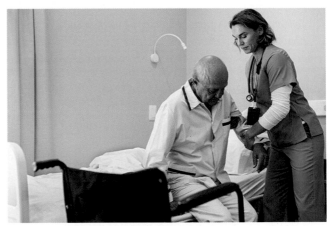

iStock.com/Ridofranz/1316202028

QUESTIONS FOR THOUGHT AND REFLECTION

1. How was Claudette able to change her life despite many early challenges in her life?
2. What role did education play in Claudette's life?
3. What role do you think a positive mental attitude played in Claudette's life and career?
4. Why did Claudette decide to become a nurse? List three reasons.
5. Do you agree with Claudette's decision to resign? How else could she have handled this situation?

A Different Path

Frank Kinsey was just about fed up. Ever since the physical therapy practice was bought by one of those giant for-profit hospital corporations, there had been one change after another. "I've been through a lot of these changes already," he would say, "and I've been against every one of them." Now, it had just been announced that the physical therapy practice was going to be moved to a location closer to the hospital, next to the Rehab Center. This would mean a longer commute for Frank and he knew more changes were likely.

In their staff meetings, Frank raised a lot of questions and concerns. He asked how many people would have a longer commute, and about half the hands went up. "What about the move itself?" he asked. "How many days is that going to take? How many of our clients are going to have to miss sessions? The medical records will probably get messed up. The company wants to make money, but they'll lose money. Think about the cost of the new building, and just the move itself. The phones, the computers—what a mess! I'm afraid we're going to lose some good people."

The practice manager, Pam Bergner, listened to Frank carefully, noting that nobody else was as vocal as Frank about the problems the move was going to cause. Still, she had not thought of some of the issues that Frank was giving voice to. She asked the Human Resources assistant, Melissa, to create a map that showed where all the employees lived and the old and the new locations, so she could see how the move would affect commutes. She saw that the commute would be longer for about half of the people and shorter for the other half. But Pam shared Frank's concern that they could lose some good people. Pam made sure she knew which employees had longer commutes, and she spoke with each one to make sure the burden would not be unreasonable or a reason to quit.

Pam arranged for a tour of the new building with all the employees when it neared completion. Frank raised more concerns. "I don't know if our equipment is going to fit here," he said. "The waiting room is too big. Our clients are going to feel like faceless people being treated by a big faceless corporation." He went on, "These tall ceilings are going to make the place noisy. The elevator is slow—it's going to take forever to get around here. I'll bet they're going to charge us for parking here. Pam, are they going to charge us for parking?"

"I'm not sure yet," said Pam, "but I know that's being discussed and considered."

"Well, there's another downside," Frank said to everyone.

Pam scheduled a meeting with Frank. "You know, Frank, I'm not the one who decided to make this move."

"I know, Pam," Frank said sympathetically. "It's a corporate move."

"Still," Pam said, "I'm responsible for the success of this move. I'm happy to discuss your concerns, and I'm glad you're raising these concerns, and they're valid. But we need to focus on how we can be successful in our move. So, in addition to raising these concerns, it would be helpful to me if you could also suggest some ideas and solutions. Otherwise, people are already concerned about the move and they'll just get more worried."

"I get it, Pam. I'll try to be more constructive," he said with a laugh.

The move went more smoothly than anyone had anticipated; even Frank was impressed. "It's a good thing I brought up that issue about the billing. I actually think they didn't lose too much money."

A few months later, the corporation decided to merge all their systems together, which was going to mean more changes for the physical therapy group.

"What a mess," said Frank. "Can't these people leave anything alone? This whole operation is going to crash."

Pam decided to call a staff meeting. She said, "We're going to go around the table, and I would like everyone to raise one issue that concerns them about the systems integration. If you don't have an issue, you can pass. Elliott, will you take notes? And Frank, just one concern per person, please," and everybody laughed.

QUESTIONS FOR THOUGHT AND REFLECTION

1. What was Frank's likely effect on morale?
2. How did Frank help Pam? How did he make Pam's job harder?
3. What could Frank have done differently to get his concerns across?
4. Why do you think Pam changed the process for identifying concerns during the systems integration? What effect did that have?

1. **Visualize an upcoming event you will attend.** If possible, imagine details using your five senses: sight, sound, taste, smell, and touch. What do you think you will you see, hear, or smell around you? What food or drink will you taste? What will you feel or touch? When you attend the event, compare your visualizations with your actual experiences. How closely did they match up? How did visualizing the event before attending affect your experiences?

2. **Think of something someone did recently that angered, annoyed, or upset you in the past.** What were some of the reasons for your emotion? How did you behave or react as a result of it? Would you do anything differently?

◎ CROSS CURRENTS WITH OTHER SOFT SKILLS

SETTING GOALS AND PLANNING ACTIONS: Now that you are equipped with a positive mental attitude, give yourself some direction. Set goals and make plans to achieve them. Your attitude means you can achieve anything, if you can conceive and believe it (Chapter 2).

AIMING TO BE ADAPTABLE AND FLEXIBLE: Your attitude enables you to adopt adaptability as an effective change strategy (Chapter 7).

MODELING PROFESSIONAL BEHAVIOR: Your attitude affects the way you treat patients and co-workers (Chapter 6).

DEALING WITH DIFFICULT PEOPLE: You will learn some tactics for this skill, but you must bring a constructive attitude to the table (Chapters 5 and 6).

EXUDING OPTIMISM, ENTHUSIASM, AND POSITIVITY: The first part of this book has focused on orienting your attitude. The last part will help you fully realize the benefits of all your hard work (Chapters 14 and 15).

Managing Your Time and Organizing Your Life

The key is in not spending time, but in investing it.
—Stephen R. Covey

LEARNING OBJECTIVE 2:
MANAGING YOUR TIME AND ORGANIZING YOUR LIFE

- Visualize your day ahead of time.
- Identify daily priorities with an appropriate sense of what is most important and a realistic sense of the time demand involved.

- Organize plans in a holistic and detailed manner.
- Choose and use some form of manual or electronic time management system that includes daily goals and a daily to-do list that puts priorities in order.
- Maintain an organized work environment.

❓ WHAT IF?

What if everything happened all at once? It's 11:00 a.m., and you have several important tasks to complete, such as ordering insulin syringes, setting up a room for a minor in-office procedure at 11:30, and preparing blood and urinalysis laboratory work for an afternoon pickup. At the last minute, the pharmacy is on the telephone trying to confirm the amount of amoxicillin to dispense to a patient.

1. What are the criteria you would use for selecting what gets completed first?
2. What if you had a reception room full of patients and one patient was having trouble breathing? Where would you fit this in the scheme of your task organization?

Organization and Time Management

If someone were to ask you to rate your organizational skills and your time management skills, would you say, "What's the difference?" Lots of people would. However, organization and time management are two different, but complementary, skills. Organization is tied to efficiency and how smoothly a job or task gets completed, whereas time management is more about prioritizing and managing tasks, thereby using time effectively. Some people can complete a task in half the time it would take another person simply because of the effective use of their time and their ability to remain organized.

Organizing From the Inside Out

Organization begins on the inside or as an internal process: learning to think in an organized fashion about a goal. This involves thinking ahead before starting a task or project, perhaps by creating lists, prioritizing tasks, and planning for the activity.

Organization is thought to be a function of the left side of the brain, whereas creativity is believed to be a function of the right side of the brain. Depending on your particular brain dominance, organization may come naturally to you, or you may struggle with

BOX 1.3

Tips for Remaining Organized and Managing Your Day

- Start your workday with the big picture in mind.
- Divide your workday into hours and schedule your goals and tasks according to the time allotted.
- Be aware of those times when you are taken off task by interruptions.
- Use the systems that are in place for organizing papers; avoid allowing piles of papers to accumulate in your area.
- Focus on working on one thing at a time. Be present with what you are working on or who you are working with.
- Practice anticipating the next move of the dentist, physician, nurse, or pharmacist by having things prepared ahead of time and ready to be administered according to the circumstance.

efficiently managing tasks, projects, and meeting deadlines. Box 1.3 offers some tips for organizing and managing your day.

Either you run the day, or the day runs you.

—Jim Rohn

 JOURNALING 1.2

Keep track this week of where the bulk of your time is going by logging your daily activities in a journal. Be sure to include the amount of time involved with each activity. Separate each activity into two columns: proactive and reactive. Write about whether your day turned out the way you visualized it or whether your day "just happened to you." How does a day that you visualized differ from one that you did not visualize? For example, do you feel more purposeful and accomplished at the end of a day you began with visualization?

Organize Your Work Environment

Working in an organized and efficient manner requires a workspace and environment that is neat and organized, so that everything has a logical place and is easily accessible. For example, patient records in a private practice should be located in cabinets that are secure and accessible to the front office staff, so they can be retrieved when patients call. These records should also be in order either by patient account or last name. With the transition to electronic medical records, this has made organization and storage much more efficient. Similarly, medical supplies should also be stored according to a logical system, so that items can be retrieved quickly and accurately from the same cabinet or shelf every time. To maintain this, reordering and restocking these supplies should be systematic, perhaps on the same day each month or on a quarterly basis, so that you never run out. In addition, avoid constantly moving items; stock and return items to the same location so the rest of your team can find them. If you share a workstation, be sure you put things exactly where you found them so that your co-worker can access them after you.

Whether you work in a cubicle, a hospital workstation, or an office of your own, strive to keep your inbox empty, whether on your desk or in your email. Once you read mail, either take immediate action or categorize it for follow-up action. Taking care of simple tasks immediately will save time in the long run and prevent forgetting to act. If you allow mail or email to pile up, you will feel overwhelmed with trying to catch up. You will most likely spend more time sorting tasks instead of using that time to move forward with completing tasks.

Be sure to label your files appropriately. For example, label your email folders so they correspond to the subject of the email that is in the folder. Finally, keep only current projects on your desk. This will prevent you from being distracted or starting several projects at once.

 JOURNALING 1.3

Write about a time when you were so distracted by interruptions that it caused you to forget something or someone else. What were the repercussions of forgetting? What could you have done differently to prevent the outcome?

A Time Management Strategy

Time management strategies go back to the early 1900s when Frederick Taylor, an American engineer, conducted time management studies in factories to boost worker productivity and output, later publishing *Principles of Scientific Management* in 1911. Since then, there have been many strategies and models for time management. Regardless, the basic principles are mostly the same.

The first step in time management is to collect all your tasks in one central place. Whether you record everything awaiting your attention in a notebook, on sticky notes, on your computer, or even in a voice recording, the task is to get everything you must do *off your mind* and into a central location. You might spend an hour or so collecting all these "to-do's" initially, and then get in the habit of recording or documenting them whenever they come up or occur to you.

Next, you will need to review and evaluate all these undone tasks and obligations. You do this by asking yourself, "What is the next thing I have to do to move this undone task toward getting done?" Once you know the answer to this question, then you have something concrete and specific that you can insert into your time flow.

Now you are ready to place your "next actions" into your calendar and organize your life and your time. If something must happen at a specific time, such as an appointment, schedule it for that time. If something must happen on a particular day, such as paying a bill, enter it into that day. If you are waiting on something before you can take the action, such as filing a laboratory test result in a patient's chart, enter into your calendar when you can expect to receive what you are waiting for so you will not forget about it and can check on it if it is late. If a next action is not time-critical, put it on your to-do list.

Schedule review periods daily and weekly to keep your schedule up to date. Every day, review and prioritize the day's events, scheduling time to prepare for them as well. Every week, collect your incomplete tasks, identify their next actions, and schedule these tasks.

Finally, the most important part of your time management system is to *do* your tasks. This should be much easier to do now that you have organized all your tasks. Anything that takes less than 2 minutes to do, such as emailing some laboratory results, should be done immediately. You do not want to wonder if you took care of a minor detail that could cause problems for you or your supervisor, co-worker, or patient later if it is not taken care of. Anything that is scheduled should be prepared for and done at the time allotted. Always have your to-do list on hand, so you know what to work on next. The steps involved in a time management system are presented in Box 1.4.

If everything you need to do is off your mind and transferred instead to your calendar or a list you constantly refer to, your time will be much less stressful, and things will get done, with little risk of falling through the cracks.

BOX 1.4

Summary of Time Management System Steps

- Collect all your undone and incomplete tasks in one central place, so they are written down rather than being a distraction in the back of your mind.
- Determine and write the next action for each one of your tasks to make it crystal clear what it will take to complete each one.
- Schedule these next actions in your life. Appointments and other time-sensitive actions should go into your calendar at specific times or days. Record everything else on your to-do list.
- Spend a few minutes organizing every day, using your calendar, your to-do lists, and your anticipation and visualization skills.
- Always have your next appointment or highest priority task teed up, so you will automatically know what to work on next to keep your life effectively managed.

Learning to Prioritize

I have two kinds of problems, the urgent and the important. The urgent are not important, and the important are never urgent.

—Dwight Eisenhower

An important aspect of time management and the process you learned above is learning how to prioritize. Health care professionals are frequently interrupted throughout the day. Therefore, it is critical to learn to prioritize tasks and know when to say, "I will get back to you within 24 hours." In other words, you need to identify what is urgent (a "now" priority) and what is important (a "later" priority). Know when you should stop what you are doing in the face of an interruption and when you should not. Sometimes, this is apparent; other times, it is not. For example, imagine drawing blood from a patient and then leaving that patient with the needle in their arm so that you could answer the phone or tend to a patient waiting at the counter. You have left the "now" priority to tend to a "later" priority. This is dangerous, and you run the risk of forgetting the first patient if you become caught up in a new task.

An effective method is using a time management matrix. A popular one was created by President Dwight Eisenhower, now called the "Eisenhower Principle," and it was how he organized his workload and priorities. He recognized that great time management means being effective as well as efficient. In other words, we must spend our time on things that are important and not just the ones that are urgent. To use the Eisenhower Principle, you need to categorize your tasks into: important and urgent; important but not urgent; not important but urgent; and not important and not urgent. The principle can be formatted into a decision matrix (Figure 1.4).

Urgent tasks require your immediate attention. When something is urgent, it must be done now, and there are clear consequences if you do not complete these tasks within a certain timeline. These are tasks you cannot avoid, and the longer you delay these tasks, the more stress you will likely experience. Important tasks may not require immediate attention, but these tasks help you achieve your long-term goals. However, just because these tasks are less urgent does not mean they do not matter or do not need to be completed. You will need to thoughtfully plan for these tasks so you can use your resources efficiently.

It is important to note that prioritizing tasks is not to be confused with procrastination. Procrastination is about putting off what needs to be done today and waiting until the last minute, usually because of an aversion to the task. Prioritizing is about sorting tasks according to urgency and importance, considering the goals for the day. Remain focused on the task you are handling, especially during direct patient care.

Here is the prime condition of success: concentrate your energy, thought, and capital exclusively upon the business in which you are engaged.
—Andrew Carnegie

Choose a Planner

There is a saying: The longest memory is shorter than the shortest pencil. That is why you need a planner to record all your appointments, commitments, notes, ideas, and aspirations. There is an endless supply of paper and electronic options.

The advantage of a paper planner is that you can always take it with you and update it easily, whenever you need to, without having to turn it on or off or charging it. They come in different formats, but most allow you to record your daily appointments, manage a to-do list, and make notes about the day's events, along with future appointment planning. The variety is so great that you can find one to fit your needs and budget.

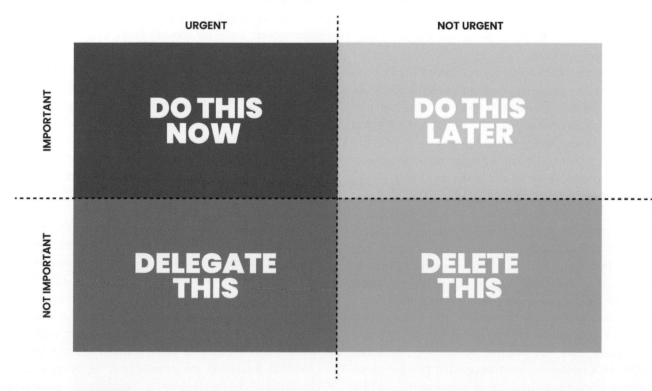

THE EISENHOWER BOX
HOW THIS DECISION MATRIX CAN HELP YOU SUCCEED

	URGENT	NOT URGENT
IMPORTANT	DO THIS NOW	DO THIS LATER
NOT IMPORTANT	DELEGATE THIS	DELETE THIS

FIGURE 1.4 The Eisenhower Principle. (iStock.com/Chavapong Prateep Na Thalang/1358702775.)

On the other hand, electronic planners are highly portable as well but make it easier to switch appointments, order and reorder priorities, and do some brainstorming. Data can also be transferred or synched to a computer or another mobile electronic device.

For health care professionals with varying work schedules, a daily planner is essential. Choose a planner that fits your lifestyle and choose one that you will *use*!

CASE STUDY 1.2
The Balancing Act

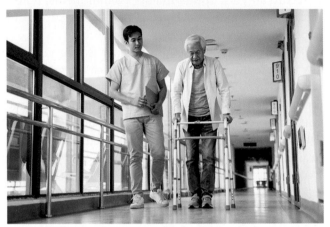

iStock.com/imtmphoto/1210903899

Robert was having a hard time adjusting to his new position as an occupational therapist. He had gotten married to Maria just a few months before he began his career in occupational therapy. Taking on these new life challenges, he is feeling overwhelmed.

Robert was quickly hired right out of college. His Upstate New York employer was delighted with Robert's education and credentials and immediately filled his schedule with new patient appointments. Robert did not want a job that required him to work overtime, but he never seemed to get home before 7:00 p.m. He had so many notes and documentations to compile at the end of the day that it always took him longer than he thought. He had planned to do the documentation in the 15 minutes between his appointments but ended up spending this time getting to know his co-workers instead. As the new person, he thought it was important to connect with the other members of the clinic staff and get to know them. As he got to know his new co-workers, he enjoyed the time he spent with them.

Regardless, Maria, who had initially tried to be patient with Robert as he started his new career, was now becoming frustrated. She had resolved to develop her cooking skills as a newlywed, even though her position as an operations manager at Great Lakes Shipping had its own demands. Now, her creative dishes got cold in front of her as she awaited Robert's arrival, which seemed to get later every day. Clearly, she thought—and Robert agreed—he needed to manage his time better.

Robert had been giving a lot of thought to what he might do to better manage his time at work and had already come up with some strategies. He was going to speak to the clinic director, LaMarsha, about limiting his appointments to only seven patients a day. He also decided that he would complete his documentation between his sessions and would eat lunch with his co-workers so he could continue staying connected to them. However, Robert did not think these steps would be enough to be effective and worried that they would not work. He needed to have a strategy.

Robert set aside two hours to collect all his uncompleted tasks, from trivial things like getting his oil changed to major things like planning their first Christmas holiday together as a married couple. He also included work-related tasks, such as reviewing the new assessment tools and ordering toys for his child clients. He also added, "Speak to LaMarsha about workload." Soon, he had a long list of tasks.

Next, he added a "next action" to every one of the uncompleted tasks he had identified, even adding a few more as they occurred to him. He took out his Day-Timer and scheduled every next action he could and then put the rest on a list. He made a special list for projects—tasks that were more complicated and would take multiple steps to achieve, like lining up internships with local employers for his clients. Finally, he grouped his tasks by location. There were tasks he could do only at work or only at home, tasks he needed to do with his computer, and tasks that could be batched and completed in less than 2 minutes each. He also batched his Saturday errands.

The following Tuesday, he met with LaMarsha about his appointment load. Instead of just dumping the problem in her lap, he offered several ideas and proposals. Robert proposed that the occupational therapy assistant, Ernie, could take some of the patient load. Some of the appointments could be reduced from 45 minutes to 25 minutes, because they were just check-ins, so Robert could see two clients in the time he would normally see one. He and LaMarsha discussed the possibility of recruiting another occupational therapist with a specialty in pediatrics, because children were becoming a larger part of the practice. In the end, they agreed on some short-term solutions and some longer-term solutions. "I'm married with three kids," she told him. "I understand the situation, and I appreciate your being proactive."

That evening, Robert was home by 5:15 p.m., even before Maria. He was even able to have dinner ready for her when she arrived home.

QUESTIONS FOR THOUGHT AND REFLECTION

1. What time management tools did Robert use?
2. Why was Robert unable to anticipate how long his work would take him?
3. What other priorities emerged at work that Robert might not have considered?
4. What will Robert have to do to make these time management improvements stick in his life?

A Different Path

Natalie is a dental assistant with a few years of experience, and she works for a busy private dental practice. She has good dental skills, but she is often distracted and inconsistent. One day, she rolled in late to work to find her employer, Dr. Cho, frantically setting up the room for the first patient. When Natalie arrived, she put her purse and lunch away and then seated the patient, who was waiting in the reception room.

For the rest of the day, the team was a bit frantic, with the team running 30 to 45 minutes behind on each patient because Natalie had not come in 30 minutes before the start of the day to set up all the procedure trays and run the autoclave to sterilize all the instruments. In addition, they did not have enough bits for the dental drill because they were not sterilized and were not ready to be used on patients. The dentist had to assist Natalie the entire day in order to catch up. The team was not able to take a lunch break, because they still had patients scheduled at specific times.

At 3:00 p.m., a patient arrived to have his gold crown permanently cemented; however, the crown was not back from the laboratory. Natalie approached the receptionist, Karen, to inquire about the laboratory case. Karen said she had confirmed the patient's appointment without knowing whether the crown had been returned from the laboratory. Natalie informed Dr. Cho about the situation, who was upset. He did not know what to do about the patient because he was leaving on a trip. When he informed the patient that the crown was not done yet, the patient was upset. He asked why they confirmed his appointment if they did not have the crown back. "This has just been a waste of my time!" he murmured as he rescheduled his appointment.

The dentist let the patient know that he would give him a discount for the inconvenience. Although the patient appreciated the gesture, he was still upset that he had to fight traffic to arrive on time, only to have to return later for the same treatment.

The next patient was seated while the previous one rescheduled his appointment. This patient was in a wheelchair and required nitrous oxide sedation. To transfer the patient from the wheelchair into the treatment chair, it took several people, including the patient's wife. Once the patient was in the treatment chair, the patient's wife left for an hour to shop while he underwent treatment. However, when they turned on the nitrous oxide tank, it was empty, and there was no backup tank. Dr. Cho asked the staff what happened, and Natalie said she had forgotten to order another one. She admitted she did not have a system for ordering and for monitoring when the tanks got low. As a result, the dentist had to explain to the patient that he could not treat him. The patient had to sit there for an hour until his wife returned.

On most days, the staff leave at about 5:00 p.m. However, on this day due to so many issues, the day ended at 6:20 p.m. Everyone left stressed, frustrated, and reactive to everything going on around them.

The next day, Natalie came in on time in the morning but returned from lunch 30 minutes late. Natalie's boss, Dr. Cho, decided to discuss Natalie's performance. He decided to wait until the end of the day, so that all the patients were treated, and their conversation did not affect the outcome of the day. Dr. Cho met with Natalie to discuss her behavior and its effect on his practice. She apologized and explained that she had been partying one of the nights and was hungover, which led her to be unfocused at work. The other night she had a problem with her boyfriend. Although Dr. Cho was concerned about his assistant's life, he was more concerned about his practice and the care of his patients. He gave her a verbal warning about her behavior and told her in no uncertain terms that it had to improve, or she would be terminated.

QUESTIONS FOR THOUGHT AND REFLECTION

1. How did Natalie's lack of self-management affect the team?
2. How would you resolve the two situations where the patient arrived, but nothing was ready?
3. How could the events of this day have been avoided?
4. What are some organizational and time management tools that Natalie could use?

1. **Identify and write on the board or a piece of paper anything you believe is an issue that could possibly affect your work and the outcome of your day at work,** including personal and professional issues. Separate on the board those things you believe are within your control and those you believe are not.

2. **Role-play in pairs, with one person being a doctor and another person being an assistant. For the doctor, how would you address the disorganization of the assistant?** Discuss how this affects patient care. For the assistant, how would you react in this situation?

3. **Define the following terms and provide a personal example for each:**
   a. Procrastination
   b. Distraction
   c. Interruption

4. **Contact a nursing facility and ask for a tour.** At the end of your tour, think about whether you would have a family member stay there. Consider the level of organization of the facility and whether the appropriate systems and processes are in place for patient care. Would you recommend this facility for care? Why or why not?

5. **Think about a time when something in your personal life affected your work at a job or at school.** How did it affect your job or schooling? In retrospect, was there anything you could have done to prevent it?

🌀 CROSS CURRENTS WITH OTHER SOFT SKILLS

SETTING GOALS AND PLANNING ACTIONS: Knowing how much time and energy you must spend on your daily tasks and how long tasks will take will help you to allocate your time and energy effectively to achieve target goals (Chapter 8).

GAINING ENERGY, PERSISTENCE, AND PERSEVERANCE: Being able to manage your time and organize your life will allow you to attack your work with renewed vigor (Chapter 3).

MANAGING STRESS: Nothing eases stress like being organized and knowing what to do next (Chapter 8).

SEPARATING YOUR WORK AND PERSONAL PROBLEMS: An integrated time management system will improve balance in your life. It will make it clear that you can take care of work-related problems only when you are at work and home-related problems when you are not at work (Chapters 7 and 13).

Being Adaptable and Flexible

Adaptability is the simple secret of survival.
—Jessica Hagedorn

LEARNING OBJECTIVE 3: BEING ADAPTABLE AND FLEXIBLE

- Apply an adaptive behavior to a new situation.
- Be prepared to be flexible in the face of an emergency or unplanned event.
- Adapt to new technology and products introduced into your facility.
- Develop a methodology for accepting and implementing disruptive changes.
- Understand how to use teams and colleagues to manage change.

A young behavioral health technician tells his friends that what he likes about his job is that he never knows what to expect from day to day: "It could be quiet one day and it could be crazy on another day. You never know. But it's never quiet or crazy in the same way twice. You always have to think on your feet and expect the unexpected." Although psychiatric facilities may be more unpredictable than other workplace settings, the fact is that unexpected changes and surprises occur frequently in all health care facilities. To deal with this unpredictability, health care professionals must be flexible and adaptable.

The difference between adaptability and flexibility is in their permanence. When we adapt, we make a permanent change from the old way to the new way, such as from using x-ray film to digital x-rays. In comparison, flexibility is a quality that enables you to make adjustments on the fly, like filling in for a co-worker or managing an emergency case. Whereas adaptability focuses on the skills one needs to respond to disruptive change, flexibility is a personality trait that reflects your willingness to make last-minute changes to support the broader goals of an organization.

It is not enough to merely tolerate change; you must embrace it if you want to keep up with the fast-paced environment of health care. A group of health care students were asked what they thought being adaptable and flexible meant as a future health care professional. A few of their responses are included in Box 1.5.

Adaptability enforces creativity, and creativity is adaptability.

—Pearl Zhu

Drivers of the Need to Adapt and Be Flexible

As discussed earlier, one of the chief drivers of large-scale change is technology. Along with new technology, changes in policies, laws, regulations, and processes often create the need to adapt. Large-scale changes often affect a broad population and tend to be more permanent, and they often require adaptation. In contrast, small-scale changes typically affect a much smaller population of people, and their effects are often temporary; this type of change commonly necessitates flexibility. These more small-scale changes may be more difficult to anticipate, however. For instance, health care professionals may be affected by small-scale changes, such as schedule adjustments or patient emergencies that will require them to cooperate with their co-workers to accommodate changes to their daily routine.

Changes in Technology

Technological changes affecting health care professions can include innovations in medical equipment, new imaging techniques, more accurate instruments, and new medical and surgical treatments and procedures. Once a technological innovation is introduced to the market, there is pressure for all hospitals and health care facilities to adopt it as soon as possible to remain competitive. However, a cost-benefit analysis must be done before the acquisition of new technologies.

Patients, insurance companies, and federal programs, such as Medicare and Medicaid, can be billed more for tests and procedures involving newer equipment. In some cases, new equipment could deliver reductions in cost. For instance, the current push to rely on electronic medical records instead of paper records will save money by eliminating duplicate tests, reducing physical storage needs, and requiring less manual maintenance. In addition, as a central repository for a patient's medical records from all providers, electronic medical records systems enable easy access to a complete view of a patient's medical history. Technological advances often offer health care professionals better information and greater efficiency, leading to improved diagnostics and patient care.

Health Care Laws and Regulations

A myriad of laws and regulations govern the practice of health care, including health care providers and professionals. Regulations and laws are created and implemented at all levels of government from federal to state and local. Additionally, each state has its own laws and regulations that affect how health care and professionals are managed in that state. For example, the licensing of many health care professionals is handled at the state level. Local health ordinances and regulations also govern factors such as traffic and parking, noise levels, fire codes, and safety. All these rules can affect you as an individual health care professional, and changes in them require you to adapt.

Some of these changes can be significant. For example, federal laws such as the Patient Protection and Affordable Care Act of 2010 have resulted in changes in the delivery of health care that will have an effect for years to come. The Health Insurance Portability and Accountability Act of 1996 (HIPAA) created significant changes in the way patient health information is handled by health care professionals. Whereas Congress passes federal laws, they authorize federal agencies to put those laws into effect through the creation and enforcement of these regulations.

New Policies, New Management, and Managerial Initiatives

In addition to federal, state, and local laws and regulations, each health care facility and organization has its own systems of governance, which may be its owners, board of directors, executives, and managers. These administrators make decisions on how the facility will be organized, managed, and operated to ensure that all applicable laws and regulations are being complied with. They will act to make their organization more competitive and attractive to their customers and clients. They will also manage capital expenditures while establishing checks and balances to control costs.

Whether in a nonprofit or for-profit business, managers and business leaders are always working to increase efficiency and reduce costs. As an organization undertakes improvement measures and initiatives, you may see many changes, such as revamped performance review procedures, new ways to measure productivity, new security procedures, new construction, new medical records systems, and new strategic initiatives. As a health care professional, you will have to find ways to adapt to these changes.

? WHAT IF?

What if your medical practice has decided to sell vitamins and other supplementals to patients to improve their health and increase revenue? What steps would you take to prepare for this change to ensure it is successful? How would you prepare the facility? How would you prepare the staff?

Effects of Disruptive and Unexpected Changes

All these complexities and rapid and pervasive changes can complicate and challenge your ability to provide care to your patients. Without a proper strategy and preparation, health care professionals can experience significant stress. In severe cases, the effects can lead to illness and burnout.

Stress is a physiological response to changes in the environment, involving the body's autonomic nervous system and hormonal changes. Managing stress is discussed in more detail in Chapter 3.

In addition, we have all experienced anxiety, but anxiety at work is particularly uncomfortable and disruptive. As anxiety impairs critical thinking and decision-making abilities, it can stop you from completing necessary tasks in a timely manner. In emergency situations, this can be dangerous. Strategies for controlling anxiety will be discussed in detail in Chapter 3.

Strategies for Being Adaptable and Flexible

Adaptability and flexibility will contribute to successful performance in a changing health care environment. Focus, problem solving, critical thinking skills, and cooperation are all important aspects of being both adaptable and flexible.

Change can transport us into unfamiliar territory. Go slowly. It will help to understand the impetus or motivation for the change. Consider what it will mean for you, your workflow, your patients, and your facility. You may need to build new skills, which takes time and patience. If possible, work from a plan. This can be particularly helpful if you are asked to make a significant change. For example, you may want a quick tutorial on the use of new equipment or training on a new medical procedure. Positive outcomes are more likely if you adequately prepare for the change.

Once you have made an analysis and a plan of what it will take for you to successfully manage change, focus on the big picture: the relationship between the change and the organization's mission and goals. It is much easier to embrace and implement a change if you see its purpose and goal.

Enjoying success requires the ability to adapt. Only by being open to change will you have a true opportunity to get the most from your talent.

—Nolan Ryan

Focus on how you can help your supervisors achieve their goals. Although they are ultimately responsible for seeing that the change is successfully implemented, you can support them in that endeavor. There is no greater feeling than receiving appreciation and acknowledgment from your supervisors, who recognize what a great job you did in helping during an emergency or a time of unexpected need.

Finally, look ahead, not back. In times of rapid or unexpected change, safety is ahead of you, not behind you. Box 1.6 summarizes a change methodology you may find helpful in your career.

CASE STUDY 1.3
Two Faces of Lisa

Dr. Wu and his associates have recently taken on two partners in their medical practice, Dr. Janklowicz and Dr. Roberts. As neither of the new physicians has their own certified medical assistant (CMA), the practice manager has had to make some staffing adjustments in the assistants' schedules to ensure that the physicians have at least one assistant working with them. With the addition of two new physicians but no new CMAs, the ratio of CMAs to physicians has decreased. Before, the clinic would have two CMAs available for complicated procedures, but now they will mostly have to make do with just one CMA. The practice manager has planned for the change by coming up with a system for cross-training the other CMAs with at least two physicians to ensure they have adequate coverage in case a CMA is on vacation or out sick. However, they have not yet completed this training.

Lisa, Dr. Wu's CMA, shows up to work her new shift. As she is preparing her day and reading through the patient charts and day's procedures, the practice manager comes in and tells her that Dr. Janklowicz's CMA will not be in that morning. "You will have to assist for both physicians today, Lisa." Unlike some of her peers, who are troubled by the recent changes in the practice, Lisa has adapted rather well.

Although she must wake up a bit earlier to accommodate her new schedule, she gets to leave earlier in the evening, allowing her to attend a yoga or Zumba class before going home. She also sees the benefit of getting to work with and assist several different physicians, as she thinks it will offer her more exposure to different procedures, techniques, and work styles.

Even though she is not familiar with the patient, procedure, or equipment, Lisa is ready to problem solve and ensure that everything is taken care of. She reads through Dr. Janklowicz's schedule and does as much as she can to be ready for her first patient.

When Dr. Wu gets to the office, Lisa explains the morning to him and how she will be working with the two physicians for the next 4 hours until her CMA arrives. Lisa assures both physicians that she will be able to manage the situation, as she has familiarized herself with the procedures and has looked over both of their schedules. By coordinating the procedures and times between them, she has prioritized the tasks and will schedule her time around the physician that needs her the most at that time. Even though Lisa will be doing double the workload and running back and forth a lot, she will do her best to make the situation as "normal" and comfortable as possible for everyone. She understands that unexpected issues can arise, and she knows that flexibility will help her manage them.

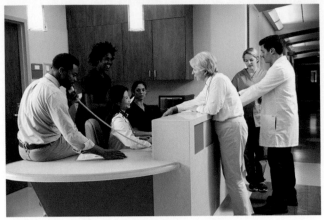

iStock.com/monkeybusinessimages/504702882

QUESTIONS FOR THOUGHT AND REFLECTION

1. What effect do you think Lisa's attitude toward the recent changes in the practice had on how she handled having to assist Dr. Janklowicz?
2. In what ways did Lisa demonstrate flexibility during this unexpected situation?
3. How do you think Lisa's behavior and attitude affected the physicians, the practice manager, and the patients?
4. What do you suppose would have happened if Lisa had complained and been unwilling to assist Dr. Janklowicz?
5. How would you have handled this situation? What, if anything, would you have done differently?

A Different Path

Let's examine Case Study 1.3 again and consider what could have happened without the adaptable and flexible behavior that Lisa demonstrated.

Angela, Dr. Wu's CMA, shows up to work her new shift. As she is preparing her day and reading through the various procedures and patient charts, the practice manager comes and tells her that Dr. Janklowicz's assistant will not be in that morning. "You will have to assist for both dentists today, Angela." Like some of her peers, Angela has had trouble adapting to the recent changes in the practice. She resents that she now must wake up earlier to accommodate her new schedule. She is also unsure how she will like working with more than one physician because she is used to working with just her own physician.

Angela immediately panics and tells the practice manager, "There is no way I can do that. I haven't trained with Dr. Janklowicz." The practice manager reminds Angela that many changes were implemented and that they all need to be flexible, and every staff member will need to step in when necessary. With a sour look, Angela begrudgingly agrees.

Angela gets her morning coffee and reads a magazine until Dr. Wu's first patient arrives. When Dr. Wu gets to the office, Angela seats the patient and then goes back to her desk to finish reading her magazine. Meanwhile, Dr. Janklowicz arrives and goes into her office to wait for her first patient.

Dr. Wu is ready to start on his patient, and he uses the "call bell" to alert Angela that he is ready. During the procedure, Angela has to run to the supply room because Dr. Wu is missing an item from the procedure he is performing. While in the supply room, the practice manager asks Angela why the patient room is not set up for the patient seated for Dr. Janklowicz. The patient has been in the waiting room for at least 20 minutes.

Angela tells the practice manager, "Well, ... uhm, I've been helping Dr. Wu. I'll get the patient set up as soon as I can." Angela retrieves the item for Dr. Wu and tells him that she will be right back and leaves him in the middle of the procedure. She then runs around frantically, setting up the room for Dr. Janklowicz, and trying to figure out what the first procedure is and what supplies and equipment she will need for the procedure.

The patient has now been out in the waiting room for 30 minutes and is angry and complaining to the practice manager. Dr. Janklowicz comes out of her office to find out what is going on, only to discover that her CMA will not be there for the morning and that Angela has not prepared the room or the patient for the procedure.

QUESTIONS FOR THOUGHT AND REFLECTION

1. How does this second scenario differ from the first? What part of Angela's behavior in this story is adaptable or flexible?
2. How did Angela's response affect the physicians, the practice manager, and the patients?
3. Compare the two scenarios, listing the actions that Angela could have controlled to improve the situation.
4. Has this changed how you would handle or think about the situation if it were you?
5. How would you have handled the situation if you were the practice manager?

EXPERIENTIAL EXERCISES

1. This week, while in class, see if you can identify a time when you, your classmates, or your instructor had to adapt to a situation. What was the problem? How did you adapt? How did this help you or the class?
2. Can you think of a time when you had to be flexible in a situation? What was the situation? What might have happened if you were not flexible? Who might have been affected and in what ways?
3. Over the next couple of days, see if you can find a situation in which you might be flexible. Write down each of these times and how you were flexible, how this helped in the situation, and who benefited from it.

CROSS CURRENTS WITH OTHER SOFT SKILLS

MODELING PROFESSIONAL BEHAVIOR: Business etiquette mandates that you at least mask your biases with pleasant behavior, the first step toward overcoming them (Chapter 5).
SHOWING EMPATHY, SENSITIVITY, AND CARING: Seeing issues from the point of view of others is an effective way to overcome biases and prejudices (Chapters 5 and 6).
LISTENING ACTIVELY: The way to crush a bias is to get to know the person behind the label. Engaging with people who are different from you and learning about their experiences with an open mind can help do that (Chapters 5 and 7).
PRACTICING PATIENCE: Biases are rigid and take years to form, so overcoming them will take time and patience (Chapter 5).

Being Dependable

The while we keep a man waiting, he reflects on our shortcomings.

—French Proverb

LEARNING OBJECTIVE 4: BEING DEPENDABLE

- Provide examples of dependability.
- Determine the dependability skills you have and those that you want to work on.
- Establish how your personal ethics, habits, or beliefs affect your personal dependability.
- Display dependable behavior with your co-workers.

Dependability is a critical skill for all employees, including those in health care who are responsible for others' well-being. Think about what being dependable means in the health care field. Ask yourself how you would rate your current level of dependability while on the job, in school, or during your interactions with others. Is it at the level you would expect from others? How can you become more dependable? How does dependability affect your ability to do well in your future career?

JOURNALING 1.6

Think about a situation in which you depended on someone, and they let you down. Or can you think of an instance when you disappointed someone by being undependable? How did you feel? How did that affect your day?

Generally, being dependable can be viewed in terms of how much and how well an employee can be counted on to perform their job. Can the employee work as a valued team member and follow rules and laws that govern the health care worker's job? Developing a reputation for being dependable will be recognized by your employer and can increase your income and help you advance in your career. Health care students were asked what they thought being dependable means, and some of their responses are shown in Box 1.7.

Diamonds are only chunks of coal that stuck to their jobs.

—Minnie Richard Smith

Behaviors of Dependable People

A reputation for dependability takes time to develop, as it is typically based on repeated and consistent behavior and performance over a period of time. What are the behaviors associated with dependability? The key to building dependability is summarized in Box 1.8.

Punctuality

Punctuality is the act of being on time. Few people enjoy being late, but many people are (Figure 1.5). Being late or waiting on someone who is late can make you anxious and stressed. In your social life, tardiness may be easily forgiven; but in the workplace, punctuality is essential.

BOX 1.7

Definitions of Dependable from Health Care Students

- "Being dependable means showing up to work and on time."
- "I think being dependable means taking good care of your patients; they depend on your care."
- "Being dependable means knowing your job and doing it well."
- "When I am working, I think I am being dependable by helping out my co-workers when they are busy or in a tight spot."
- "Your company depends on you to ethically take care of your patients, following the rules like HIPAA, or working within your scope of practice."

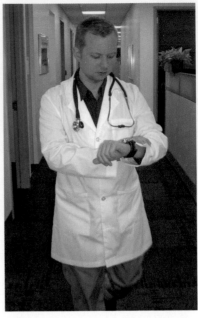

FIGURE 1.5 A health professional practices good time management skills through punctuality.

BOX 1.8

Steps to Building Trust and Dependability

1. Overdeliver in routine tasks.
2. Come to work prepared.
3. Be on time for work and meetings; reply to requests or communications in a timely manner.
4. Follow through on your commitments.
5. Aim for consistency in your results.
6. Be honest about your mistakes and admit them.
7. Practice listening twice as much as you speak.
8. Check your intentions; be sure you do things for the right reasons.
9. Avoid gossiping about others.
10. Do what you say and say what you do; aim for consistency in your life.

Efficient delivery of health care depends on everything starting on time, from shifts to treatments to meetings to patient appointments. Punctuality is particularly important if you work shifts and are being paid based on time. Just as important, punctuality communicates your respect of your job and to your co-workers and patients. For example, when you run late, it is likely that your co-workers will have to cover your tasks until you arrive. Patients may have to wait beyond their appointment times when they may have had to take time off of work or made childcare arrangements for the appointment. Being punctual helps establish your reputation as a dependable and consistent worker.

Some people see punctuality as a time management issue, and others see it as a respect issue. Research suggests that those who chronically run late may have difficulty estimating how long tasks will take. If this sounds familiar to you, try to make note of how long it takes you to complete routine tasks, such as getting ready for work, commuting to work from door to door, writing patient notes, or taking vital signs. Then, when you have to be somewhere by a certain time, you will be better able to plan the time you need to arrive on time or to complete specific tasks.

Here are two easy tricks and reminders you can use to develop this essential habit: Always assume that getting there will take longer than you think and set your alarm early. Respecting the time of your patients and co-workers, as well as your own time, means you need to arrive on time.

Being Trustworthy and Reliable

It sounds simple: do what you say you will do. However, not everyone does. Though there may be many reasons why that is the case, a common one is that many people have trouble saying "no." They want to be seen as cooperative, helpful, and agreeable. Similarly, others have good intentions but fail to estimate how long things will take or what other obligations they have. The result is that people commit to doing something but fail to follow through.

Instead of being seen as cooperative and helpful when you fail to do what you say, you may be viewed as untrustworthy and unreliable. Before you say "yes" to an invitation or a request to help, consider carefully whether you can deliver on your commitment. Be okay with saying "no" when you need to. It is usually wiser to underpromise and then overdeliver rather than to overpromise and underdeliver.

Being a Positive Example

Stop to identify the positive role models in your life. It is also important to look for a good role models at work to whom you might look for advice and guidance in difficult situations. Think about how they conduct themselves and treat others at work, and then consider ways you can model your behavior after theirs. When you model your behavior on someone you respect and admire, you can become a positive example to someone else (Figure 1.6).

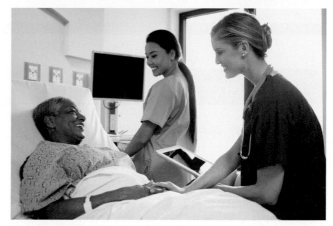

FIGURE 1.6 Empathetic hospital workers interact with an elderly patient. (Copyright © istock.com.)

CASE STUDY 1.4
Mr. Smith Goes to the Dentist

Monday is a very busy day, and Sonia, a medical assistant, has a special patient coming in, Mr. Smith. Mr. Smith is a 90-year-old man who does not have a personal caregiver and walks to his appointment on his own. He is a sweet, elderly man who requires a lot of attention when he comes to the office. But he brings the staff flowers from his yard and sometimes cookies or candy. Because she knows Mr. Smith is on the schedule, Sonia plans her morning to allow her the time to give Mr. Smith the extra care and guidance he will require for his appointment. Mr. Smith often needs help reading his forms and understanding the procedures. Because of his age, he often gets confused and disoriented, but he recognizes Sonia. She is able to keep him calm and comfortable, and he trusts her.

On the day of his appointment, Mr. Smith arrives a bit out of breath from his morning walk. He has a big grin on his face and a bunch of large pink flowers in his hand from his yard. Sonia greets him with a smile. She takes the flowers and puts them in a vase, while she has him take a seat in the waiting room. Another patient in the waiting room and several of the physician's comment on Sonia's ability to care for Mr. Smith and to make sure he is comfortable despite how time-consuming it can be.

When the physician is ready, Sonia takes time from her regular duties to get Mr. Smith and take him to the patient room. Mr. Smith forgets why he is at the office, and Sonia spends time reminding him of where he is and why he is at the clinic. Once he is comfortable, she leaves him with a magazine and says she will be back to check on him.

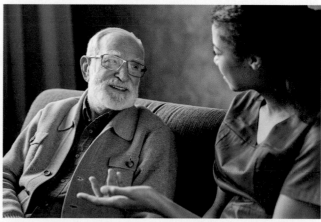

iStock.com/Inside Creative House/1313904397

QUESTIONS FOR THOUGHT AND REFLECTION

1. Which of Sonia's behaviors would be considered dependable?
2. How did Sonia's actions affect Mr. Smith? How did it affect others?
3. How might Mr. Smith's experience have been different if Sonia were not there?
4. Would you be able to handle such a patient? Why or why not?
5. Think of a time when you made extra effort for someone. What was it, and how did it affect that person?

A Different Path

Let's revisit Case Study 1.4 with Sonia taking different actions:

Monday is a very busy day. The office opens at 8:00 a.m., and Sonia is scheduled to be there at 7:30 a.m. to open the office. However, Sonia is running late but does not call or text anyone until 8:30 a.m. to let them know.

At the office, the first patient of the day, Mr. Smith, has arrived. He is a very nice 90-year-old man, who usually walks to his appointment and brings flowers to the staff. When he arrives there 15 minutes early, the office is locked, and the building is dark. Mr. Smith begins to second-guess himself. "Was I supposed to be here today?" he wonders. But he is tired from his walk, so he figures he will rest a bit before heading back home. Fortunately, the front desk receptionist arrives and greets Mr. Smith and has him seated in the waiting room. She tells him to hold on to the flowers.

Mr. Smith is becoming a bit worried and slightly agitated. Natasha, another medical assistant, does not usually have to come in until 9:00 a.m., but she arrives early after receiving a text from Sonia that she will be arriving late. To come in early, Natasha had to ask her mother to take her two kids to school. Because she is rushed and somewhat upset that she had to make arrangements to arrive earlier than her scheduled time today, she does not really have the time to talk to Mr. Smith. After he repeatedly asks, "Where is Sonia?" she tells him, "Sit tight, Mr. Smith. Someone will be with you as soon as possible." By now, Mr. Smith is getting confused and is starting to feel unwell.

Mr. Smith's physician arrives and tells Natasha to bring him to the patient room so he can get started. While waiting for the physician, Mr. Smith asks her why he is there and asks where Sonia is. Natasha tells him Sonia should be arriving soon but that she did not know the purpose of his visit since she was just helping until she arrives. Mr. Smith starts to panic and begins pacing the waiting room and repeatedly asking where he is and why he is there. He is so agitated that Natasha is unable to take his vital signs. It takes the physician more than 20 minutes to calm him down and reassure him. Now, the physician will be behind all morning and the entire office will be behind due to Sonia arriving late.

QUESTIONS FOR THOUGHT AND REFLECTION

1. What were the repercussions of Sonia's lack of dependability?
2. What does Sonia's behavior say about her personal values? How about her work ethic?
3. Although not her fault, could Natasha do anything else in this situation to improve it?
4. Should there be any consequences for Sonia's actions? What should the physician do? What should her co-workers do?

⭐ EXPERIENTIAL EXERCISES

1. During the next few weeks, identify others who display dependability in your work, school, or even your personal life. What do they do to project dependability? What effect does this have on those around you?
2. For 1 week, look for ways in which you can practice being dependable. Write down what the situation was, what you did, and the effect it caused. Did it help others? Did others take notice and remark on it? How did you feel? Was this easy or hard to do? Why?
3. Make a list of role models you admire in your life. Observe the behaviors or characteristics that make them a role model for you. Note how you might adopt some of those behaviors in your life and imagine the impact that would have.

Achieving Honesty and Integrity

In looking for people to hire, you look for three qualities: integrity, intelligence, and energy. And if they don't have the first, the other two will kill you.

—Warren Buffett

LEARNING OBJECTIVE 5: ACHIEVING HONESTY AND INTEGRITY

- Define the relationship between honesty and integrity.
- Recognize why people are tempted to lie or be dishonest.
- Develop a plan for maintaining your integrity.
- Identify ethical dilemmas in the workplace and how to deal with them.

The world presents itself in shades of gray. It is not always clear what is the right thing to do all the time. Nowhere is this more evident than in the world of health care. Patients, health care providers, and the insurance company may have different opinions about what the right thing is in an ethical dilemma. However, honesty and integrity serve as guides during ethical decision-making.

Honesty is defined as "adherence to the truth." *Integrity* is defined as "adherence to moral values," of which honesty forms an integral part. Both concepts comprise fairness and incorruptibility. As health care professionals, we should adhere to the qualities of honesty and integrity to help us navigate the ethical rough waters we will sometimes find ourselves in at work.

Your Integrity at Stake

Consider the kinds of challenges to honesty and integrity that can arise in a health care setting:

* You could be involved in participating in a Medicare fraud scheme by falsifying records.

* You could access confidential medical information about someone you know personally.
* Someone could lie about their religion to get time off.
* You might observe a patient being mistreated by a co-worker.
* A colleague might have falsified her resume to get her job.
* You might have an infectious disease but consider going to work anyway.
* Your certification might have lapsed, but your employer has not noticed.
* Your co-worker might have signed up for a conference but just took the day off instead of attending.
* You might observe a co-worker pocket some cash he found in a pair of jeans from a patient in the emergency room.

As you can see, there are innumerable opportunities that may challenge your integrity, ethics, and honesty in the health care setting. In many cases, the dishonest person may never be caught; however, the chances of a dishonest person getting caught increase because a person acting dishonestly just once is rare.

Real integrity is doing the right thing, knowing that nobody's going to know whether you did it or not.

—Oprah Winfrey

As a health care professional, it is your duty to resist temptations and to strive to do the right thing in all circumstances. In most situations, being honest should be easy for you, although there may be a few extreme circumstances that may require mustering up your courage. The habit of speaking truthfully needs to come easily to you. It is said that lying is a habit, but so is telling the truth.

Challenges to Integrity

A half-truth is a whole lie.

—Yiddish Proverb

The benefits of telling the truth and acting with integrity are so obvious that few people need to be convinced of that virtue. Yet there are people who frequently lie. There are many reasons why someone may lie, such as being ashamed of what they did; fear of retribution, revenge, or being punished; wanting to be seen in a positive light; or hating being wrong.

There are many kinds of lies, however, including lies of kindness or "white lies." For instance, a physician may decide not to tell a patient with Alzheimer's disease calling out for his wife that she has been dead for more than 10 years. The physician may feel it is unkind to plunge the poor man into renewed grief every single day. Nor would you go out of your way to hurt someone's feelings by telling the truth about inconsequential things, such as how bad their new haircut is.

In other cases, people avoid telling the truth by remaining silent when they should not. If you have information that is needed to make a good decision, correct a mistake, or prevent bad behavior and you make the choice not to disclose it, you have essentially lied by omission. Another type of lie is the half-truth: disclosing information selectively to give the wrong impression or misdirect someone's attention away from a more serious matter.

You can see that the challenge in being truthful comes when you have something to lose by acting with integrity, such as a co-worker becoming hostile toward you or a patient being angry if you tell them the truth. There may be real consequences for acting honestly and with integrity: you could lose your job; other people could lose their jobs; or your employer could be sued. Even highly ethical people might hesitate before taking action consistent with their personal integrity when serious consequences are the likely result. However, even when faced with moral dilemmas or grave consequences for their honesty, ethical people will remember the consequence of failing to tell the truth and to act with integrity. They stand to lose their sense of honor and their good reputation. Once a person's professional reputation is damaged, it is difficult to repair.

You often cannot control when you will be faced with an ethical dilemma. Often, you will be suddenly confronted with circumstances you did not anticipate. Taking time to imagine dilemmas that may arise in the future will help you think about your options and the best course of action, so you will be well prepared to make ethical decisions when the time comes.

❓ WHAT IF?

What if you saw a co-worker remove a $20 bill from an open cash drawer?

Strengthening Your Integrity

You can strengthen your integrity muscles, so to speak, by developing skills and strategies to serve you in times of crisis. For example, since you have chosen a career in health care, it is likely that you already have a highly developed sense of empathy, which is the ability to deeply understand the feelings of others.

When you can put yourself in your patients' situation, you are better able to improve health outcomes and patient satisfaction and to have better communication and interactions with patients.

Our emotions are part of what makes us human. However, it is important to not let our emotions always guide our actions at work. Instead, learn how to cope with challenges in a constructive, respectful, and civil manner. Developing the ability to check your emotions will help you deliver a more measured, crafted response when faced with challenges. If the circumstances you find yourself in make you feel angry, disappointed, frustrated, or regretful, acting on your emotions would likely make the situation worse. Take a moment to acknowledge your feelings. Take a deep breath and then decide on the most logical next steps. For instance, when faced with a demanding patient, you might tell yourself, "I am getting frustrated and angry." Take a second to breathe and reflect on the situation. Maybe they are simply tired and cranky. Perhaps the patient feels scared and is making demands to gain a sense of control over something that feels out of their control. In any case, you should approach the situation calmly and rationally. Instead of snapping at the patient, you can gently explain the procedure, why it needs to be performed, and then manage their concerns and expectations.

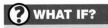 JOURNALING 1.7

Do you act the same way when you are by yourself as you do in front of other people? Think of an instance where you made a difficult but ethical decision, even though nobody else knew about it. Record this incident in your journal and reflect on how your actions made you feel.

Confronting Ethical Dilemmas

Ethical dilemmas at work can place you in a delicate situation. You may face an uncomfortable conversation; you may have to disclose information you would rather keep private; you may have to put something you value, like your job or friendships, on the line. Although these situations may be uncommon, some foresight and planning will help you skillfully handle these situations should they arise.

When your integrity is challenged in some way, check your emotions and get all the facts you can. Try to focus more on the problem and its solutions and less on the people involved. For example, imagine that a co-worker is very busy and asks you to document that she gave a patient a bed bath when you are not sure she did. This presents an ethical dilemma. You have the patient's chart, and your co-worker asks you to do this in an offhand way, since you are already doing your own documentation in the chart anyway. Your first reaction might be to be offended. This person is asking you to lie and take legal responsibility for it. Before you react and say the first thing on your mind, you should get the facts. You might want to ask, "Did you really give her a bath?" If the co-worker insists that she did, you should request that she document it herself. If and only if you can confirm that the patient was given a bath can you ethically document it, and your documentation should be "Mary states she gave Mrs. Parsons a bath, and Mrs. Parsons confirmed it." Gathering as many of the facts as you can helps you handle the situation more effectively.

A more difficult situation is when you cannot confirm what your co-worker has claimed. In this case, you would need to confront your co-worker. You might say, "It doesn't seem that this patient received a bed bath this evening, Mary, so I can't document that in her chart." It may help to choose language that does not directly accuse your co-worker but states the facts and your ethical responsibility clearly. Even if you know that this co-worker frequently asks other people to do her documentation for her, do not point that out and get into that discussion. If you do not have the facts, past behavior is off the point and could lead to a different and unproductive discussion. Instead, focus on the current problem, stick with the facts, and take the action that preserves your integrity.

If your co-worker argues with you, you will just have to repeat your position and make it clear you are sticking to your principles. "I can't document what I can't verify." At this point, your co-worker may be angry or annoyed with you, but that is a small price to pay for your integrity and to protect you legally.

In any case, you have not accused or blamed her. You have stated what you can or cannot do, and you have given your co-worker a chance to respond. Suppose she says, "I'm sorry I put you in that position. I've been so busy, and I just didn't have time to give her a bath, although I know she needs one." At that point, after your co-worker has admitted her mistake, you can help resolve the situation by focusing on the solution and not on your co-worker's poor decision and behavior. You might say, "I'll help you give her a bath right now" or "Let's ask Alicia to give her a bath when she gets in." The priority is to act with integrity and then preserve your relationship with your co-worker if you can.

Guidelines for Acting With Integrity in the Health Care Workplace

* Be on time. Health care facilities depend on promptness and punctuality.
* Treat every patient's medical information with discretion. Do not talk about patients with other people—both inside and outside the clinic—not directly involved with their care. Act to protect their privacy.
* Do not gossip. If you get information you cannot trust, verify it rather than spreading it.
* Complete your work and clean up afterward.
* If you say you are going to do something, follow through and do it, so others know they can depend on you.
* Document patient care accurately and in a timely, professional manner.

Honesty is the best policy. If I lose mine honor, I lose myself.
—William Shakespeare

Importance of Humility

Humility is another useful quality to develop. Humility is being modest, humble, and having an appreciation of your own significance and insignificance. It puts your ego in the background and allows you to remain more open to feedback, guidance, and acceptance of responsibility.

Imagine you just started a new job, and one of your co-workers introduces herself and tells you to let her know if you have any questions or if there is anything she can help you with. Your ego might lead you to think that you do not need her help, as you are perfectly capable of handling things on your own. Although that may be true, a sense of humility would help you see that your new co-worker likely offered to help you out of professionalism and wanting to help you succeed in your new position, not because she thinks you are not capable. Further, she likely *does* have things to teach you. In fact, if you stay humble and open, you will likely find your co-workers to be a great source of information and support in your work (Figure 1.7). In contrast, ego has little use in the health care professions and will prove to be a detriment to your interactions at work with your patients and co-workers.

Humility, along with honesty and integrity, will help you to accept responsibility for your actions. Blaming others accomplishes very little. It usually makes a situation worse by making others defensive, and it can create a hostile work environment. Worse, assigning

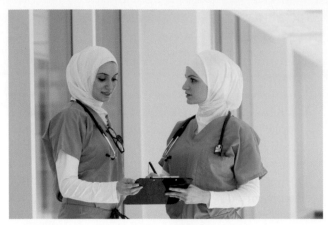

FIGURE 1.7 Two health care professionals discuss patient information. (Copyright © istock.com.)

blame tends to generate excuses, not solutions. As a person of integrity, you want to focus on solutions to morally ambiguous situations that challenge your integrity. Plus, each time you take accountability for your actions, it makes you stronger and makes it easier to do the right thing the next time. For example, a person who double-bills Medicare may seek to avoid responsibility for her actions by claiming that she was just doing what she was told to do. But, if she took personal accountability for her actions, she would see that she is ultimately responsible for her role in the fraudulent activity, and she is more likely to do the correct thing the next time a similar situation arises.

At times like these moral and ethical dilemmas, your self-confidence may come into play. If you are confident in your behavior, you will be able to exhibit the courage required when faced with an ethical dilemma. You can bolster your confidence by thinking about what other highly ethical people would do in the situation. Pick your role models and use your vision of their moral courage to support yourself in a challenging situation. Or imagine that someday your children, or someone else whose opinion of you matters, will find out what you have done, whether for better or worse. Finally, remember the big picture, keeping in mind the overriding benefits of being honest, which are briefly summarized in Box 1.9.

CASE STUDY 1.5
The Courage of Her Convictions

The last thing Isabel had ever expected to see from Mario was Medicare fraud. She had seen signs of it before, but she had pushed it to the back of her mind, not quite sure that she had seen it and perhaps not knowing what to do.

It started last August when Mr. Hemminger, a patient, asked Isabel, the senior medical assistant at the medical practice, about a Medicare claim that had been filed that he knew nothing about. Isabel copied the paperwork Mr. Hemminger brought in and later asked Mario about it. She and Mario had started together at North Central Orthopedic Associates 5 years ago. Mario had started out as a medical insurance coder, but he had been promoted over the years and now is the clinic manager.

She showed Mario the documentation and said, "Do you know what this is about?"

"Hmmm, no. Let me see that. Hmmm, I wonder if this was supposed to be for someone else. You're sure he didn't have these services performed?"

"He said no," said Isabel.

"Hmmm. Well, I'll straighten it out," he told her.

Isabel felt reassured that Mario would resolve the issue, and she never gave it a second thought until another incident arose several months later. Only this time, the person with the complaint was Dr. Fessenden, a professor emeritus at the local university. Dr. Fessenden was certain he was billed for services that he never received, and he wanted to discuss it personally with Dr. Griffiths, the physician at the practice, which Isabel encouraged him to do. Later, she saw Dr. Griffiths with Mario in his office, looking over paperwork and having a hushed conversation.

A few months passed, and then it came up again. This time, it was for Mrs. Hanson, one of Dr. Griffiths' patients at the nursing home, whose daughter brought it up. There seemed to be some bills for durable medical equipment that Mrs. Hanson never received and a bill for "foot surgery," when Dr. Griffiths had only trimmed her toenails.

Isabel took this documentation to Mario. "I can't ignore this anymore," she said.

"Ignore what?"

"These fraudulent Medicare charges."

"What? Whoa! That's a very serious allegation Isabel. Very, very serious. People go to jail for that. I'm very surprised to hear you say this, Isabel, an old friend like you."

"I can't ignore it anymore."

"I just think these must be mistakes. Maybe I billed the services to the wrong people. I'll have to research this."

He looked up and made eye contact with Isabel, who he could tell was not believing him. "Look, Isabel, we're just trying to maximize our Medicare reimbursement. You know we provide all kinds of free services here, and not everybody even takes Medicare patients anymore."

"What do you mean free services, Mario? These are serious violations, and someone could go to jail."

Mario laughed abruptly and covered his mouth with his hand. "Well, I just don't know … what to say." He laughed again and brushed his hair back vigorously. "I guess I'm in a bit of a fix here."

"You needed the money?"

Mario said nothing, staring at the documentation.

"I'm just," he said after a moment, "sort of in the middle. It's really Mark," he said, referring to Dr. Griffiths. "He asked me, uh … I'm going to tell him to stop. This is just a mistake. Let's keep this between you and me, and I'll put a stop to it."

Isabel said nothing. She rose and left the room.

Back at the front desk, Isabel was in a daze. A patient approached her, and it took her a moment to notice. She helped the patient and decided to throw herself back into her work and think about what she should do when she had a chance to give the matter her full attention. Before the end of the day, though, Mario asked her to come to his office. When she entered the office, she noticed Dr. Griffiths sitting in the chair behind the door.

"Hello, Isabel," he said with a wan smile. "Mario tells me you have some concerns about some mistaken medical bills."

"Mistaken? Yes, they were for equipment and services that weren't provided." Isabel took a very slow deep breath. This was not a situation she ever wanted to find herself in. She liked Dr. Griffiths. He had been good to her, and he was a good doctor.

"Well, that's a very serious statement, Isabel,'" said the doctor. "I'm very sorry all this was brought to your attention. It should not have been. When Dr. Fessenden came in, you rightly referred him to me, and it was all straightened out. I think this is all just a big misunderstanding, don't you? If anything of this nature ever concerns you again, you come and see me, all right?"

She nodded and stood up. Dr. Griffiths opened the door for her. "I'm glad we got this all straightened out," he told her.

That evening, Isabel went on the website of the US Department of Health and Human Services' Office of the Inspector General (OIG), the office that oversees Medicare fraud. She copied down the number, and the next morning she called it and spoke to a staff member at the OIG. As instructed, she assembled all the documentation she had copied and saved and wrote a statement of her concerns, and then she sent it to the OIG by Postal Express. When she arrived at work, she felt afraid, as she was unsure where her complaint would lead. She worried about Mario and Dr. Griffiths. When she got to work, she quietly resigned.

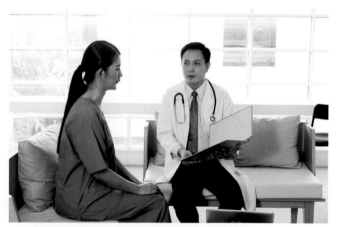

iStock.com/cocorattanakorn/1363559960

QUESTIONS FOR THOUGHT AND REFLECTION

1. What role did Isabel play in this situation? What about Mario?
2. Do you think that Isabel was correct, that Medicare fraud was taking place?
3. What potential consequences could Isabel's decision to report the fraud have?
4. What else could Isabel have done in this situation? Do you agree with her decision to resign?
5. What would you do if faced with similar circumstances?

A Different Path

Even though it was only his fourth day on the job, Carl was late again. "Traffic," he muttered.

"Why don't you leave earlier?" asked Susan. "You're always late."

"If I left earlier," he said, "I'd get here even later." He started laying out his theory of timing and the Kennedy Expressway, but most people stopped listening to him and started their day.

When Alyssa took her midmorning coffee break, Carl was already in the breakroom, paging through a magazine. "Hi," he said, "hey, have you seen these new smartphones? I was the first one to get an Android, but I kind of like the latest iPhone. I want FaceTime so I can see my brother when I call him. He's a big shot at the Chinese Embassy in Beijing. I'd be waking him up in the middle of the night, but it'd be cool to be able to see his face. Maybe it's worth the cost of a new phone."

"Can't you just use Skype or Google Duo? They're free."

"True, but then I wouldn't have the latest phone," Carl said with a laugh. "I'm really into new technology. It's kind of my thing. I just got one of those new OLED TVs. The picture is amazing. How about you? What are you into?"

"I don't know, Carl. I have a lot on my mind."

"Okay. Me too."

At 11:30 a.m., Carl asked his supervisor, Mike, if he could leave 15 minutes early for lunch. "I'm meeting a friend for a little handball, and I'll never get there on time if I don't leave early."

Mike said, "No. And try to get here on time in the future." In a little while, Mike noticed that Carl was hanging around the lobby, apparently waiting until the stroke of noon, so he could be out the door.

Later that afternoon, Susan approached Mike and said, "You're not going to believe this. I just saw the new guy, Carl, take a $20 bill from a patient and put it in his pocket."

"Susan," said Mike, with a grave look on his face. "Are you absolutely sure?"

"I wouldn't say anything if I wasn't," she said.

Mike took a few moments to compose himself and approached Carl and said, "I've been informed that you may have a $20 bill from a patient."

Carl smiled broadly. "What, somebody squealed on me?"

Mike ignored him. "Did you take cash from a patient?"

"Not really," said Carl. "It was a tip."

Mike just looked at him, not breaking eye contact or blinking.

"The guy just wanted to make sure his laboratory results would get to his doctor before his next appointment."

"We don't charge for the prompt delivery of laboratory results, Carl. What was the patient's name?"

"Well, I could probably look it up, why?"

"Because I'm going to return it to him as soon as you're out of the building."

QUESTIONS FOR THOUGHT AND REFLECTION

1. How much credibility do you think Carl has with his co-workers? Why?
2. Do you think Susan did the right thing by telling Mike about the $20 bill?
3. What do you think of the way Mike handled the situation with Carl?
4. If you were Carl's supervisor, how would you manage his behavior?

★ EXPERIENTIAL EXERCISES

1. Do you have a difficult conversation you have been putting off? Plan the conversation in advance and select the words and phrases you will use. Come back to these in the face of argument, emotional reactions, or disagreement.
2. Arrange a debate on an ethical question. Take the position that is against your own, so you can experience what it feels like to argue for something you disagree with and to see the other person's position.
3. Go see a movie that features a character you think you would admire. Think about this character the next time you face an ethical dilemma. What would they have done?

CROSS CURRENTS WITH OTHER SOFT SKILLS

BUILDING RELATIONSHIPS: Honesty and integrity are the foundations of trust (Chapter 5).

DEALING WITH DIFFICULT PEOPLE: Honesty and integrity should inform all your relationships, especially difficult ones, where your character may be challenged (Chapters 6 and 7).

BUILDING SELF-ESTEEM: Once you choose honesty and integrity as the hallmarks of your character, self-esteem will take care of itself (Chapter 3).

TAKING ACCOUNTABILITY: This is how you demonstrate your integrity (Chapter 10).

CHAPTER 2

Managing Your Emotions

BY THE END OF THIS CHAPTER, YOU WILL BE ABLE TO

- Understand Emotions and Emotional Intelligence
- Recognize When Your Work and Personal Problems Overlap
- Describe the Emotional Challenges That Personal Problems Can Cause at Work
- Explain How to Manage Your and Others' Strong Emotions
- List the Advantages and Challenges of Being Optimistic
- List the Advantages and Challenges of Being Pessimistic

Managing Your Emotions

LEARNING OBJECTIVE 1: UNDERSTANDING EMOTIONS IN THE WORKPLACE

- Understand how emotions can positively and negatively affect your work.
- Define emotional intelligence.
- Understand how emotional intelligence can affect your job performance.
- Learn how to increase your emotional intelligence.
- Explain the role of emotional and self-awareness.

Experiencing emotions and being able to express our emotions are universal experiences and fundamental to life. Emotions are reactions that human beings experience in response to events or situations. Although there are many different types of emotions, the four kinds of basic emotions are happiness, sadness, fear, and anger, which are differentially associated with three core affects: reward (happiness), punishment (sadness), and stress (fear and anger). The type of emotion a person experiences is determined by the circumstance that triggers the emotion. For example, a person experiences joy when they receive good news. A person experiences fear when they are threatened.

Emotions have a strong influence on our daily lives, both at work and at home. We make decisions based on whether we are happy, angry, sad, bored, or frustrated. We choose activities and hobbies based on the emotions they incite. Understanding emotions can help us navigate life with greater ease and stability.

Pity those who don't feel anything at all.

—Sarah J. Maas

Key Elements of Emotion

Emotions result from a series of factors. This is often called the *modal model of emotion* (Gross and Thompson, 2007) and is based on the following four components:

* the situation you are in (whatever is happening to you at that moment),
* the details you pay attention to,
* your appraisal of what the situation means for you personally, and
* your response, including the physical changes and your behaviors (like shouting or crying).

For an emotion to happen, there must be something happening around you (the situation you are in). You might be at work on a particular busy day, or in the examination room speaking with a patient. You will then only pay attention to the parts of the situation that are relevant to you. For example, multiple patients arriving for their appointments while the phone is ringing and the doctor is asking for assistance. Next, in your appraisal, you will interpret what those details mean to you. This process could be unconscious or conscious, and it will determine the feelings you experience. Based on the thought processes you have (the appraisals), you will then have a response. This emotional response involves several components. This may include your actions (yelling or standing up and leaving), expressions (frowning), and physical changes (increased heart rate, sweating).

I don't want to be at the mercy of my emotions. I want to use them, to enjoy them, and to dominate them.

—Oscar Wilde

Emotional Intelligence

Now that you understand why we have emotions, it is important to also understand how you interpret, control, and evaluate your emotions and others. This is called emotional intelligence (EI), which is the ability to understand emotions and their effect on behavior. Improving your EI improves your understanding that people have different points of view and helps you understand their points of view. Having this understanding or ability is important; otherwise, how will

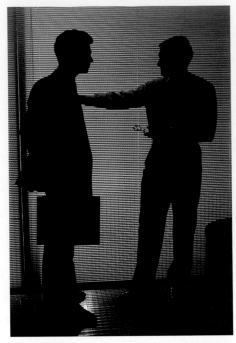

FIGURE 2.1 Emotional intelligence allows you to understand your and other people's emotions. (iStock.com/ Prostock-Studio/1374577592.)

you know when a co-worker is angry with you, or a patient is feeling scared (Figure 2.1)?

EI is vital for success in the workplace and may be just as important as "traditional" intelligence. According to psychologists John Mayer and Peter Salovey (Salovey and Mayer, 1990), who developed a comprehensive theory of the concept, there are four branches to EI:

1. Perceiving emotions in oneself and others
2. Using emotions to facilitate thinking
3. Understanding emotions and emotional meanings
4. Managing emotions

Perceiving emotions is the first step in being able to use your emotions in constructive ways and promote empathy for the feelings of others. The ability to recognize emotions in yourself and others will serve you well in both the job and your personal relationships. This equates to an emotional self-awareness, which enables you to identify what you feel and clearly communicate those emotions. Perceiving emotions is the first step in being able to use your emotions in constructive ways and promote empathy for the feelings of others.

It may seem counterintuitive to let emotions guide your thinking. However, emotions can offer powerful insights into what we value and regard as most important. This branch of EI deals with the ability of emotions to help guide thoughts and prioritize our thinking. Emotionally intelligent people know how to use their feelings to help them make decisions and

BOX 2.1

Signs and Examples of Emotional Intelligence

- An ability to identify and describe what people are feeling
- An awareness of personal strengths and limitations
- Self-confidence and self-acceptance
- The ability to let go of mistakes
- An ability to accept and embrace change
- A strong sense of curiosity, particularly about other people
- Feelings of empathy and concern for others
- Showing sensitivity to the feelings of other people
- Accepting responsibility for mistakes
- The ability to manage emotions in difficult situations

BOX 2.2

How to Practice Emotional Intelligence

- Being able to accept criticism and responsibility
- Being able to move on after making a mistake
- Being able to say no when you need to
- Being able to share your feelings with others
- Being able to solve problems in ways that work for everyone
- Having empathy for other people
- Having great listening skills
- Knowing why you do the things you do
- Not being judgmental of others

direct their cognitive focus to the things that matter most.

Emotions can reveal human needs and lead to actions and patterns of behavior. Thus, understanding emotions and their meanings is critically important for those in the health care field. Increasing your ability to interpret the messages attached to emotions will help you tremendously in your work, not only with patients but also with your supervisor and co-workers. Box 2.1 are some key signs and examples of EI.

Finally, the ability to manage your emotions is a key skill for any professional. You will likely find yourself in high-pressure situations that will require you to handle the emotions of others and your own emotions. Learning to regulate your emotions will help you to communicate your own needs more effectively and influence the emotions of others. This ability will encourage teamwork and collaboration with your co-workers and enable you to achieve your personal and professional goals more easily.

Developing Emotional Intelligence and Job Performance

While some people might come by their emotional skills naturally, some evidence suggests that this is an ability you can develop and improve. What are some steps to developing EI?

First, if you want to understand what other people are feeling, take the time to listen to what people

are trying to tell you, both verbally and non-verbally. When you sense that someone is feeling a certain way, consider the different factors that might be contributing to that emotion.

Picking up on emotions is critical, but you also need to be able to put yourself into someone else's shoes in order to truly understand their point of view. Practice empathizing with other people. Imagine how you would feel in their situation. Such activities can help you build an emotional understanding of a specific situation as well as develop stronger emotional skills in the long term.

The ability to reason with emotions is an important part of EI. Consider how your own emotions influence your decisions and behaviors. When you are thinking about how other people respond, assess the role that their emotions play. Box 2.2 lists some ways to practice EI.

Being able to use EI in your work will help improve your job performance because your moods and emotions affect those around you, including your co-workers. Emotional outbursts or inappropriate displays of emotion could damage your relationship with your co-workers. Your ability to recognize and manage your feelings at work will ensure that you maintain productive relationships, in which you collaborate with your peers, you take direction well from your superiors, and your co-workers and supervisor can freely discuss work-related issues with you without fear of exacerbating your bad mood.

It also allows professionals to effectively approach the conflict resolution process, taking into account the emotions involved among the parties concerned, and be able to separate and focus those emotional components into finding a solution. Lack of EI in the workplace can escalate conflict and cause further division among team members. Emotional decision-making in the absence of EI can widen the communication gap between opposing opinions and can damage the self-esteem of the individuals and the cohesiveness of the team.

People with high EI often make excellent leaders because they are able to effectively motivate, inspire, and earn the trust of their teams and mitigate any potential conflict before it escalates.

We will talk more about managing conflict in Chapter 7, but the sections in this chapter discuss separating work and personal problems and managing your emotions—valuable skills that will help develop your EI.

Emotional and Self-Awareness

Self-awareness is an important component of EI. Self-awareness is made up of emotional awareness, accurate self-assessment, and self-confidence. In other words, it is all about knowing your emotions, your personal strengths and weaknesses, and having a strong sense of your own worth.

Emotional awareness is an ability to recognize your own emotions, and their effects. People who have this ability will know what emotions they are feeling at any given time, and why; understand the links between their emotions and their thoughts and actions, including what they say; and understand how their feelings will therefore affect their performance. Being aware of your own emotions, and how they affect your behavior, is crucial to effective interaction with others. But it can also be crucial to your personal health and well-being.

People can find self-analysis of their emotions difficult, especially if they have suppressed them for a long time. It may be hard for people to accurately recognize their emotions and even more difficult to understand why they are feeling them. However, self-analysis is a vital skill to learn and develop for good EI.

If you are aware of your values, you can quickly see why you may have had a particularly emotional reaction to an event or person. Most importantly, you can then take action to address the issue, with a better understanding of the problem.

Understanding your own and others' emotions also requires a good understanding of your personal strengths, weaknesses, inner resources, and, perhaps most importantly, your limits. It can be particularly hard to admit to weaknesses and limits, especially if you are in a competitive and fast-moving work environment, but it is crucial for EI and your own

well-being. People who are good at self-assessment generally not only have a good understanding of their strengths and weaknesses, but they are usually very reflective, learning from experience, and open to feedback.

Another important component of self-awareness is self-confidence, which is having a strong sense of your own self-worth, and not relying on others for your valuation of yourself.

People with good self-confidence are generally able to present themselves well, prepared to voice unpopular opinions and not always "go with the flow," and are able to make good decisions grounded in their own values.

Separating the Personal From the Professional

**LEARNING OBJECTIVE 2:
SEPARATING YOUR WORK AND PERSONAL PROBLEMS**

- Identify methods to create a work-life balance.
- Recognize when a personal problem is affecting you, your behavior, and your emotions at work.
- Be aware of triggers that can spread personal problems to your workplace.
- Understand the consequences of being a problem employee.

Creating a Work-Life Balance

As the meaning of work changes, particularly in the way we work and the type of work we do, the importance of work and life changes meaning and importance. You are likely to hear the term "work-life balance" a lot more compared to several years ago, especially as a result of the COVID pandemic and more workers working remotely or at home.

Ideas or definitions about work-home balance differ among people. Thus, it has become difficult to have a universal definition since the idea about "work-home balance" is personal. Work-life balance refers to a state, where one effectively balances work or career demands with those of their personal life. Work-life balance defines how well a person prioritizes personal and career demands, and how much work is present in one's home (Figure 2.2). An individual who lacks a work-life balance has more work and home obligations, works longer hours, and lacks personal time.

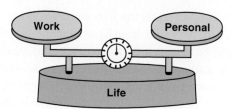

FIGURE 2.2 Balancing personal and work life. (istock.com/ LightFieldStudios/1151675546.)

As a new health care professional, it will be important for you to establish this in your own life. Often, work may take precedence over everything else in your lives, particularly as you begin a new career or a new job. The desire to succeed professionally could push you to set aside and not prioritize your own well-being or your friends and family. Creating a work-life balance does not necessarily mean an equal balance of each all the time. Trying to schedule an equal number of hours for each of your various work and personal activities is usually unrewarding and unrealistic. Life is often more fluid and what works today may be different tomorrow. People have their unique work-life balance routines. Things that work for someone else cannot or might not work for you since our priorities differ.

The key to creating a work-life balance is finding the right balance for you, which will change with time and your life circumstances. For example, the right balance for you when you are single may be different when you marry, or if you have children or a family; when you start a new career versus when you are nearing retirement. Regardless, in order to be an effective professional and to create a positive work and home environment, it will be important for you to create a work-life balance that works for you. Remember that a work-life balance is not necessarily about evenly dividing hours in your day but about having the flexibility to get things done in your professional life while still having time and energy to enjoy your personal life. Some days, you might focus more on work, while other days you might have more time and energy to pursue your hobbies or spend time with your loved ones. Box 2.3 lists some considerations for creating a work-life balance.

Keeping Your Work and Personal Life Separate

Health care presents unique challenges to its workers, who seek to balance work-life with family and personal life and try to keep problems in one area from spreading to other areas. The health care industry

BOX 2.3

Establishing a Work-Life Balance

- Accept that there is no "perfect" work-life balance.
- Do not strive for the perfect schedule; strive for a realistic one. Balance is achieved over time, not each day.
- Find a job that you love.
- Although work is a necessity of life, your career should not be restraining. You do not need to love every aspect of your job, but it needs to be exciting enough that you do not dread getting out of bed every morning.
- Prioritize your health.
- Your overall physical, emotional, and mental health should be your main concern.
- Set boundaries and work hours.
- Take time to unwind to recover from your daily and weekly stress. Avoid thinking about work and not answering work emails and phone calls when not working.
- Make time for yourself and your loved ones.
- While your job is important, it should not be your entire life. You were an individual and had interests and hobbies before taking this position, and you should prioritize them in your life.

places added demands on its workers because of the nature of the work. Patients cannot go without care, so mandatory overtime is required of some workers, and hours extend beyond the scheduled time as urgent issues demand attention. Moreover, both single parents and young parents dominate most health care professions, and many workers must balance the pressures of caring for young children with the pressures of caring for patients. With the urgent and constant care required for patients, it is easy to see how problems at work can spill over into the home, and problems at home can become stressors at work.

Separating your personal problems from work can be relatively easy if you are successfully navigating both parts of your life and are satisfied in both areas. However, when problems arise, the separation between your work and personal lives may become more permeable: You may start dwelling on personal problems while at work or carry the stress of your workday home with you. When dealing with issues in your personal life, it may be tempting to vent about them at work or seek advice from your co-workers. After all, you will likely have friends at work who you look forward to seeing, because they care about you and support you. However, these relationships should remain professional while you are at work, and you should avoid burdening your work friends with your personal problems.

If you maintain friendships with co-workers outside of the workplace, that would be a more appropriate time to share challenges you are facing at home. If you do not have contact with your co-workers outside of work, that is likely an indication that your relationship is more professional than personal, and it would be best to avoid discussing your personal problems. In fact, many people experiencing issues at home find that work is therapeutic, or at least a distraction from their personal problems. Recognize that if you cannot do anything while you are at work to fix or improve your personal problems, you can at least use work as a chance to get away from your problems for a while.

Recognizing Personal Problems at Work

Sometimes, however, your personal problems can spill over into the workplace, exacerbating the stress of work. The first step in addressing such a problem is to recognize when it is affecting your mood. Being able to assess your own mood takes work, commitment, and insight. We all bring a long, deeply ingrained history of behavior patterns to work. Understanding how you tend to behave, think, or feel physically when experiencing certain emotions will help you identify your moods more effectively. For instance, when experiencing stress, you may be less patient in your interactions with others, have racing thoughts, and feel tightness in the muscles between your shoulder blades. Identifying your moods, in turn, can help you prevent your personal problems from seeping into your work. When you recognize the cause of your behavior, you can better control it. You might not be able to help your feelings, but you are responsible for your actions.

Triggers That Cause Personal Problems at Work

Work conditions and circumstances can resonate with your personal problems or remind you of them in ways that make you feel emotional. Perhaps a difficult person at work reminds you of a difficult person

at home, and work seems like a continuation of your complicated personal life. In caring for a sick child, you might be reminded of the emotional attachments you have with your own child. If a co-worker treats you in a demeaning manner or a patient is hostile toward you, it may take all your effort to avoid reacting as you would if you were confronted with the same behavior at home.

When Work Problems Cause Personal Problems

Conversely, in today's environment in which most people carry their smartphones with them and can be reached at any time of day, it is natural for issues at work to trigger anxieties or arguments at home. Although you may be able to take a phone call or answer an email after hours, you usually cannot address work problems when you are not at work. You can only worry about work problems when you are not there. If you can, learn to use your commute as a transition period between your work and home life. Try to wrap up the problems of the workday and put them in the back of your mind. Look forward to your home environment, even if it has its own problems.

Many people think the problems of work-life balance are caused by having too little time at home. However, it is often an issue of attention. When you are home, give your relationships with partners, roommates, children, or other family members your complete and undivided attention. You will be more productive in your personal life if you can be fully present when at home, rather than dividing your focus and mentally multitasking. Trying to address the needs of your job and the demands of your personal life simultaneously can lead to burnout. Being fully engaged, whether at work or at home, will help you resolve issues in both areas more efficiently and effectively.

When Personal Problems Become Serious Matters at Work

When employees bring their personal problems to work, negative behavior patterns can settle in and affect the quality of their work. Such employees may become argumentative, sullen, rude, incommunicative, angry, uncooperative, and difficult to work with. Workplaces have definite response patterns in place to deal with these problem employees.

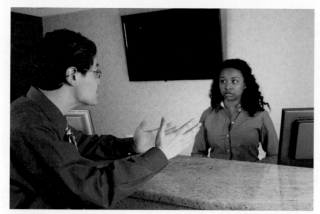

FIGURE 2.3 Employee receiving a performance improvement plan (PIP). (From Proctor DB, Adams AP: *Kinn's the medical assistant: an applied learning approach*, ed 12, St Louis, 2014, Elsevier.)

Performance Improvement Plans

Usually, problem employees will have an opportunity to correct their behavior to avoid termination. They will be presented with a performance improvement plan, often called a PIP. Usually crafted in a collaboration between the employee's manager and the human resources department (if there is one), the PIP will identify the problem behavior or performance issue, prescribe expected behavioral improvements, and establish a timeline for progress, usually 30 or 60 days. PIPs are confidential and serve as serious warnings (Figure 2.3).

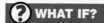
WHAT IF?

What if you were placed on a performance improvement plan? How would you respond to that?

Terminations

Employees in the vast majority of the United States are considered by law to be "employees at will." That means as long as employers do not discriminate against employees or treat them unfairly, they reserve the right to terminate them at any time. In most cases, people who lose their jobs are eligible for a certain amount of unemployment compensation. However, a person fired for reckless behavior cannot receive unemployment compensation.

In an ideal world, you will find a workplace that supports a healthy work-life balance and provides sufficient income for you to pursue your personal and family goals, achieving a work-life balance that works for you. Although there is much you can do to promote this balance, there will remain aspects of your work and home life that are out of your control. The balance between work and home responsibilities is always fluctuating, and it takes effort to maintain this healthy equilibrium,.

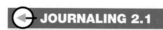
JOURNALING 2.1

Describe the work-life balance you would like to achieve.

CASE STUDY 2.1
Holiday Spirit

It had been years since Paula had to work Christmas Eve, but this year it was unavoidable. There had been a big argument about working the holidays in the staff meeting, and somebody mentioned in a fit of anger that Paula had not worked the Christmas holidays in more than 5 years. "Who keeps track of that?" she said, looking around the room to silent faces and averted eyes. "My daughter just turned 2. Christmas is a big deal for a 2-year-old." Still, no one spoke up.

After the meeting, Paula reflected on the issue. She felt a little selfish objecting to the holiday shift at the staff meeting. Paula knew her husband and daughter would be disappointed that she would not be home on Christmas Eve. But she also understood that the holidays are a busy time at the

hospital, and the employees need to share the responsibility of working over the holidays to ensure the hospital has adequate staff available. Everybody has to pitch in, and it was her turn.

At home, her husband, Terry, was more understanding than she had expected. "Don't worry," said Terry. "I'll bring Rosie over to the hospital before I put her to bed. You can spend some time with her on your break, take her down to the gift shop, and we'll all be together Christmas morning when you get home from work." That made sense to Paula, and she felt better knowing she had her husband's support.

By the time she arrived for her 3:00 p.m. shift on Christmas Eve, the snow was coming down hard. Terry called to say he did not think it would be a good idea to venture out with Rosie. Paula was disappointed, but she had to agree.

The snow kept coming as the evening wore on. The Director of Nursing asked the nurses to stay for the night shift, as none of the night nurses could get their cars out of their garages, and the streets were mostly impassible. They would try to get them relief in the morning as soon as possible.

By 2:00 a.m., Paula and all the nurses were feeling fatigued. Paula was the most senior among the nurses, so she called a meeting. She thanked everyone for staying and providing such professional care. There were four of them and plenty of empty beds. She proposed they take turns working 2 hours and sleeping 2 hours. If anyone needed help, they could wake whoever was sleeping.

Kenny volunteered to take the first shift, and the other two followed, letting Paula sleep until 6:00. "You shouldn't have let me sleep past my shift," she said, when Catherine woke her up, but Catherine said the patients were all fine and it was better to let her sleep.

The Director called at 7:00 a.m. with more bad news. They hoped to get some relief by noon, but that would be the earliest. Paula felt like crying, as this meant she would miss opening presents with her daughter. She left the nurses' station and returned to the room where she had slept, taking a moment to collect herself and shift her focus from her disappointment back to her job responsibilities. She thought to herself, a lot of the patients here would rather be home with their families, too. She took a deep breath and went to check on some patients before returning to the nurses' station.

In a few minutes, Catherine arrived with a surprise. She knew Paula was sad to miss Christmas morning with her daughter, so she arranged a video chat on her cell phone with Terry and Rosie. She thought Paula seeing her daughter's face for a few moments might help.

Rosie showed her mother all the presents that Santa had brought. When they hung up, Paula gave Catherine a big hug. "It's still early, Catherine, but you made my day!"

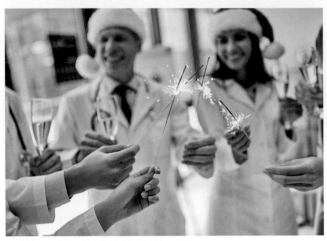

iStock.com/Vasyl Dolmatov/1084479428

QUESTIONS FOR THOUGHT AND REFLECTION

1. What personal problems did Paula experience while at work? How did these affect her work?
2. List examples of Paula's professionalism.
3. How do you think Paula's and her co-workers' actions toward each other help them get through the unexpectedly long shift?
4. How would you describe Paula's level of emotional intelligence?
5. How would you describe Catherine's level of emotional intelligence?

A Different Path

Dr. Williamson got an early flight home from the medical convention and decided to drop by the office to catch up after his 3-day absence. The receptionist greeted him nervously and glanced down the hall toward his office. Dr. Williamson unlocked his office and was surprised to see that his medical assistant, Marianne Kolodny, was sitting in his chair and talking on his phone.

"I have to go," she said, alarmed, and hung up. She stood up, as if at attention. "I … I … I was just talking to, um, my son's day care. It was private. I'm sorry but I didn't think you would mind if I used your office."

"I do mind, Marianne. This is completely inappropriate." He stood aside as Marianne rushed past him and out of the office.

"Thanks for the warning, Jill," she sharply muttered to the receptionist while walking by her.

Everybody knew that Marianne's marriage was disintegrating. Marianne talked endlessly about how difficult her husband, Marco, was. She was hoping the doctor would not be in that day so she could leave a bit early. She looked around the waiting room and only one elderly man was there.

"Do you know a good divorce lawyer?" she asked him.

He was so startled he could hardly mumble that he did not.

"Because I'm going to need one," she went on. "I have reason to suspect my husband is unfaithful," she said. "I think he's spying on me too and that's why I can only ask strangers."

Just then, Dr. Williamson entered the room with a broad smile. "Mr. Carlson, I didn't know you were here."

"Hi, Dr. Williamson. I'm just waiting for Alice. She's getting some blood drawn."

"Do you know my medical assistant, Marianne?" he asked in his courtly manner.

"Uh, … yes. I've been getting to know her?" said Carl.

"Well, come on back and wait in my office, if you like, and tell me how your retirement has been going."

In a few minutes, the men returned to the lobby, along with Alice. When he came back in from walking them to their car, Dr. Williamson asked to speak with Marianne in his office.

The next morning, everyone was surprised to see that Dr. Williamson was already there. He usually came in at 9:00 on the dot. When everyone had arrived, he asked the staff to join him in the conference room. "I just wanted to let you all know, before you heard it elsewhere, that I've decided to let Marianne go. I'm sure we all appreciated her service, but I felt that it was time for her to move on."

QUESTIONS FOR THOUGHT AND REFLECTION

1. What kind of mood did Marianne create in the office when she talked about her personal problems?
2. How do you think Dr. Williamson defined professionalism? What about Marianne's behavior might not have fit with his definition?
3. Why was Carl surprised to learn that Marianne worked in the office?
4. Did Dr. Williamson handle the news of her termination appropriately? Why or why not?

⭐ EXPERIENTIAL EXERCISES

1. Identify a colleague at work who will be candid with you. Ask your colleague to give you honest feedback on your mood, attitude, and body language.
2. During your commute, practice making the transition from home to work and from work to home.
3. Think of times when you had to overcome emotions associated with personal problems while you were at work. Was work therapeutic for you?

CROSS CURRENTS WITH OTHER SOFT SKILLS

READING AND SPEAKING BODY LANGUAGE: Pay close attention to how your emotions are reflected in your body language (Chapter 4).

DEALING WITH DIFFICULT PEOPLE: Make sure you are not the difficult person your co-workers have to deal with (Chapter 7).

CONTROLLING ANXIETY: Anxiety can take over your emotions and lead to negative outcomes (Chapter 3).

Managing Anger and Strong Emotions

Anger is a short madness.

—Horace

LEARNING OBJECTIVE 3: MANAGING ANGER AND STRONG EMOTIONS

- Understand why people become angry.
- Learn how to better manage your anger.
- Learn how to respond to others' anger and emotions.

Why People Become Angry

Everybody gets angry from time to time. Anger is not a negative emotion, but it can lead to negative actions and behaviors if not properly directed. When anger results from empathy with another person's situation or the recognition of an injustice, for example, it can be motivating and can lead to positive change. However, uncontrolled anger can damage relationships, particularly when based on resentment or jealousy, and it can take a toll on us physically and mentally. To avoid the latter, it is important to recognize the source of your anger and take responsibility for your actions.

Most of the time, people become angry because they are hurt or frustrated. They may feel they have been treated unfairly or thoughtlessly ignored, disappointed, or taken for granted. Anger, then, substitutes for a deeper hurt. At work, anger may result from a sense that others are not doing their fair share.

For instance, someone did not empty the sharps container when it was full and now someone got injured from a needlestick. Sometimes problems arise that do not have immediate or obvious solutions, and they cause a great deal of frustration.

Anger is only one letter short of danger.

—Eleanor Roosevelt

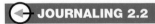 **JOURNALING 2.2**

Describe an occasion when you became angry at work. How did your anger affect your actions? Based on your actions, would an objective observer think you were justified or that you overreacted? How would you handle the incident differently if you could do it over again?

Controlling Your Anger

Even though anger is a common emotion, it rarely solves problems rarely does it make you feel better to indulge in your anger. As soon as you feel your anger rising, try to moderate it with one or more of the following strategies:

* *Try relaxation techniques.* Breathe deeply and visualize a peaceful image. Do some gentle stretches.
* *Try reframing the situation.* Try not to jump to conclusions or use extreme language, such as always, never, worst, or impossible. Try to examine the situation rationally and in context. It probably is not the *worst* day of your life. Perhaps your co-worker did not intend to question your abilities when she offered to help you. Instead, state the problem accurately and without assessing blame on anyone. For example, "I am upset because this is the third weekend in a row I have had to work."
* *Refocus with problem-solving techniques.* Complicated problems can be frustrating, especially if you are in a hurry. For example, a pediatric medication dosage may not always be easy to calculate. You do not know how to spell the term you are researching, so it is taking you a long time to find information about it. Combine deep breathing with a step-by-step approach, talking yourself through a complicated calculation or seeing if you can break the tricky term down into known word parts from your medical terminology courses.
* *Adopt positive communication strategies.* When we are angry, being heard and understood often helps. Likewise, it is important to be a good listener. By listening, we are less likely to say something that escalates the conflict. Do not forget to listen to yourself, too. Angry people often jump to unwarranted conclusions, so be careful not to voice those before you have had a chance to calm down. Despite what you might be thinking, expressing your thoughts in the heat of the moment might make things worse. Try to convey understanding when having a difficult conversation.
* *Combine humor with insight to defuse anger.* Sometimes, self-deprecating humor can defuse your anger and help you to gain a new perspective. Humor must be used delicately, however. Never use sarcasm or cynicism in an angry situation.
* *Change your environment.* Often, a change of scene can defuse anger. Try leaving the area where you became angry to reflect and regain your perspective.

Confronting Others' Anger

Angry people can be very intimidating. That is often part of the destructive power of anger. How you respond when confronted by an intimidating, angry person can determine whether the situation gets better or worse.

Some people "take the bait" of an angry person and respond with anger. Suddenly, it becomes a competition of who is the angriest or the most intimidating. Although strong emotions can be contagious, it is a mistake to meet anger with anger. Such a response escalates a conflict, rather than defusing it. Confrontation, no matter how well intentioned, is rarely a constructive approach to an angry person.

Speak when you are angry, and you will make the best speech you will ever regret.

—Ambrose Bierce

Dealing With Angry Patients

With most people, and particularly in response to angry patients, it is best to be empathetic and comforting (Figure 2.4). Try to listen and ask nonconfrontational questions or objective questions, such as "When did this happen?" or "What did she tell you then?"

As a health professional, your aim should be to defuse their anger and attempt to address any issues in a constructive manner. Recognize that people who appear angry may actually feel hurt, disappointed, or disrespected. If possible, sympathize with the patient to validate that they have a right to their emotions. Seeing that someone understands and respects

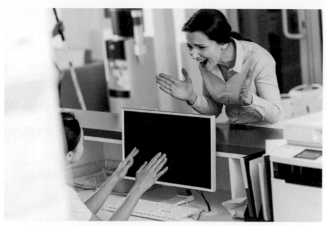

FIGURE 2.4 A receptionist listens to a complaining patient. (Copyright © istock.com.)

their feelings may go a long way toward assuaging their anger.

You never understand a person until you consider things from his point of view.

—Harper Lee

JOURNALING 2.3

Describe a time when you dealt effectively with an angry patient or co-worker. What happened? What actions did you take to control the situation?

Dealing With Angry Co-Workers

Co-workers who exhibit professionalism and manners learn to separate their work problems from their personal problems and rarely display anger at work. Unfortunately, you may encounter co-workers who behave in a less-professional manner. One effective technique for dealing with difficult or emotional co-workers is to find out what is at the center of their feelings.

Even if co-workers act unprofessionally toward you, their anger may have nothing to do with you. Asking a constructive question about the source of their anger may be all that is needed to help your co-worker refocus on their work. For instance, you might ask, "You seem upset. Did something happen?" If your co-worker is upset with you for some reason, your question will get the matter out in the open, so it can be addressed effectively. Box 2.4 offers some helpful questions to use for initiating productive conversations with angry or frustrated co-workers.

Dealing With an Angry Supervisor

Sometimes, supervisors think it is their right as the boss to express inappropriate anger toward their team. Some may even think anger is an appropriate management strategy or a motivational tool. However, anger is an emotion, not a management tool. Those in charge of others should try to keep their emotions in check when interacting with their team members and staff. Instead, focus on the goal of your interaction; what do you want to change?

It is tempting, if the only tool you have is a hammer, to treat everything as if it were a nail.

—Abraham Maslow

As professionals, we may sometimes be confronted by an angry supervisor. If a supervisor's angry behavior is highly unusual, the most constructive approach would likely be to treat them with empathy. Recognize that your supervisor is a human being and may get angry sometimes, just like everybody else. Your supervisor may be under a lot of pressure from their supervisor or some other reason unbeknownst to you. Try to listen and respond in the same way you would respond to an angry patient, and see where you might be helpful to them.

If your supervisor is frequently angry or seems especially angry toward you, you may need to try a different strategy. Confrontation is not recommended, particularly in a public place, and arguing with a supervisor may get you in trouble. Instead, try to discern the source of the supervisor's anger by listening to what they say in meetings or in interactions that precede an outburst. It may be that what you perceive as anger is really frustration with an employee's behavior or quality of work.

If you have an ongoing concern about the way your supervisor treats you in particular, schedule a meeting with them and give them the same direct feedback you would offer to a co-worker. This tactic may be enough to address your concerns. At the very least, it will lead to a frank discussion of the issues your supervisor may have with you. Be prepared to receive constructive criticism. If it is your behavior or the quality of your work is the issue, use that as an opportunity to try to improve. If you feel your supervisor's expectations are unrealistic, share that concern. Have an honest, respectful conversation with them to manage expectations and set realistic goals.

However, if your supervisor's behavior is hostile, aggressive, bullying, or otherwise inappropriate, you should report this behavior to Human Resources. If possible, document any interactions you have with them in order to support your case. Keep emails or voicemail messages that reflect the hostile behavior, for instance, or take note of the date and time of inappropriate or threatening conversations, as well as what was said.

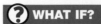 **WHAT IF?**

What if your supervisor embarrassed you in public? How would you respond?

For every minute you are angry, you lose sixty seconds of happiness.

—**Ralph Waldo Emerson**

CASE STUDY **2.2**
Lifetime Achievement

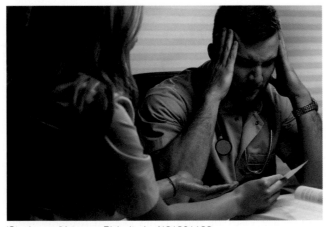

iStock.com/KatarzynaBialasiewicz/481801122

Molly Griffin is a speech therapist, and she was having a difficult time communicating with the medical administrative assistant, Lou. He had received a poor performance evaluation from the office manager, Kenosha Cooper, and still seemed mad about it. One area of improvement that they discussed was for him to improve his communication with co-workers.

During their lunch break, Lou complained about his evaluation to Molly. "Can you believe that?" When Molly did not say anything, he got upset and said, "Do you agree with her or something?" Molly cautiously replied, "I don't know but I think that's a discussion between you and Kenosha." They ate the rest of their lunch in silence.

A few days later, Molly is reviewing the patient schedule for tomorrow. She notices that the 10:30 a.m. slot is double booked. She discovers that Lou was the one to schedule that appointment. When asked, he said, "Oh, yeah. I scheduled Mr. Hanaway for the 10:30 a.m. appointment. I forgot to call him to reschedule his appointment since Ms. Gerrick was already scheduled for that time."

"Well, have you called Mr. Hanaway yet?" Molly asked.

"Uh, not yet. But I'm planning to," Lou stammered.

"Lou! His appointment is tomorrow! You needed to let him know a lot sooner. This is really too short notice to cancel the appointment."

"Okay, well, I'll call him right now and let him know."

Later that week, Kenosha asks Molly to conduct the weekly inventory of medical supplies. As she was reviewing the list, she noticed that it was already done. She noticed that Lou's initials were on the inventory list. Molly decided to confirm with Lou.

"Hi, Lou. Kenosha asked me to do the inventory of the medical supplies, but I see your initials on it. Did you already do it?" Molly asked.

"Yeah, I did it last week."

"Well, did you inform Kenosha that you were doing it?" Molly asks, exasperated.

"No. I didn't," Lou answers sheepishly.

"Oh, Lou, you've got to tell people when you do things. Otherwise, we're tripping over each other," Molly says.

"Are you my supervisor too now?" Lou says angrily. "Why don't you mind your own business next time. I don't need your help," he adds as he storms off.

Molly is speechless as she watches Lou walk away upset. She was not expecting such an emotional reaction from him since all she was trying to do was do her job and do what Kenosha, her supervisor, asked of her. She was going to go after Lou and give him a piece of her mind, but she stopped herself. She took a deep breath and thought about why Lou would react that way. She understood that he had some difficult conversations with Kenosha, which is surely making it a stressful situation for him. Molly decides to let Lou calm down before talking to him about their interaction.

Later that week, Molly sees Lou eating alone in the breakroom. She approaches him and asks if she can sit down. He nods.

"I think we should talk about what happened earlier this week. I appreciate you and I want us to work well together. Wouldn't you agree?" she asks.

Lou nods and says, "I do. I guess I was just getting frustrated."

"I should've known that, and I should've been more sensitive about that. But, you know, I was only doing my job, like you. I know you're stressed and frustrated, but it's better for you to try to express that more constructively. Not everyone is going to know what a good person you are and how hard you try," Molly said.

"I appreciate that you said that. I do try, but it always seem like I'm getting in trouble."

"Maybe I can help you with ways to stay organized and to improve your communication," Molly offered.

QUESTIONS FOR THOUGHT AND REFLECTION

1. What challenges did Lou have at his job?
2. Why do you think Lou reacted the way he did toward Molly?
3. What would have happened if Molly reacted in the same way as Lou did to her?
4. What are some effective tools that Molly can provide Lou for him to be better at time management and communication?

A Different Path

Management at the assisted living facility brought in a new director, Peter Harmon, to cut costs and streamline operations. Peter is in charge of both the facilities and reporting to the owner, Dr. Houdek. "Everybody's job is on the line," he announced in his first meeting with the staff.

He flashed a notebook and a red pen. "Now, I want to get everyone's views on what we can do to reduce costs and increase services. Say what's on your mind." No one spoke.

Pretty soon, however, a voice came over the speakerphone. It was Jeff, the recreational therapist at the Greene Street facility. He was advocating for combined field trips because there was plenty of room on the bus, and it would be a good social opportunity for the two facilities. Pretty soon, Peter was rolling his eyes. Finally, he jammed the mute button on the phone as Jeff continued outlining his ideas. "I really can't make out what that guy is saying," said Peter, "but he's clearly clueless." He interrupted Jeff. "Field trips cost money. We're not doing that. Anyone else have other ideas?"

Eve spoke up and said, "I didn't think that was such a bad idea."

"Oh, you don't, Miss …?" said Peter.

"Deming," she said. "Eve Deming."

"So, what's *your* big idea?" said Peter.

"I don't have an idea. I just thought Jeff …."

Peter interrupted her. "Miss Deming, no ideas? Anyone else?"

"Excuse me, but I wasn't done speaking. I think this process would be more effective if you were more open to ideas," she pressed on.

"Oh, you don't have any ideas and you don't like my process," he said. "Well, here's the deal, *Ms*. Deming. We're going to make some big changes around here."

QUESTIONS FOR THOUGHT AND REFLECTION

1. How would you describe Peter's demeanor toward the staff?
2. What do you think Peter's goal was in the meeting? How might he behave differently to achieve that goal more effectively?
3. Do you think Eve's response was appropriate?
4. In your opinion, what should Jeff, Eve, and the other employees in the meeting have done? What were their options?

1. Keep track of the number of negative thoughts, inaccurate assessments, unkind evaluations, and mental insults you make about other people during an entire day. If you can, write them down so you can look at them and reevaluate them the next day. What did you learn from this?
2. What kind of anger would you tolerate from someone else? Does it matter who the person is? At what point would you walk away from the person, refusing to subject yourself to further abuse? Where do you draw the line, personally?
3. Pretend to get angry and shout at yourself in a mirror. What do you see? Would you be intimidating to others? Unpleasant? Ugly? Scary?
4. Avoid challenging an angry person by locking eye contact with him, by focusing at a spot low on his forehead just between his eyes. Try this out with a friend. Tell each other what it felt like.

 CROSS CURRENTS WITH OTHER SOFT SKILLS

MODELING BUSINESS ETIQUETTE: A well-mannered employee can command respect in the workplace without ever being angry or difficult (Chapter 13).
SHOWING EMPATHY, SENSITIVITY, AND CARING: Empathy is the best way to disarm an angry patient or co-worker (Chapters 3 and 5).
DEALING WITH DIFFICULT PEOPLE: Emotional people can be difficult (Chapter 7).
PRACTICING PATIENCE: A thoughtful, patient, considered response defuses many emotional situations (Chapter 3).

Optimism, Pessimism, and Realism

I wish I could show you, when you are lonely or in darkness, the astonishing light of your own being.

—Hafiz of Shiraz

LEARNING OBJECTIVE 4: EXUDING OPTIMISM, ENTHUSIASM, AND POSITIVITY

- State the benefits of optimism.
- Connect optimism with good health.
- Relate goal achievement to optimism.
- Understand the limitations and strengths of pessimism.

We can view optimism and pessimism as ways to interpret the events of life. Optimists typically believe that the world is good at its core and good things await us in the end, despite any difficulties we may encounter. They believe things will work out, and if things go wrong, they will get better. Pessimists, on the other hand, take a different perspective. They often see the world as a hostile place, with danger lurking everywhere. They see the negative possibilities and believe if things can go wrong, they will.

When you believe things will go wrong, they often do. When you believe things will work out, they often seem to. These differences are largely due to perspective, or what a person chooses to focus on. It is not that a pessimist experiences more difficult or trying situations and optimists have more good things happen to them, but that a pessimist focuses on the negative, whereas an optimist focuses on the positive. These attitudes influence the small and large outcomes in your life.

Both optimism and pessimism, however, can be self-fulfilling prophesies and potentially limiting. Realism, on the other hand, is understanding how the world works and willing to accept it. Realists are the people who believe that the world is not perfect and that there will be problems. They are not idealistic and have few unrealistic expectations. A realist accepts and gets on with life for better or worse. They don't see the world in black and white, but rather in shades of gray.

← JOURNALING 2.4

Write about two instances in your life—one when you gave up more easily than you should have, and one when you were resilient in the face of a challenge. Which characteristics did you display in each of these situations? What were the differences and similarities in both situations that resulted in different actions?

Optimism

Benefits of Optimism

Optimists believe in the power of positive thinking. They are often happy and see the glass as half full. Optimists are people who believe that everything will be all right in the end. They believe that there is always hope for the future, even if things are not going well in the present. Box 2.5 lists the many benefits of being optimistic.

BOX 2.5

Benefits of Optimism

- It enables you to generate an alternative, more hopeful explanation for difficulties experienced.
- It reduces your level of stress.
- It increases longevity.
- It promotes happiness.
- It forges persistence, which is an essential trait for achieving success.
- It creates a sense of fulfillment and satisfaction.
- It promotes healthy living.
- It creates a positive anticipation of the future.
- It allows you to deal with failure and mistakes constructively.
- It enables you to counteract any negative thoughts that arise.
- It increases the likelihood of effective problem solving.
- It creates a positive attitude.
- It increases your level of motivation.
- It promotes laughter.
- It welcomes any form of constructive change.
- It creates positive expectations.
- It sets your mood for the day.
- It promotes positive relationships.
- It builds resilience in the face of adversity.
- It promotes self-confidence and boosts self-esteem.
- It improves your social life.
- It increases your mental flexibility.
- It is therapeutic.

Affects on Health

Research shows that an optimistic outlook can strengthen the immune system. As optimistic people believe their fate is in their own hands, they may be more motivated to pursue healthier lifestyles, including eating a balanced diet and exercising regularly.

They are more likely to seek help from health care professionals when they have health concerns, and they seek support from friends when they are dealing with problems. By being proactive about their health, optimists achieve physical resiliency and positive health outcomes.

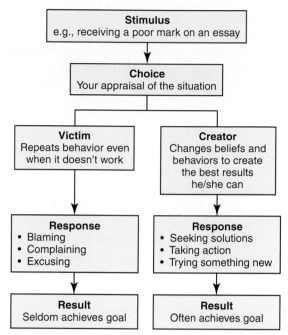

FIGURE 2.5 How two responses to an event can influence the outcome. (Modified from LaFair S: *Don't bring it to work*, San Francisco, 2009, Jossey Bass.)

Resilience and Perseverance

Optimists tend not to take failures personally. This may create a blind spot, as focusing on internal factors within one's control can help a person learn from their failures. However, they also do not view setbacks as permanent, which can lead to greater resilience in the face of challenges.

If optimists try to learn from their experiences, greeting disappointments with renewed hope, energy, and informed strategies, they can overcome even big obstacles that greet them in the future. Simply put, optimism enhances resilience and perseverance, and resilience and perseverance fuel success. Different stimuli and factors can influence outcomes (Figure 2.5).

How to Be a Realistic Optimist

The hardest challenge is to be yourself in a world where everyone is trying to make you be somebody else.

—E. E. Cummings

Talk Like an Optimist

What you say when you talk to yourself matters tremendously. Pessimism often involves negative self-talk, littered with absolutes such as "you never get anything right" or "it will never work out for you."

Being a realistic optimistic involves choosing to focus on the positive and adjusting your behavior and self-talk accordingly. You can recognize when things go wrong and take ownership, while still maintaining a positive outlook. Positivity keeps your focus on the future you want to achieve, and positive expectations often lead to positive results. Just because things went wrong this time does not mean things will always go wrong for you. Rather than blaming or berating yourself for making a mistake, focus instead on what you can learn from it. If something does not work the first time, try another approach. Talk to others about your plans and positive expectations. People tend to like positive people and want to help them.

Sharing your optimistic perspective and approach to a problem will not only spread positivity but also attract the help and support of those around you. It may also help you get valuable feedback that can help you plan more effectively.

Pessimism

If it wasn't for bad luck, I wouldn't have no luck at all.

—William Bell

Martin Seligman (Seligman and Csikszentmihalyi, 2000), a researcher from the University of Pennsylvania and past president of the American Psychological Association, wrote about some of the dangers of being pessimistic. His research showed that pessimistic people are eight times more likely to suffer from depression than optimistic people. In addition, pessimists lead shorter lives than optimists and suffer from more illnesses. The cause of this gap is still being researched, but existing research indicates that depression lowers immune system function. Other studies suggest that people who feel helpless are more susceptible to cancer and fare much more poorly in fighting disease and infection. This may also be attributed to pessimists being less likely to seek medical help sooner. Thus, although pessimism can help people anticipate problems or potential complications, it may also promote a sense of fatalism when things do go wrong, preventing people from believing that things will improve.

You can either be an actor in your own life, or a reactor in somebody else's.

—Hillary Rodham Clinton

BOX 2.6

What Optimists Can Learn From Pessimists

- Analyze situations to uncover risks and obstacles.
- Evaluate risks realistically.
- Know when to cut your losses and move on.
- Pay attention to safety-related issues.
- Be open-minded.
- Be flexible.
- Sympathize with those going through hard times.

Benefits of Pessimism

Although pessimism is often seen as a negative, studies show that pessimists tend to be more realistic in their assessment of a situation than optimists. This means that optimists sometimes overlook obstacles when making and pursuing plans. Optimists can learn from their pessimistic counterparts by analyzing all sides of a situation carefully, listening with an open mind to opposing views, and being skeptical when appropriate. A balanced view of what optimists can learn from pessimists is shown in Box 2.6.

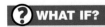 **WHAT IF?**

What if you accomplished something great, but you overheard someone say you did not deserve it? What would you say to yourself or that person?

Plan Like a Pessimist

An honest assessment of your circumstances and the scope of an issue will enable you to set realistic goals, make plans that account for possible obstacles, and make steady improvements in your performance. As discussed previously, optimistic people tend to be less realistic in their plans, as they can fail to account for potential problems. Pessimists, expecting that things will go wrong, tend to plan for those possibilities and are thus better prepared if something does go awry.

Optimists need not adopt a pessimistic attitude but would be well served by learning to plan like a pessimist. For example, if you must give a slide presentation, first imagine all the things that could go wrong: you might trip on the computer cords walking up to the podium, your presentation might not load properly, or you might forget what you want to say. How you can you plan for these things without expecting to fail? You can prepare for them by making a mental note to watch out for cords when walking up to the podium, saving your presentation on two different thumb drives and emailing yourself a copy, and printing out notes in case you forget what you want to say. Then, tell yourself that your preparation for any setbacks will ensure that things go smoothly. Now that you are well prepared, you can anticipate a positive outcome. If things do not go well, you can use that experience to help you plan better the next time.

Whether you think you can, or whether you think you can't, you're right.

—Henry Ford

 EXPERIENTIAL EXERCISES

1. See a health care professional, such as a dentist, a massage therapist, or a pharmacist, as soon as possible about a health concern you have been putting off.
2. Volunteer somewhere that interests you.
3. Dispute a pessimistic belief that you have.

 CROSS CURRENTS WITH OTHER SOFT SKILLS

ADOPTING A POSITIVE MENTAL ATTITUDE: An optimist attitude can lead to positive results (Chapter 3).

THINKING CRITICALLY: Critical thinking will help you reap the benefits of optimism, while avoiding its pitfalls (Chapter 6).

SETTING GOALS AND PLANNING ACTIONS: Optimism, along with realistic planning, makes significant goal achievement possible (Chapter 15).

STRENGTHENING RESILIENCE: Any attitude that strengthens your immune system strengthens your resilience (Chapter 3).

References

Gross JJ, Thompson RA. Emotion regulation: conceptual foundations. In: Gross JJ, ed. *Handbook of emotion regulation*. The Guilford Press; 2007:3–24.

Salovey P, Mayer JD. Emotional intelligence. *Imagin Cogn Pers.* 1990;9(3):185–211. https://doi.org/10.2190/DUGG-P24E-52WK-6CDG.

Seligman MEP, Csikszentmihalyi M. Positive psychology: an introduction. *American Psychologist.* 2000;55(1):5–14. https://doi.org/10.1037/0003-066X.55.1.5.

CHAPTER 3

Building Emotional Strength

BY THE END OF THIS CHAPTER, YOU WILL BE ABLE TO	
	■ Understand and Evaluate the State of Your Self-Esteem.
	■ Create a Plan to Boost and Sustain Your Self-Esteem
	■ Know How to Manage Anxiety
	■ Connect Patience to Long-Term Results
	■ Identify Different Stressors in Your Personal and Professional Life
	■ Determine Different Methods to Maintain Emotional and Physical Health. Building Self-Esteem

Don't let anyone speak for you, and don't rely on others to fight for you.

—Michelle Obama

LEARNING OBJECTIVE 1: BUILDING SELF-ESTEEM

■ Defining what is self-esteem.
■ Set goals to increase your self-esteem.
■ Bring more positive influences into your life.

Importance of Self-Esteem

Self-esteem describes a person's overall subjective sense of personal worth or value. In other words, self-esteem may be defined as how much you appreciate and like yourself regardless of the circumstances. There are many elements of self-esteem, such as self-confidence, feelings of security, sense of belonging, and feel of competence.

Self-esteem is important because it impacts your ability to make good decisions, your relationships, and your emotional health and overall well-being. It also influences motivation, as people with a healthy, positive view of themselves understand their potential and may feel inspired to take on new challenges.

People with low self-esteem tend to feel less sure of their abilities and may doubt their decision-making process. They may not feel motivated to try novel things because they do not believe they can reach their goals. Those with low self-esteem may have issues with relationships and expressing their needs. They may also experience low levels of confidence and feel unlovable and unworthy.

However, people with overly high self-esteem may overestimate their skills and may feel entitled to success, even without the abilities to back up their belief in themselves. They may struggle with relationship issues and block themselves from self-improvement because they are so fixated on seeing themselves as perfect.

Feelings of high or low self-worth often start in childhood. In fact, self-esteem tends to be lowest in childhood and increases during adolescence, as well as adulthood, eventually reaching a fairly stable and enduring level. Many factors influence one's self-esteem, such as age, family, socioeconomic status, physical ability and disability, genetics, and life experiences. For example, racism, sexism, and other types of discrimination often have negative effects on self-esteem. It is often our experiences that form the basis for overall self-esteem. For example, low self-esteem might be caused by overly critical or negative assessments from family and friends. Those who experience unconditional positive regard will be more likely to have healthy self-esteem. Box 3.1 lists the key characteristics of healthy self-esteem.

Being saddled with low self-esteem is like being prejudiced against yourself. Only you can place a value, high or low, on the way you view yourself. No one can make you feel inferior without your consent.

—Eleanor Roosevelt

Building Healthy Self-Esteem

Although some of your self-esteem has already been developed by the time you reach adulthood, you are still able to control it. Your self-esteem is based on your interpretation of your actions over time. Although self-esteem evolves, you may still carry feelings associated with childhood experiences. Recognize that those circumstances were likely beyond your control as a child, but you have more agency to guide your experiences as an adult. You can also choose how you view yourself and your response to different experiences and events in your life. By taking control of your thoughts, you can improve your self-esteem.

There are several steps that you can take to address problems with your perceptions of yourself to create healthier self-esteem. First, beware of what can create negative self-esteem (Box 3.2). Learn to identify the negative thoughts and thinking patterns and counter those with more positive and realistic ones. Use positive self-talk and practice reciting positive affirmations to yourself. Finally, practice self-compassion. Remind yourself that you should not expect to be perfect and that you will make mistakes. Forgive yourself for past mistakes, learn from them, and move forward.

By paying attention to your actions and behaviors, as well as your interactions with others, you can take steps to become a healthier, more confident person. In fact, your work performance is a great opportunity for building and molding your self-esteem. For one thing,

? WHAT IF?

What if a patient yells at you for something that is not your fault? How would you respond?

BOX 3.1

Characteristics of Healthy Self-Esteem

- A firm understanding of one's knowledge and skills
- The ability to maintain healthy relationships with others as a result of having a healthy relationship with oneself
- Realistic and appropriate personal expectations
- An understanding of one's needs and the ability to express those needs

BOX 3.2

Factors That Contribute to Low Self-Esteem

- Trying to impress others
- Seeking approval from others
- Comparing yourself to others
- Envy
- Always giving in or compromising
- Cringing at criticism
- Worrying
- Being fearful of trying something new
- Never stepping outside of your comfort zone
- Striving for perfection or unrealistic goals
- Lashing out, being abusive, or bullying
- Silently putting yourself down
- Lacking control over your life and decisions
- Isolating yourself socially
- Boasting

you can learn to abandon the practices discussed that result in low self-esteem.

Everyone struggles with self-esteem at one time or another. An individual's self-esteem can fluctuate moment by moment in response to events, perceptions, self-talk, and feedback. Our self-esteem can be especially vulnerable when we experience change, whether it is an extremely challenging patient, a new piece of medical equipment or software, or a different supervisor. Such changes often require new skills and may put us into unfamiliar situations we have little experience with. As we struggle to gain proficiency and learn to manage the new circumstances effectively, we may lose confidence in our abilities.

It ain't what they call you, it's what you answer to.

—**W.C. Fields**

Set the Right Goals

One of the worst things you can do for your self-esteem is to compare yourself to others. There will always be someone who is smarter, faster, younger, stronger, funnier, fitter, or better looking than you. At the same time, you will outperform others in different ways at different times. You may excel at things others struggle with. In fact, merely by getting a job, you have succeeded where someone else failed. Even though it is okay to feel good about these successes and to acknowledge areas in which you have room to grow, constant comparisons with other people are counterproductive and can injure your confidence.

Rather than comparing yourself with others, compare your present self with your former self. Are you getting better? Do you have a plan to develop your abilities so that you have a brighter future? Instead of trying to impress or seek the approval of others, focus on improving your own opinion of yourself. Your opinion matters most.

Setting realistic goals will set you on the path to a better life and improved self-esteem. If you know what you want to achieve in life and you feel you are working on a plan to achieve those goals, your self-esteem will rise. Visualize a future full of meaning, success, and satisfaction. Imagine it as vividly as you can, using all your senses to think about all the areas of your life.

Do not let past failures and disappointments interfere with your opinion of yourself. Those mistakes are over and should be used as learning opportunities. Move forward. Embrace the present—the only place where you can be effective—and take actions that move you closer to the future that you envision and desire.

There is nothing noble about being superior to some other man. The true nobility is in being superior to your previous self.

—**Hindu proverb**

Focus on Your Strengths

Do you give yourself permission to celebrate your accomplishments? Recognize your strengths and work on developing them. Do not be afraid to give yourself credit for your achievements (Figure. 3.1).

What about your weaknesses? We all have limitations. You should work to minimize the effects of these limitations, but you will be happier and more successful if you concentrate on your strengths and accept your limitations. Do not exaggerate or invent limitations through negative self-talk and false beliefs.

You yourself, as much as anybody in the entire universe, deserve your love and affection.

—**Buddha**

Build the Positive Into Your Life

Nurturing your self-esteem can be a daily struggle. You are constantly being evaluated, challenged, and offered feedback you may not even want. Pursuing actions every day that support your positive self-esteem will help you accept and process criticism.

For starters, make it a point to associate with positive people. Humans need social interaction and acceptance, and you can make this an extremely positive part of your daily life if you choose who you spend your time with. Avoid taking in unnecessary negativity by surrounding yourself with positive people.

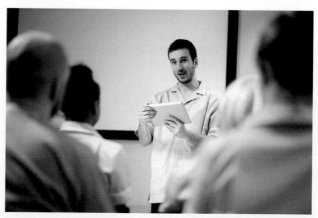

Figure 3.1 A confident health care professional gives a presentation. (Copyright © istock.com.)

When you are alone, take time to do activities that make you feel good. Meditate. Practice yoga. Detach yourself from your daily stressors, even if it means stepping into a quiet room or taking some deep breaths. The more you know how to protect yourself from stress, the better you will feel about yourself.

Project confidence with your body language. To *feel* confident, *act as if* you are confident. In other words, "fake it until you make it." A confident mindset is the strongest pathway to achieving healthy self-esteem. Finally, accept praise and criticism with a simple "Thank you." Even those who criticize you give you something to think about. If you do not agree with their critique, simply smile, thank them, and say you will give some thought to their comment or the help they are offering. When you receive a compliment, a simple thank you acknowledges the kind comment. Put the praise in your gratitude journal (see Journaling 3.1).

JOURNALING 3.1

Make a section of your journal a "gratitude journal." At the end of every day, describe an instance that you are grateful for.

Challenge Yourself

Challenging yourself is the surest way to improve and to raise your self-esteem. The thing to remember when approaching a new challenge is not to let fear get in your way. Although some fears are based on real threats, many are irrational and counterproductive. The latter tend to disappear or at least recede when met head-on. For instance, if you fear approaching new people, you will usually find that it is not as scary as you thought if you challenge your fear, and it will become easier the more you do it.

Consider ways you could increase your self-esteem at work if you were not being held back by fears. Once you identify a fear that is holding you back, make a plan to confront the fear and master the behavior. You will be more effective at your job and possess a solid level of positive self-esteem. When you step outside of your comfort zone, it will feel a little dangerous at first, but persist. Soon, your comfort zone will expand to encompass more and more skills and experiences. Keep pushing the boundaries.

Surround yourself with people who are better than you at what you want to learn. Think about playing a sport. If you play against someone who is equal in skill or much worse than you, your skills may stagnate. By the same token, if you play against someone who is better than you, you will improve your game. This philosophy applies to any activity or role. You learn best from those who are more advanced than you, so seek these people out when you want to improve your abilities. In the end, you will improve your self-esteem, as well.

Once your efforts to improve your self-esteem start to pay off, continue developing your skills. Assertiveness, for example, is a great skill to cultivate. Being assertive means showing confidence and being able to act and say what is on your mind. However, there is a proper time and place for asserting yourself, and assertive is not the same as aggressive or defensive. As noted previously, listen respectfully when others offer constructive criticism, even if you do not agree with them, and avoid acting defensive. You should use assertiveness to defend the policies and rules of your workplace, the safety and professionalism of your practice, and the standards of behavior you expect from co-workers and clients. However, you should avoid aggressively demanding that others do things your way or agree with your opinions. Seek to build positive relationships with others by standing up for what you think is right, while listening to and respecting the views of others.

CASE STUDY 3.1
The Diploma

Christine Sarkasian had been working as a professional coder on cardiology units for 3 years. She had already earned her Certified Professional Coder (CPC) certification, and she had a goal of making a yearly salary of at least $50,000 within 2 years. She had advanced knowledge of cardiac coding,

and she thought she would try for the Certified Cardiology Coder (CCC) credential. She submitted the required two letters of recommendation and signed up for a test date. As an American Academy of Professional Coders (AAPC) member, she qualified for a reduced fee and one retake.

The examination did not go as well as Christine had anticipated. The 150 multiple-choice questions covered many situations she had never encountered, and she had to guess on many of them.

The week-long wait for her score was excruciating. Christine had told many of her colleagues, friends, and family members that she was going for the CCC credential. Finally, she went online and learned that she had failed.

At first, she was angry. How could she fail the examination with all her experience? How was she going to tell her friends and colleagues? Christine started beating herself up about her score. "I'm just stupid," she told herself. "I'm not cut out for this." That night, she had trouble sleeping.

When she awoke, she called her friend Marsha, who was an instructor with a CPC-I certification and taught at the college Christine had attended. "You should have called me *before* you took that test," Marsha said. "That examination is super hard. I could have given you some prep tips."

"I didn't prep at all," Christine said. "I'm so stupid."

"It was a mistake not to prep, but you're not stupid," Marsha said. "You just made an error in judgment."

After speaking with Marsha, Christine put together a plan for retaking the examination. She asked her colleague, Dr. Bachmann, for help with her cardiac catheterization procedures. He agreed to help her devise a study plan. Christine registered for online practice examinations at the AAPC site. With her membership, she could register for less than $30. Plus, the practice examinations included rationales, and she could take them as often as she wanted. She asked her colleagues about their CCC examination experiences, as well.

After 4 weeks of preparation, Christine took advantage of the examination retake. She figured out that she had 2 minutes and 15 seconds to answer each question. She left the test site that afternoon feeling confident about her effort.

Due to all her hard work, Christine passed the examination. Ten days after taking it, she received the certificate diploma. She framed it and hung it in her office cubicle.

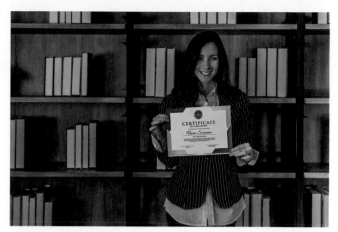

iStock.com/Mongkolchon Akesin/1302191259

QUESTIONS FOR THOUGHT AND REFLECTION

1. What do you think would have happened if Christine had succumbed to low self-esteem?
2. How did Christine's conversation with Marsha help her?
3. What was different about the first time Christine took the test and the second time?
4. What else could Christine have done to prepare for the retake?

A Different Path

Ava had been a surgical technologist for 2 years, but she had never had trouble like this. She had been hauled into a meeting of the surgical oncology team for a review of a recent surgery that had gone wrong. The patient had lung cancer but developed sepsis shortly after the lobectomy. He is now in a coma and not expected to live.

"For one thing, Ava, we don't seem to have the patient's informed consent for the surgery on file," said Dr. Hector, his face a pale shade of purple. "You did get the informed consent, didn't you?"

"Yes. You initialed it," she said.

"Good. Then, where is it?" he thundered.

Ava muttered that she would look for it. She was bad at filing. She hated it. But it must be somewhere in the stack on her desk.

"It's only a matter of time before lawyers are sifting through that chart. Mr. Longoria won't be signing another one, so I want that consent form in the chart immediately. Go ahead and look for it right now and let me know once you do."

A few minutes later, Ava found the consent form. "What an idiot I am," she thought to herself. "I'm making problems for myself." She put the form in Mr. Longoria's chart and went to let the doctors know.

"Great. Now, what about the infection? What can you tell us about your autoclaving of the instruments?"

Ava's heart sank. She thought she had properly sterilized the instruments, but it seemed now as though they were blaming her. "Well, I think I followed all the steps."

"You think or you know you? Did you or did you not sterilize them properly?"

"Yes. I sterilized the instruments. I've done it many times before," she replied, as she was getting more anxious and irritated.

"Well, I have to tell you that you will be asked about this by the attorney. You'll really need to think about if you did or not and how you'll respond," Dr. Hector said.

Ava went home angry at herself and the doctors. She flopped on the bed. All that time to become a surgical technologist, and for what? She wondered whether she should look for another line of work. Maybe she was not cut out for this type of high-pressure, highly detailed job.

⭐ EXPERIENTIAL EXERCISES

1. Review the journal you have kept for this book and look for signs of your self-esteem.
2. Pick out a positive self-affirmation you can always use silently to yourself when your self-esteem is challenged.
3. Make a list of your "greatest hits," the things you have accomplished in your life that you are most proud of.
4. Make a list of all your weaknesses. Now, cross out all of those that do not really hold you back from achieving your goals and feeling content. If there are any left uncrossed, make a plan to correct them to the level that they stop holding you back. Then, return to your strengths.
5. Wear a rubber band around your wrist. Whenever you notice that your self-talk is negative, snap the rubber band against the inside of your wrist. Notice how many times you snap the rubber band.

CROSS CURRENTS WITH OTHER SOFT SKILLS

ADOPTING A POSITIVE MENTAL ATTITUDE: When you choose to be positive and enthusiastic, your self-esteem rises (Chapter 2).

MANAGING STRESS: Many of the strategies and techniques you use to manage stress can contribute to your healthy self-esteem (Chapter 15).

SHOWING EMPATHY, SENSITIVITY, AND CARING: When your focus is on others, you are also being kind to yourself (Chapter 5).

READING AND SPEAKING BODY LANGUAGE: Let your body language project confidence to the outside world, and your inner world will follow (Chapter 6).

SETTING GOALS AND PLANNING ACTIONS: When you work on achieving your personal goals, you strengthen your self-esteem (Chapter 15).

QUESTIONS FOR THOUGHT AND REFLECTION

1. Do you think Ava's response to Dr. Hector was appropriate? What about Dr. Hector's comments?
2. What could Ava have done to better protect her self-esteem?
3. How do you think Ava will behave when and if she returns to work? What words of encouragement would you give her?

Controlling Anxiety

LEARNING OBJECTIVE 2: CONTROLLING ANXIETY

- Explain anxiety and its affect.
- Manage internal thought processes to control anxiety.
- Understand the role of anxiety on health outcomes.

What Is Anxiety?

Anxiety is the feeling you get when your well-being is threatened. You or a loved one could be in physical danger. Perhaps something challenges your self-esteem. Maybe you feel your status is being threatened because you are criticized in public. Maybe you had a falling out with a friend that threatens the relationship. Maybe your supervisor micromanages you at work, and it feels as if you have lost control of your time and activities. Maybe you are treated unfairly. When you have something to fear or lose, anxiety can dominate your feelings.

Anxiety occurs on a continuum from mild to debilitating. Mild anxiety can actually improve your performance by motivating you to concentrate on the activity that has raised your feelings of anxiety (Figure. 3.2). For instance, you may be extra cautious when drawing blood from someone who intimidates you. You may focus more intently on your job when assisting a dentist you may not know very well. Anxiety like this can still be uncomfortable, but it can also help improve your performance by forcing you to plan and concentrate.

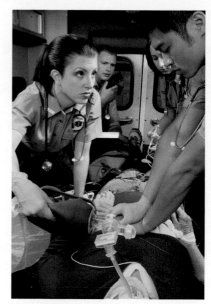

Figure 3.2 Emergency medical technicians quickly and efficiently respond to the immediate medical needs of an injured man. (Copyright © istock.com.)

Most anxiety associated with work is temporary. It may be triggered by a past negative experience, such as losing a job or interacting with a difficult patient. The more anxiety you experience, the more poorly you may perform, which can create additional anxiety. For that reason, an effective strategy is to identify and minimize your anxiety.

When anxiety goes beyond mild, it can impair performance. A higher anxiety level triggers the stress response. It clouds your thinking process; creates rapid, shallow breathing; raises your heart rate; and imposes a sense of panic. More severe cases of anxiety may be chronic anxiety, which is a constant and general feeling of dread about everything. Intense anxiety may also result in phobias, which are anxieties in response to specific triggers, such as spiders (arachnophobia) or closed spaces (claustrophobia). If you suffer from chronic anxiety or phobias, you may need to seek medical treatment to prevent these from interfering with the quality of your life, affecting your performance at work, and impeding your goals.

Anxiety is a thin stream of fear trickling through the mind. If encouraged, it cuts a stream through which all other thoughts are drained.

—Arthur Somers Roche

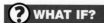 **WHAT IF?**

What if your entire life were anxiety-free? You did not worry about bills being paid, the children being safe, getting in a car accident, not graduating, or not having a job. What would it feel like?

In contrast, what if your day was filled with anxious thoughts about everything in your life? What physical symptoms do you think this would manifest if you continued being anxious from one moment to the next?

Factors Contributing to Anxiety

When anxiety is not effectively addressed, it can leave you with an irrational bias that affects your professional behavior. For example, a medical assistant may avoid screaming children due to a stressful interaction. They may develop an unfounded belief, such as, "I am not good with children. I always make them cry." However, they may not be the cause of the outburst, and it does not mean that the same reaction will happen every time. It is important to take time to challenge the original negative thought before it develops into a bias.

Sometimes, when a profound incident occurs, we develop stories to justify why we perceived the event as negative instead of neutral. For example, almost every medical office assistant will encounter a patient who is upset about a billing error sooner or later. One person may handle the situation and not attach any meaning to it, whereas another person might avoid handling any future billing questions. They think, "I always mess up patients' accounts. Someone who is better at math should handle all the billing questions."

If an incident causes you to avoid an activity, this can interfere with your work and the work of your co-workers. For example, suppose a patient vomited after a dental assistant took x-rays of their teeth. The assistant may believe that they caused the patient to gag and vomit, and may not be good at taking x-rays. As a result, they may avoid taking x-rays of future patients, which creates hardships for their co-workers and may even affect job performance. Avoidance limits your usefulness on the job and creates obstacles to your progress. Try instead to use such experiences as learning opportunities to improve your performance.

JOURNALING 3.2

Write about something or someone you avoid at work because of a past negative experience. What thoughts and feelings did you choose to associate with this event or person? What story did you create to justify avoiding future encounters? Rewrite the story with a new, positive, and realistic outcome.

Controlling Anxiety

It is not always possible to control anxiety, especially if it is serious and becomes a medical condition. There are times we can control it, and learning how to effectively manage your anxiety is crucial to your overall and day-to-day success at work. It is important to catch anxious thinking early, before it evolves into fearful behavior. To do so, you will have to be skilled in identifying when those anxious feelings arise and take steps to employ strategies to try to overcome them. You cannot always control external events, especially those causing anxiety, or your internal reactions to these external events. But you can try to recognize when they happen and control your responses or how you behave because of them.

We cannot direct the wind, but we can adjust our sails.

— Bertha Calloway

Choose Your Thoughts

Believe it or not, you can control your thoughts. You stand at the gate of your conscious mind, so to speak, and you get to determine what passes through and what is cast down. When you guard your thinking, you can refute some of the thoughts that do not align with reality. For example, if you are administering an IV for a patient in the hospital and you think, "What if I give the patient the wrong medication?" In that moment, when you become aware of the thought, stop and refute it by checking the medication order before it develops into fear. You can do this with any negative thought by:

1. Identifying the concerning thought.
2. Analyzing whether it is a logical thought.
3. Refuting the thought or challenging its validity.
4. Carefully completing the action you had the anxious thought about.

Cognitive psychology, which is a field of psychology, offers effective approaches you can use to alleviate your anxiety. These approaches help you realize that the reality you experience is based on your thinking, your thoughts, and your interpretation of events and circumstances. When you challenge irrational thoughts that counter anxiety, you can replace them with rational thoughts that tend to reduce or eliminate the anxiety out of the situation. Box 3.3 offers a series of reminders to combat and alleviate anxiety.

 JOURNALING 3.3

Do you harbor irrational beliefs? For example, it is irrational to think that everything is directed at you personally. List as many as you can think of. Then, write out a statement to refute each of them.

Preventing Avoidance Behaviors

To conquer avoidance, you must have enough courage to take a small step toward countering your fear. For example, the dental assistant anxious about taking x-rays can use a process called "gradual exposure" to combat the feared stimulus (taking x-rays) until it no longer produces anxiety. They can start by developing the films for another assistant who has taken x-rays and then mount the films. Next, when they are confident that they can complete this task, they can move to setting up the films and film holders for the other assistant and seating patients. Then, they can hand the other assistant the film holder for placement in the patient's mouth. This process will provide enough positive experiences to nullify the "all or nothing" thinking developed by the negative experience and allow for resolution and alleviation of the anxiety.

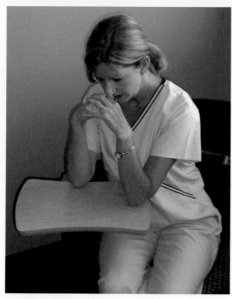

Figure 3.3 A health care professional regaining her composure.

Learn to Relax

Relaxation is a learned behavior; it is knowledge you should have in your battle against anxiety. Many techniques, such as deep breathing or meditation, are simple and require little time. Other strategies, such as recomposing yourself in private, require a more focused approach (Figure. 3.3). Other relaxation strategies appear in Box 3.4.

Forgiving Yourself

We can be amazingly hard on ourselves. Negative self-talk, low self-esteem, anxiety, uncontrolled emotions, impatience, intolerance, and even self-hatred are common ways we beat ourselves up. If you are your own worst enemy, bring yourself immediate peace of mind simply by recognizing how hard you have been on yourself. Next, try to be kind to yourself. Recognize that mistakes are normal. You are compassionate toward your patients. Why not be compassionate toward yourself?

Anxiety and Your Health

Finally, use your own health as strong motivation for controlling anxiety. Remember that anxiety can cause physical symptoms, including heart palpitations, sweating, shortness of breath, stomach pains, nausea, muscular tension, shakiness, and dizziness. Many of these symptoms can interrupt a normal workday and even cause biochemical changes in the body, which can create illness.

If you feel anxious, try some of the anti-anxiety techniques listed in Box 3.5. It is much easier to prevent severe anxiety than to address it once it gets out of control. If anxiety becomes chronic or severe, you may need medication and mental health care to effectively manage it.

Heavy thoughts bring on physical maladies; when the soul is oppressed, so is the body.

—Martin Luther

CASE STUDY 3.2
The King Exception

Martha had been a dental assistant for about 5 years. She knew the clinical side well, but she was too timid for the front office. There were so many different duties and responsibilities, and you often had to deal with multiple people at the same time. The thought of this made Martha very anxious.

To push herself to be more assertive, she asked to work the front office one day a week. She is assisting Mr. King, a longtime patient, and notices that he has an outstanding balance on his account.

"It looks like you have a balance, Mr. King. Would you like to pay that in full now?"

Mr. King replied that he usually gets billed, but Martha was not aware of that arrangement, stating, "Unfortunately, this is the policy. We'll need to receive payment for the full balance now."

After a few more minutes of back-and-forth, Mr. King fumbled for a credit card and slammed it on the counter. "Here! Put the entire balance on this." Martha was, at first, startled by his outburst but calmed herself. She thanked him and gave him his receipt. Mr. King grabbed it angrily and walked out, muttering, "You can cancel my next appointment...I won't be returning."

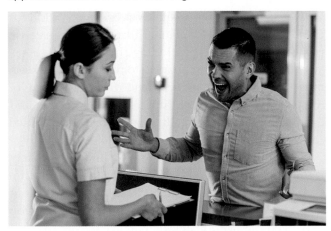

iStock.com/LightFieldStudios/1151675522

Martha felt a bit shaken. She began to feel her heart beating faster and her breathing quicken. She had not intended to make the patient angry. She was just trying to do her job and follow policy. She felt a pang in her stomach, thinking of all the possible consequences of her actions. She was afraid Dr. Singh, the dentist, would be upset at her for losing a patient. She was afraid she would lose her job over this, and—"Stop!" she said to herself out loud.

"Stop what?" asked Muriel, Martha's co-worker, startled.

"I was just talking to myself," Martha laughed. "I didn't mean to say it out loud."

"What are you trying to stop?" Muriel asked.

"Well, Mr. King canceled his next appointment and left in a huff because I made him pay his bill in full."

"Ahh, he's a difficult patient," Muriel said. "He insists on being billed. I should have told you that."

Martha felt a little better, but she still wanted to discuss it with Dr. Singh. "Oh, he is a demanding patient, that one," Dr. Singh said, "but we can make an exception to the policy and bill him. But it's good that you were able to collect from him."

Martha decided to call Mr. King that afternoon to explain the misunderstanding.

"Mr. King, I made a mistake in not billing you," she said. "We can make arrangements for you to be billed moving forward if you like."

"Yeah? What happened to your policy," he said sarcastically.

"Well, it is our office policy to be paid at the point of service," she told him cheerfully. "But, for longtime patients like you, we are happy to make an exception. I wasn't aware that you have a special arrangement."

"Okay. I guess I understand that" grumbled Mr. King.

"Can I confirm your next appointment, on May 7?"

"Yeah, I'll be there," Mr. King said.

QUESTIONS FOR THOUGHT AND REFLECTION

1. Describe the symptoms of anxiety that Martha was experiencing.
2. How did she manage to control her anxiety? What steps did she take?
3. What do you think Martha learned about herself?

A Different Path

Kathy and Peter are dental assistants at a busy cosmetic practice in a highly affluent area. Kathy was the assistant for the owner, Dr. Cromwell, and Peter was the assistant of the associate dentist, Dr. Gerald. Peter was new to the practice, but he and Kathy were already not getting along. Kathy just did not like Peter, and Peter did not care what Kathy's opinion of him was. Peter knew that both dentists appreciated his hard work, and this seemed to make Kathy jealous. Kathy took her time when she worked, but Peter moved quickly and efficiently. It did not help that both dentists always spoke highly of Peter but said little about Kathy, even though she had been there longer.

As time passed, both assistants avoided each other. After a few months, Kathy left her keys on Dr. Cromwell's desk with a short note: "You think Peter is so great. You can have him. I quit."

The following Monday, everyone found out that Kathy quit without notice. There was a lot of murmuring about why she quit and how much everyone liked her. Peter stayed silent but felt it was because of him. He suddenly felt anxious. He never expected Kathy to quit. His anxiety escalated throughout the day as he ran between the two dentists, trying to assist them both. He felt responsible for the office drama.

Peter's thoughts continued to take shape in a negative direction. He could not help but think, "Maybe it was my fault. Now, everyone is going to blame me for her leaving. I'm going to get fired because of what happened." He found himself perspiring and dropping instruments. As soon as he made one mistake, more cascaded.

"Calm down, Peter," said Dr. Cromwell, as he watched him fumble instruments. "Everything is fine. Take a minute."

Peter still found it difficult to calm down. It seemed to him that people stopped talking when he arrived, as if they were talking about him. He just wanted to be a dental assistant, not the center of a work crisis. That night, he lay awake in bed. How was he ever going to get through another day of work?

QUESTIONS FOR THOUGHT AND REFLECTION

1. Do you think Kathy quit because of Peter?
2. Could Peter have done anything to improve the situation with Kathy? What could he have done?
3. What effect did Peter's negative thoughts have on his performance?
4. What is an instance of positive self-talk that Peter could have used to neutralize his negative self-talk?

⭐ EXPERIENTIAL EXERCISES

1. The next time you feel anxious, see if deep breathing makes you feel better.
2. Identify a traumatic or profound past incident that still makes you feel anxious today when you think of it; what can you do to lower or eliminate the anxiety it still causes you?
3. List tasks or duties at work that you prefer to avoid or that make you feel anxious.
4. How do you relax?

CROSS CURRENTS WITH OTHER SOFT SKILLS

MANAGING YOUR TIME AND ORGANIZING YOUR LIFE: This eliminates a major source of anxiety in everyone's life (Chapter 1).
MANAGING AND RESOLVING CONFLICT: Conflict will not go away by itself; it will cause anxiety until it is satisfactorily resolved (Chapter 7).
FOLLOWING RULES AND REGULATIONS: Knowing what is expected and what is permissible helps alleviate anxiety (Chapter 14).

Practicing Patience

How poor are they that have not patience! What wound did ever heal but by degrees?

—**William Shakespeare**

LEARNING OBJECTIVE 3: PRACTICING PATIENCE

- Understand the importance of patience.
- Manage stressors to increase patience. Learn to be slow and methodical. Identify your triggers that may cause impatience.
- Relate patience to emotions.

As communication has become instantaneous, we are sometimes expected to be in two places at once and produce or perform at increasingly faster rates. Everyone wants immediate results and instant gratification. However, this need to be available all the time and to have instantaneous feedback can make us anxious.

Many of the important things in life take time and patience: health, education, meaningful relationships, raising children, being promoted, or buying your first home. With impatience, however, we risk missing out on the fun and meaningful parts of life and work. Being stretched too thin might result in depression, anxiety, or anhedonia (the inability to experience pleasure).

Patience means enduring provocation, delay, or annoyance without becoming upset or agitated. When practiced regularly, patience can help prevent anxiety by managing our reactions to external stressors. Patience offers the clearest pathway to the big things that matter. Fortunately, patience can be learned and made a habit. Developing patience can be a slow process but also a step-by-step approach to attaining things that matter.

How to Gain Patience

Patience demonstrates respect and care. Whether with elderly people or children, people with communication disorders, or with a friend who wants to talk about her problems, you can show your respect and concern for them by maintaining patience. Further, people who give respect tend to get respect in return. You will build stronger relationships by treating others how you would like to be treated.

Health care professionals often need great reserves of patience. Some work will be tedious but necessary. On other occasions, you may have to spend a lot of time with patients in nursing homes, psychiatric facilities, or surgical units. You must build up your patience reserve. Start small. Exercise patience in a line, in traffic, or in a meeting. Build the patience demanded for the important things in life and work.

Delays, waiting, and unexpected events are all part of life. Try to remain flexible and avoid becoming too attached to your original plans. Be ready to make new ones when the need arises. There are also multiple strategies and techniques that you can employ to develop your patience.

Pace Yourself

At work and at home, we are encouraged to get things done quickly. It may be a paradox but going slowly is sometimes the best way to go fast. If you slow down, you are less likely to make mistakes and avoid having to do as many tasks over again. Making a little extra time now, when things are not rushed, can make a big difference later, when things become hectic. For instance, take a few minutes to clean up examination rooms or dental stations after seeing a patient to get them ready before the next patient comes in.

Many activities in health care require precision. You want to go slowly when you are calibrating an IV drip, mixing dental cement, or positioning a patient for a radiograph. Making deliberate decisions and movements are often standard best practices in the health care field.

Going slowly and giving adequate time to each task can also build rapport with patients. For instance, a health care professional focusing attention on the patient and not being distracted will most likely have better treatment adherence from the patient (Figure. 3.4).

Keep Your Cool

Build a toolkit of techniques to help you keep your patience (Box 3.6). Chief among these techniques is deep breathing. Take a deep breath from your diaphragm. You should be able to see your abdomen

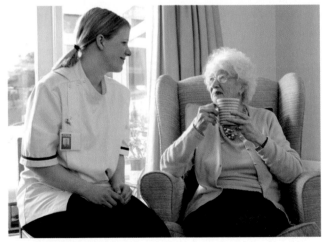

Figure 3.4 A health care professional spending time with a nursing home patient. (Copyright © istock.com.)

BOX 3.6

Tips for Maintaining Patience

- Avoid staring at clocks.
- Savor a quiet moment; they are hard to come by.
- Practice yoga.
- Breathe deeply.
- Reflect before acting or reacting.
- Be nonjudgmental.
- View waiting as a positive experience.

expand as you fill your lungs with oxygen. Inhale slowly, and then exhale even more slowly. Take your mind off whatever is making you feel impatient and focus just on your breath. After several breaths, you will be able to reassert your patience, and choose a rational, healthy response to whatever is provoking you.

In addition to deep breathing, adopt some simple activities you enjoy as a stopgap against impatience. Sometimes it is a matter of physically removing yourself from the irritation you are experiencing. Exercise or take a drive if you have the time. If time is limited, just step outside or look out a window. A change of scenery often takes your mind away from your impatience and helps you restore equilibrium. Meditate to regain your patience and better judgment. Empty your mind. When challenged by something you cannot change, accept it and let it go.

Identify the triggers that make you impatient, such as crying children, crashed computers, thoughtless coworkers, or unscheduled interruptions. Anticipating triggers before they occur will help you remind yourself that you have a choice in how you react.

◀ JOURNALING 3.4

List the people, places, situations, circumstances, and times that cause you to lose your patience. This will help you become aware of these triggers. Next, list tips to help you remain patient when faced with these triggers.

★ EXPERIENTIAL EXERCISES

1. Take some deep breaths the next time you are annoyed or frustrated. How did that feel?
2. The next time you are waiting in a line, try to focus on something else besides how fast the line is moving or why it is moving so slowly. See if by concentrating on something, the line seems to go faster. Try this strategy in other situations, such as being stuck in traffic.
3. Empty your mind of all thoughts for 1 minute. When a thought comes to mind, acknowledge it with patience and send it on its way. Practice this twice a day for 10 days.
4. Try a new activity that takes concentration, like sewing, ice skating, or a musical instrument. Go slowly. Challenge yourself to be exact.
5. Do something you like and that you are good at. See if you can experience a state of flow, where you lose track of time.

⊘ CROSS CURRENTS WITH OTHER SOFT SKILLS

MANAGING STRESS: Learning to become patient can become a tool to combat stress (Chapter 15).
SHOWING EMPATHY, SENSITIVITY, AND CARING: How does patience as a learned skill complement patient care? (Chapter 6)
LISTENING ACTIVELY: Is listening thoughtfully possible without patience? (Chapter 6)
SETTING GOALS AND PLANNING ACTIONS: Goals can only be achieved little by little, working patiently every day (Chapter 1).

Strengthening Resiliency

Inside of a ring or out, ain't nothing wrong with going down. It's staying down that's wrong.

—Muhammad Ali

LEARNING OBJECTIVE 4: STRENGTHENING RESILIENCY

- Understand the relationship between stress and resilience.
- Understand the relationship between resilience and problem solving.
- Describe the internal locus of control.
- Understand the relationship between resilience and optimism.

Resilience is the upside of stress. It is the ability to bounce back when you are knocked down. Resilient people have what is called an "internal locus of control" (Figure. 3.5). They feel that, ultimately, they have control over their life. They do not believe that they must submit to external circumstances. For instance, they might move to Arizona if they cannot stand the cold of Alaska. They might decide to get divorced after trying everything to make their marriage work. They will change jobs if they are mistreated. They will

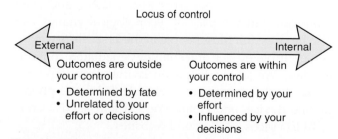

Figure 3.5 Locus of control.

make decisions to change their circumstances, instead of allowing the circumstances to control their life.

How do people change their locus of control? You need to recognize that there is almost always a choice. When faced with a problem that feels out of your control, brainstorm things you could do that would have an effect on the situation, even if you do not think they would completely solve the problem. Write down all your possible choices, no matter how outlandish they may seem. If necessary, ask a friend to help. Avoid judging individual choices until you have the longest list you can think of. Then, decide which choices are good and, among these, which is best. The choices you select represent your first course of action and alternative courses of action. After a while, you may find that identifying the choices you have in your life becomes a habit and easier to do.

For now, try to meet challenges as they arise. What you do when confronted by a stressor determines how difficult the stressful event or situation turns out to be. Remember that good outcomes can result from bad beginnings.

JOURNALING 3.5

Record three crises or stressors you have encountered in the past month. Then, briefly describe anything positive that could or did come from these events.

Sources of Stress

The rate of change in society and the workplace is increasing at an unprecedented pace, as new technological advances transform the way we live and work. The resulting demands placed on us can intensify existing stressors as we struggle to keep pace with the changes. It can feel like stress is coming at us from virtually all directions.

Technology, Addictions, and Productivity Demands

Technology makes our lives easier, faster, and even more fun, but the pace of technological change can also be stressful. Most people in the 21st century manage multiple modes of technology-mediated communication. We follow people on Twitter, Facebook, and LinkedIn. We remain reachable 24/7 by cell phone, mobile device, and email. We text and send friends links to videos, photos, and websites.

Although new devices and software enhance our lives in many ways, they also require continual learning as we figure out how to operate and optimize these new technologies. Moreover, face-to-face human connections decrease as communication becomes more mediated by technology, depriving us of important social interaction. As productivity demands increase at work and at home, we often turn to television, video games, the Internet, and social media to escape from the world around us.

You can't have everything. Where would you put it?

—**Stephen Wright**

JOURNALING 3.6

Make a list of the technology you use every day. Consider how these devices may add to your stress. Brainstorm ideas to reduce your time using these devices to reduce your stress level.

Multitasking

Many people respond to these demands by resorting to multitasking, but this strategy can backfire. Whereas computers can execute multiple tasks without stress, your brain does not operate the same way. Although habitual tasks may require less of your attention, you can only concentrate on one complex task at a time (Figure. 3.6). For instance, you may be able to sign routine documents while talking on the phone. However, if you try to answer your email while you talk on the phone, you might miss subtle details in an email or have to ask your caller to repeat themselves. Switching between these more complex tasks has a cost, as it takes your brain longer to switch to a new task than to continue or complete the same task, and this may result in more errors. In many cases, it is best to tackle more complex tasks individually. Otherwise, you may

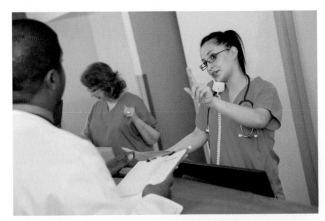

Figure 3.6 Responding to multiple demands can be overwhelming. When you cannot effectively multitask, it is best to prioritize your work and concentrate on one issue at a time. (Copyright © istock.com.)

end up taking longer to complete the tasks or you will have to go back and correct mistakes.

Worrying

Other animals respond only to immediate dangers and then return to their normal state, but humans can generate the stress response about events that have not even occurred, maintaining a constant stress level. Comedian and stress expert Loretta LaRoche describes severe worrying as "catastrophizing," fixating on the absolute worst thing that could possibly happen. In fact, approximately 90% of the outcomes that people worry about never come to pass. Worrying about the future will not make it better, but it can damage your well-being. Box 3.7 offers a strategy to reduce or eliminate worry.

I am an old man and have known a great many troubles, but most of them never happened.

—Mark Twain

BOX 3.7

A Strategy for Reducing Worry

1. Catch yourself when you worry.
2. Identify what you are worrying about:
   a. Is it a realistic problem, or part of the 90% of worries that will never come to pass?
   b. If it is a realistic problem, can you do anything about it *right now*?
3. Imagine that your worry scenario is a DVD you are watching. Eject it and replace it with a positive DVD.
4. Convert worry to concern, replacing something negative and unproductive with something positive and productive. Once a worry is a concern, pose solutions that are actionable. Determine when you will be able to perform those actions, schedule them, and move on.
5. Put your problems into perspective by helping someone else. This will allow you to play the role of an objective third party and formulate tips to apply to your own problems later. Plus, you will have connected deeply with another person, one of the most effective ways to relieve your stress.

Managing Stress

Stressors often generate emotional responses. Your immediate response may be difficult to control. We are all human, and our brains have powerful limbic systems that govern our emotions. However, many people project their feelings by lashing out at others when something else altogether is bothering them. Knowing the cause of your emotions is the first step in dealing with the situation. When you understand what precipitated your feelings, you can better control your actions. Box 3.8 lists responses that may exacerbate stress and anxiety.

The human body goes into the stress response only when it *perceives* a stressor. If you can deflect the perception of stress, even in the face of an objective threat, you can prevent the physiological stress response and simultaneously respond much more resiliently to the stressor. This chapter has offered you an array of tools for reframing the threat, such as seeking the bright side of a problem or viewing it in a larger context. Ask yourself, "Will this still matter in 24 hours?"

As with anxiety, you can address many stressors using straightforward analysis. Do you see any patterns in the stressor? Has this happened before? Is this just one more obstacle you have encountered along your path? Which strategy do you think will help you deal with this? For instance, if you receive a poor score on a test, you probably already know you could have done more to prepare. Now you can use the poor score as a lesson to turn things around by preparing more for the next test.

A stressor is usually just a problem that you allow to upset you. The sooner you switch to problem-solving mode, the less the stressor will overcome you in any way.

When I knew better, I did better.

—Maya Angelou

BOX 3.8

Factors Increasing Stress and Anxiety

- Personalizing
- Catastrophizing
- Isolation
- Worry
- Blame
- Victimization
- Self-pity
- Immobilization

Practicing Resiliency

Finally, remember that life throws all kinds of challenges at us, large and small. Try to see obstacles as opportunities. Practice building your resilience when small issues crop up. Return the unpleasant phone call. Schedule that dental appointment. Apologize to your co-worker. Get over your team's big loss. Decline the invitation. Resilient people figure out the appropriate response to a problem and carry it out immediately rather than allowing problems to pile up.

Think of how good you will feel when you have solved your problem and put it behind you. Box 3.9 suggests sources to strengthen your resilience.

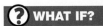

? WHAT IF?

What if you oversleep and are late to work? How will you manage this minor crisis and stressor?

BOX 3.9

Sources of Resilience

- Love
- Truth
- Humor
- Forgiveness
- Exercise and recreation
- Vacation and breaks
- Sleep and rest
- Music
- Friends
- Family
- Deep breathing and meditation
- Reframing perceptions

CASE STUDY 3.3
Skittles and Bits

Karalee had a pounding headache by the time she got to work at Pediatric Associates, and the parking lot was full of patients waiting for the clinic to open. The health care providers would not be there for another half hour. She unlocked the doors and let the patients fill the waiting room. When she went into the back room to put away her belongings, the other medical assistants, Mindy and Carlos, were already there, drinking coffee.

"Why didn't you guys open up?" she said. They just looked at her as though no reply was necessary. Karalee was relatively new compared with them, so she decided not to press the issue. She took some ibuprofen for her headache and put a smile on her face as she headed out to the reception desk, followed by Mindy and Carlos a few minutes later.

As if in a wave, the patients rose from their seats and approached the reception desk. Karalee took a deep breath and greeted a mother and her two children, who were first in line. Karalee could not help but notice that she was processing patients at about the same rate as her two colleagues put together, but she just assumed their patients had more complex issues.

Once the patients were checked in, Karalee pulled all the charts for the day's appointments. Pretty soon, Dr. Vang came out and demanded to know who pulled the charts. Karalee told her she did. "Well, this is the wrong 'Murphy,' Karalee. Let's try to be more careful moving forward."

Her ears burned as she overheard Carlos referring to her as "Karaless." But she closed her eyes for a moment and took more deep breaths. Everybody makes mistakes, she told herself. I will be more careful next time.

Then she approached her co-workers. "Wow," she said, "that was embarrassing. I need to be more careful."

"Don't worry," said Mindy. "It was a simple mistake."

"Thanks. I appreciate your saying that."

Just then, there was a commotion in the waiting room. "Allie, Allie!" screamed a woman's voice. Karalee ran to the waiting room and saw a woman kneeling over a child, whose face was turning blue, especially around her lips. "She's choking on a Skittle," the mother screamed.

"Go get one of the doctors," Karalee said to Mindy, who ran off. "Carlos, get everybody back. We need some room here." She gently turned Allie around and placed the heel of her hand on her sternum, careful to ensure it was in the right spot. She gave her the Heimlich maneuver, but nothing happened. Carlos had created some space around the scene, gesturing people back and moving some chairs out of the way. Karalee gave the toddler another Heimlich, harder this time, but no response. She could hear that Allie was not breathing or gasping for air. Just as Dr. Levin and Mindy rushed into the room together, Karalee gave it another try, and out flew the Skittle. Allie sucked in a deep breath and let it out with the loudest, best-sounding cry Karalee had ever heard.

The mother cried out in joy and picked Allie up. The mother and daughter followed Dr. Levin to an examination room.

Other people in the waiting room started to crowd around. "Wow, that was crazy," said one of the parents. "That was so scary! What if it didn't come out?" said another. "Well, at least it happened in a doctor's office, with trained professionals around."

"Thank you for everyone's help and for staying calm," Karalee addressing the patients in the waiting room. "Please give us a few minutes and we'll start bringing people back."

The rest of the day went without any other incidences. As Karalee was getting ready to leave for the day, Dr. Levin pulled her into an office with Dr. Patel. "I talked to Mrs. Sallah, Allie's mom," Dr. Levin told her. "You showed great skill today, Karalee. You stayed calm and showed greater leadership. You really took command of a very serious situation."

"Thank you," said Karalee. "I just took a deep breath and relied on my training."

"Well, we both wanted to thank you and Mrs. Salla wanted to thank you too."

That evening, Karalee finally got a chance to reflect on the day. It was stressful, but she managed it well. She loved that Dr. Levin said she showed leadership. From now on, she was going to think of herself as a leader too.

QUESTIONS FOR THOUGHT AND REFLECTION

1. What actions did Karalee take to keep her stress in check?
2. What do you think of how Karalee interacted with her co-workers? Would you have handled things differently?
3. How did Karalee manage the patients and her co-workers?
4. Why do you think Dr. Levin thought Karalee showed leadership? What actions do you think demonstrated her ability as a leader?

A Different Path

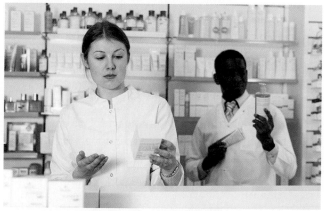
Istock.com/JackF/947938382

Brenna was in a foul mood. She had just learned that her sister got engaged to be married.

"You're not happy for her?" asked Nick, one of the other pharmacy technicians. "Why? Don't you like the guy?"

"The guy's fine ... for her. I wouldn't marry him. I mean, I am happy for her that she's engaged. It's just that she's younger than me, and I'm the pretty one. I should be the one getting married first."

"In other words, you're jealous," Eleanor, another pharmacy technician said, laughing.

Brenna glared at her. "I've dated plenty of men. I just wouldn't marry any of them, that's all."

"Have any asked?" said Eleanor. Brenna gave her another look. She did not like that girl.

Ralph, one of the pharmacists, stuck his head in. "Brenna, is that Hobson script ready yet?"

"You made me lose count!" she shouted, forgetting whom she was speaking to. "Oh, sorry. What?"

"The Hobson script. I told you to get it out here right away. Where is it?"

"The Hobson script?" She blankly stared at Ralph.

"Brenna, if you didn't spend so much time chatting, I wouldn't have to tell you twice." She found the prescription and started filling it. "Like he doesn't stop and talk with people," she muttered, counting out the 200 mg pills. "What, am I supposed to be silent all day long?"

Ralph stuck his head in again to check on the progress of the prescription. "Those are 200s, Brenna. Read the prescription. They're for 100s," he shouted, startling Brenna, who knocked over the big jug and dumped 200s everywhere. "And after you're done, I want you to count every one of these 200s when you pick them up and sign off on them." Brenna immediately stooped down and started scooping up the 200s. "I said *after*," said Ralph. "I need the Hobson script now." Brenna stood, but she was immobilized. Ralph threw up his hands and left. She could hear Ralph apologizing to Mrs. Hobson.

"She'll get her script," Brenna muttered to herself and looked up to see Eleanor and Nick watching her. "I could use some help here," she snapped at them.

Brenna's cell phone rang. "Oh hi," she said. "I'm OK. I'm just working with idiots, that's all." She saw Eleanor pass by and roll her eyes just as she said that. "Look, I can't talk. Wait 'till you hear the news, though. I'll call you back." She could see Ralph waiting near the doorway. "Let's see, 100s, 100s." She stepped on more 200s as she finally delivered the script to Ralph.

"Is this 90?" he said.

"Oh, man, she wants 90?"

"Yes," said Ralph. "The doctor who ordered the medication for Mrs. Hobson wants 90. It's on the script," Ralph said with obvious frustration. "Eleanor, would you please fill this script for Mrs. Hobson. And recount these to make sure you have 30 to start with."

QUESTIONS FOR THOUGHT AND REFLECTION

1. In what ways is Brenna contributing to her own stress?
2. What do you think about the interaction between Brenna and her co-workers? What can she do to improve it?
3. How would you assess Brenna's focus at work?
4. If you were Brenna, what would you do in response to Ralph telling Eleanor to fill the prescription?

★ EXPERIENTIAL EXERCISES

1. Keep track of everything you do for 24 hours. Do you have any regrets about how you spent your time? Is there something else you wish you had done, or done more of?
2. Take a yoga class. If you already practice yoga, try a new dance or exercise class.
3. Pick a pleasurable, relaxing place you have been to in the past. Visualize it, and use your sense of sight, sound, smell, taste, and touch. Recall the feelings you experienced when you were in this place. Visualize this relaxing place so that you can call upon it at will when you need to relax and meditate.
4. Start a collection of videos you find hilarious and remember to watch them in times of acute stress.
5. Focus on your breathing. Try to deepen and lengthen your breaths. See if you can feel the sense of calm this gives you. Do this repeatedly until you make deep breathing a habit and always have it as a remedy in times of stress and anxiety.

◎ CROSS CURRENTS WITH OTHER SOFT SKILLS

BEING DEPENDABLE: If you are dependable, you have removed many stressors, like being late, from your life (Chapter 1).

MANAGING AND RESOLVING CONFLICT: You cannot eliminate conflict from your life, but you can manage it effectively to minimize the stress associated with it (Chapter 7).

CONTROLLING ANXIETY: Anxiety is caused by stress; if you can combat anxiety, you can combat stress (Chapter 15).

EXUDING OPTIMISM, ENTHUSIASM, AND POSITIVITY: These traits can be effective in shielding you from stress (Chapter 2).

Maintaining Health

LEARNING OBJECTIVE 5: GAINING ENERGY, PERSISTENCE, AND PERSEVERANCE

- Understand the sources of human energy.
- Maintain a balanced diet to stay healthy.
- Know how to stay active and get enough sleep.
- Explain the role of socializing in maintaining health.

In addition to emotional health, establishing and maintaining physical health is just as critical. Health professions are physically and mentally demanding. The fast-paced environment is full of problems to solve and decisions to make. The work requires good judgment because answers are rarely black and white. A lot is at stake, including lives. It takes a lot of energy and persistence to be a health care professional (Figure. 3.7).

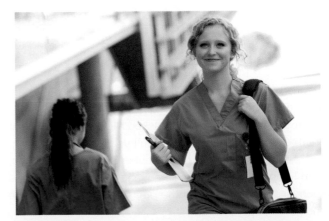

Figure 3.7 With energy and persistence, a student can overcome obstacles and become a confident, competent medical professional. (Copyright © istock.com.)

Think about the many challenges a health care professional faces on a typical day that take persistence to overcome. You may have to:

* Guide a confused and fragile patient
* Find an artery to take blood
* Keep a small child busy
* Communicate with someone who speaks little English or who is deaf
* Document a difficult incident
* Make sense of a cluster of laboratory results
* Prepare to administer an injection to a fearful patient
* Enter reimbursement codes for patients with multiple diagnoses and treatments

If you feel that you suffer chronically from low energy, some long-term changes could help improve your energy levels. Embracing healthy habits is one of the most effective changes you could make. These include maintaining a healthy weight; eating healthful, nutritious food; reducing stress; and getting the recommended amount of sleep. As a result, you need strategies to build, maintain, and boost your energy.

Sources of Energy

How many times have you heard that your body needs fuel? Although this is true, it is just one piece of the puzzle. Energy requires a balanced diet, physical activity, adequate sleep, fulfilling work, and opportunities for positive interaction. Not meeting all of these demands may negatively affect your health and energy levels.

Maintaining a Balanced Diet

As food serves as the primary source of energy, good nutrition is key to maintaining sufficient energy levels. To function well daily, you need to choose food that produces stable blood sugar and provides vital nutrients throughout the day. Eating a healthy breakfast is important to your energy, as well as keeping your weight in check. A mix of protein, healthy fats, and carbohydrates low on the glycemic scale will help you to start your day alert and will keep you energized until lunch. Hydration is also necessary for maintaining healthy circulation and normal brain function.

In many health care settings, there are days when you will have little or no time for lunch. A supply of low-glycemic snacks stashed away in your purse, backpack, or desk may come in handy on these days. Nuts, dried fruit, or energy bars are easy to store and eat whenever you have a spare moment or need to energize yourself.

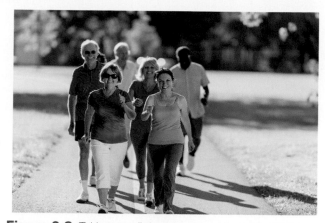

Figure 3.8 Taking a walk is a good way to reduce stress and regain energy. (Copyright © istock.com.)

Getting Active

It may seem like a paradox, but exercise is energizing. Although it is true that *too much* exercise can tire you out, physical activity that gets you moving will increase your energy. Many jobs require a person to sit all day, often staring at a computer screen. This will make anyone tired. If your job is sedentary, you should plan activity throughout the day. Taking the stairs, volunteering for errands, or checking on patients will all keep you moving and keep your energy up.

In addition, regular exercise will help improve your heart and lung health, which will increase your energy and your metabolism (Figure. 3.8). Whether you prefer a trip to the gym before work, a long walk in nature, or a few quick laps around the parking lot, incorporating exercise into your regular routine will give you the energy you need to tackle your day.

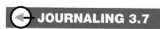 JOURNALING 3.7

Outline times or periods during the day when you are most energetic or have the most awareness; this is called your energy cycle. Align your typical daily activities with your energy cycle.

Getting Sufficient Sleep

Neuroscientists still have much to learn about the exact biological processes that occur during sleep, but we do know that sleep significantly impacts brain function and physical health. Research suggests that sleep helps the body reproduce and repair cells, and the brain uses sleep to store memories and integrate experience and learning in the form of neural connections. Your body needs a minimum amount of sleep to perform these functions.

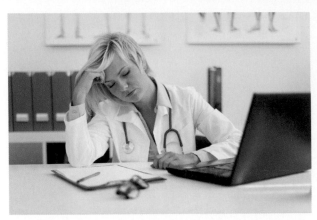

Figure 3.9 Sleep deprivation interferes with a health professional's ability to focus. (Copyright © istock.com.)

The necessary amount varies, but healthy adults typically need between 7 and 9 hours. Adolescents need about 9 or 10 hours of sleep to thrive, toddlers and young children should get between 10 and 14 hours, and doctors recommend infants and newborns get between 14 and 17 hours of sleep per day.

However, most children and adults get less than the recommended number of hours of sleep. The consequences of too little sleep, especially on a prolonged basis, can be devastating to your state of mind and energy level (Figure. 3.9). Your critical thinking skills deteriorate, leading to poor decision-making and bad judgment. Your alertness is dulled, leading you to overlook important cues when communicating and treating patients. You may become more susceptible to mood swings and depression, making you less able to cope with stressful situations and interpersonal conflict. For health care professionals, sleep deprivation can have serious consequences.

The worst thing in the world is to try to sleep and not to.
— F. Scott Fitzgerald

If you often have difficulty falling asleep or sleeping through the night, try to find out why and make adjustments. Most of the time, going to bed and waking up at the same time every night can help significantly, as your body will grow accustomed to the routine. Develop a nighttime and morning routine to create a positive sleep habit and help your body know when it is time to sleep. For instance, before bed, you might read for half an hour, record your thoughts in a notebook to clear your mind, take a hot bath, drink herbal tea, or use relaxing scents like lavender to help prepare you for sleep. In the morning, open the curtains to let in a lot of light, use lamps or a light therapy box if you wake up when it is still dark outside, and eat breakfast before going to work.

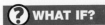

WHAT IF?

What if you did not get enough sleep last night? What will you do to manage the workday ahead? What actions will you take to correct the lack of sleep you got?

If you tend to watch TV late at night or use your phone, computer, or tablet right before bed, you may want to try turning off these devices at least 1 to 2 hours before bed. The blue light emitted from electronic device screens can interfere with your circadian rhythm and suppress the body's production of melatonin, a hormone that regulates the sleep-wake cycle. If turning off these devices is unrealistic for you, another option is to use blue light-filtering software and apps that reduce blue light exposure during evening hours and shift to warmer, redder light. Making your bedroom dark, quiet, and cool can also help optimize the brain's ability to sleep.

Getting regular exercise during the day can also help you sleep better at night. However, you should plan to complete vigorous workouts within 3 hours of bedtime. In addition, pay attention to what you eat and drink. Avoid caffeinated beverages in the late afternoon and evening. Limit your intake of alcohol near bedtime, as well; although it may help you relax, alcohol is a stimulant and can interfere with your sleep.

If you snore, wake up with headaches, or feel exhausted despite sleeping all night, you might have sleep apnea. People who suffer from sleep apnea frequently stop breathing during the night, which deprives the brain of oxygen and stresses the heart. Seek help at a sleep clinic, where the clinician may recommend polysomnography (sleep study) and possibly prescribe a continuous positive airway pressure (CPAP) device. In rare cases, you may need to take a thyroid test to make sure you do not have hypothyroidism, which can cause fatigue. Finally, if stress and anxiety are giving you insomnia, pursue some of the remedies discussed later in this chapter.

JOURNALING 3.8

Record your sleep habits. What time do you go to bed? How long does it take you to fall asleep? How deeply do you sleep? Do you wake up feeling refreshed or just as tired as you were going to bed? Do you have a routine before you go to bed or after you get up? What works best about your sleep-related behavior? What would you like to improve, and how would you do that?

Understanding Nutrition

If you are chronically tired, your diet may not include enough of the right kinds of food. Heavy meals can make you feel lethargic as your blood is diverted from supplying your brain with oxygen to digesting your food. Foods high in sugar can spike your blood sugar, creating a short burst of energy followed by a long crash. Ideally, you want a consistent supply of nutrients that keeps your blood sugar steady and your brain supplied with glucose—the only substance it can burn-all day long.

Breakfast is an important part of such a program because it "breaks" the "fast" of sleeping all night, giving your body a much-needed injection of blood sugar to start your day off right. Select protein, healthy fats, and carbohydrates that are low on the glycemic index and full of soluble and insoluble fiber (Box 3.10). Low-glycemic carbohydrates release sugars slowly and promote a feeling of fullness. Adding these foods to your diet will help to prevent blood sugar spikes and insulin surges that deplete sugars from the blood and prepare them for storage as fat. Even making small changes—such as eliminating or cutting back on sodas or other sugary drinks, choosing whole grain bread and pasta instead of white bread or refined pasta, choosing lean meats over high-fat meats, and adding leafy greens to your meals whenever possible—can make a big impact on how you feel.

Fatigue may also be a symptom of dehydration. Your body is about 60% water, and water mediates virtually all your bodily functions, including brain function and metabolism. For instance, water regulates body temperature; enables cells to grow, reproduce, and survive; allows the brain to regulate hormones and neurotransmitters; and helps deliver oxygen throughout your body.

The amount of water you need to stay adequately hydrated depends on your age, weight, gender, and activity level. In general, men should drink about 13 cups of water per day, whereas women should drink around 9 cups. However, highly active people or women who are pregnant or breastfeeding should get more than that amount. Figure out the right amount for you and make plans to keep yourself well hydrated. Other nutritional tools include the following:

* Eat snacks that release energy slowly, like yogurt, cheese, trail mix, nuts, berries, or peanut butter on an apple or banana.
* Avoid sweets, junk food, and energy drinks that contain excessive sugar.
* Use caffeine sparingly but strategically. Try green tea for its antioxidant properties. Or eat a small piece of dark chocolate for the caffeine and endorphin stimulation.
* Finally, take a daily multivitamin rich in B vitamins, vitamin C, and vitamin D.

Importance of Socializing

Health care professions offer a unique blend of challenges and rewards; the job can be physically and emotionally demanding yet provide gratifying social connection and deep spiritual meaning. Human beings are wired to interact with other people. Take advantage of this human need to create and build energy and engage with all aspects of your job. A conversation, a discussion, a sharing of interests, the solving of a problem, a group decision, a feeling of connection in a crisis—these are all energy-building experiences because they fulfill our need for social connection. Introduce yourself to co-workers you do not know or learn more about those you do not know well. Have lunch with different people. Learn a new skill and share it with others. Your job as a health care professional will provide you with countless opportunities to connect with people. Taking advantage of these opportunities will help you thrive in your career.

Social Tools

Few things restore energy faster than a good laugh, especially if you can share it with a co-worker (Figure. 3.10). For extroverts, social interaction can make them feel more energized. Try these social strategies when you need a boost:

BOX 3.10

Low-Glycemic Foods

- Most fruits, especially grapes, grapefruit, cantaloupe, honeydew, raspberries, strawberries, blueberries, oranges, and avocados
- Most vegetables, especially broccoli, cauliflower, green beans, spinach, peppers, and squash
- Whole grains
- Fructose
- Most beans and legumes
- Most nuts

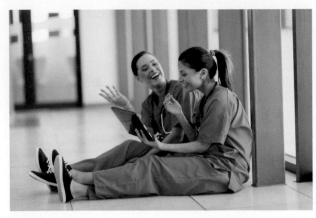

* Try to schedule isolated, routine tasks like paper-work between more social or active tasks, like meetings and interactions with patients. Break up periods of more monotonous tasks with social activity or interactions with your co-workers.
* Have a short social conversation with a co-worker who is good at putting things in perspective.
* When you have a spare moment, offer to help a co-worker with a task.
* If possible, ask a co-worker to join you on a break and do something active together, such as take a walk outside or stretch.

Figure 3.10 Co-workers take a break and laugh together. (Copyright © istock.com.)

CASE STUDY 3.4
Picker-Upper

Penelope Pagonis added a lot of fun to the hospital pharmacy where she worked as a pharmacy technician. She had a big personality, a big family, and a big social life. She was high energy and never had any trouble getting her work done. In fact, she eagerly volunteered to help when others felt overwhelmed, making medication deliveries to the units, working overtime to fill prescriptions, and starting new lines of customers to get everything moving faster.

One Monday morning, Penny did not seem like herself. Her father, Gus, was a roofer and he had fallen off a ladder. Fortunately, he only broke his leg, but it still put him out of work. With a heavy sigh, Penny started filling prescriptions at half of her usual pace.

Later that day, an irritated customer started speaking harshly to Penny. "If you can read, Penelope," he said, reading her name tag, "the doctor wants me to take 40 milligrams now, not 20." Penny calmly apologized to the man, but Lane, the pharmacy manager, noticed that Penny was breathing deeply. After a few minutes, he said, "Penny, when you have a minute, I want to introduce you to our new epidemiologist."

Lane took Penny to the conference room and introduced her to George Papas, a dark-haired young man hovering over a keyboard. "I don't know how to do this," he told Penny. "I'm studying off-label uses of atypical antipsychotics, and I can't figure out how to access the data." Penny sat down as George explained the criteria he was searching for. "I can show you how to do that," she said. "Probably the easiest method is to use cross tabs. Here, let me show you."

After an hour, George had what he needed. "Thank you, Penny. You're a life saver. I'll probably need your expertise again with SAS. How can I reach you?"

Penny returned to the pharmacy with a familiar pep in her step.

QUESTIONS FOR THOUGHT AND REFLECTION

1. What effects did Penny's down mood have on her performance at her job?
2. Why was Lane's intervention effective?
3. Why do you think Penny hit it off with the epidemiologist?
4. Can you see a pattern in Penny's energy?

A Different Path

Anthony had spent practically the whole night at the Italian Festival, and he was dazed when he arrived for his 7:00 a.m. shift on Sunday. As a patient services clerk, he never knew how busy his days were going to be at the public hospital he worked at downtown. Sundays were usually slower, but that was not always the case. As he took his seat in his cubicle, he felt like he could sleep right there, sitting up.

But there was no time for that. A middle-aged man sat down at his station, and Anthony drearily started collecting the information from him. Apart from the standard questions, Anthony barely acknowledged the man until he said he forgot his insurance card. Anthony looked up from his computer screen, making eye contact with the man. "How are we supposed to treat you, sir, if you can't give us your insurance information?"

"I know it's Aetna," said the man. "I'm a regular patient here. Do you think you could look it up?"

"Sir, how am I supposed to look it up? Do I look like Google to you?" The volume of his voice started to rise.

"Maybe you have it on file. I've been a patient here before," the man said again.

"Then you should know to bring your insurance card with you!" said Anthony, almost shouting.

"Is there a problem here?" asked Ranni, who came over when she heard Anthony's angry voice.

"Oh, just a little one," said Anthony, leaning back in his chair and jerking his thumb toward the man. "He forgot his insurance card and doesn't know the number."

"Excuse me, sir," she said to the man. "We can help you over here." She directed the man toward another agent, Karla, apologizing to the woman who would have been next in line for Karla. "This gentleman needs your assistance, Karla," said Ranni.

"Of course," Karla said with a smile. "How can I help you, sir?"

Ranni returned immediately to Anthony's station, before another patient could be called. "Is everything okay, Anthony? You look like a bit unkempt today," she told him. "And I'm not sure I approve of the way you handled that last patient."

"Yeah, I'm okay. But he didn't have his insurance card. How was I supposed to help him?" he said with a sneer. "Why are you blaming me?"

"I'm not blaming you for him not having an insurance card. But I do hold you responsible for the way you treated him and handled the situation," Ranni said sternly. "It's obvious you're not ready for work today. Go ahead and go home, Anthony."

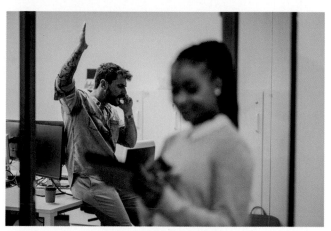

iStock.com/zamrznutitonovi/1404944782

QUESTIONS FOR THOUGHT AND REFLECTION

1. How did Anthony's lack of sleep affect his behavior? Did you think that this differed from Anthony's usual manner of speaking?
2. How did his behavior affect his co-workers?
3. How did Ranni handle the situation? If you were his supervisor, what would you have done?
4. What should Anthony do when he returns to work the next day?

⭐ EXPERIENTIAL EXERCISES

1. Create a list of activities that deplete your energy and note how and when you will stop doing them.
2. Plan a brief exercise routine, dance, or stretches you can do almost anywhere to boost your energy.
3. Prepare a list of snacks that you like and can carry with you that would boost your energy. Look up their calories and nutritional value to ensure they fit within your diet plan and will not cause sugar spikes.
4. Collect 10 jokes that you find funny and are confident others would not find offensive or off-color. Try them out on your friends. Use them at strategic times to raise somebody's spirits through laughter.
5. Perform a fine-motor skill, like writing, drawing, or eating, with your nondominant hand. Persist until you find the activity just a little bit easier.

⟳ CROSS CURRENTS WITH OTHER SOFT SKILLS

PRACTICING PATIENCE: Perseverance takes energy, as well as patience (Chapter 1).

STRENGTHENING RESILIENCE: You need resilience to overcome the obstacles that make perseverance difficult (Chapter 7).

MANAGING YOUR TIME AND ORGANIZING YOUR LIFE: If you manage minor distractions by planning your time and staying organized, you can devote your energy to the challenges of your work and personal life (Chapter 1).

EXUDING OPTIMISM, ENTHUSIASM, AND POSITIVITY: These traits will support your perseverance (Chapter 6).

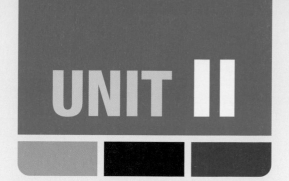

COMMUNICATION SKILLS

Mastering Professional Communication

- Understand the Importance of Professional Communication in the Health Care Setting
- Describe the Different Aspects of Professional Communication
- Leverage the Three Core Elements of Effective Speaking
- Communicate Effectively Through Writing by Using and Following Grammar and Spelling Guidelines
- Improve Your Writing Skills to Advance Your Profession

Speaking Professionally in Health Care

Good communication is the bridge between confusion and clarity.

—Nat Turner

LEARNING OBJECTIVE 1: SPEAKING PROFESSIONALLY IN THE HEALTH CARE SETTING

- Recognize the value of speaking professionally at work.
- Understand the different types of communication.
- Use language appropriate for business and health care settings.
- Learn to expand your vocabulary and use them in everyday speech in the proper context.
- Censor the content of your conversations at work.

For medical offices and health care organizations, ensuring that patients receive proper care takes more than making a diagnosis and performing procedures. Communication is a crucial component in all steps of the health care process. Whether it be a clinic accurately sharing patient information with another facility or a group of physicians, nurses, specialists, and other staff at a hospital discussing how to treat current and incoming patients, the need for concise, effective communication is critical in the health care field.

Effective speaking is one of the best tools you can develop to achieve your objectives in the workplace and at home. Effective communication helps to improve patient safety, save on costs, and increase day-to-day operating efficiency. Poor communication may result in patients not feeling safe in communicating honestly and openly, resulting in not receiving appropriate medical services and treatment. For example, a patient who feels embarrassed about a rash will likely feel more safe mentioning this to a health care provider who is compassionate, patient, and has a professional demeanor.

Right or wrong, we are often judged by the way we speak. Our language affects how others perceive and relate to us. When you use proper grammar, tone, and vocabulary for work-related conversations, you improve your chance of being heard, respected, and understood. Thus, one of the best ways to become successful in your field is to use the language of your profession appropriately, such as correctly using and pronouncing medical terms, and to speak professionally.

Consider all the different types of speaking you engage in at work and estimate how much time you spend talking, listening, and interacting. You communicate in different ways all day long. You interact with your supervisor and co-workers to learn, exchange information, and advance your causes and concerns. In meetings, you will be called upon to offer your ideas and input regarding the issues of the day. You may be called upon to make presentations. You may present a patient's case or explain your ideas and proposals. Most importantly, you interact with patients by welcoming them, collecting their information, assessing their needs, preparing them for treatments, explaining procedures, and scheduling their appointments (Figure. 4.1). Thus, speaking well at work is key to your effectiveness, success, and career growth.

Mend your speech a little lest you mar your fortunes.

—**William Shakespeare**

Effective speaking is the art of combining the four main types of communication:

* Verbal communication
* Nonverbal communication
* Written communication
* Visual communication

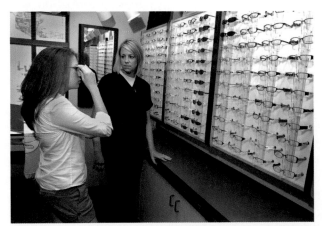

Figure 4.1 An optician helps a patient choose a pair of glasses. (Copyright © istock.com.)

Verbal Communication

The words you use contribute to your success, or lack of success, every day. If you want more influence, connection, or opportunities to come your way, practice speaking in ways that bring out your best. The world often mirrors how you represent yourself. If you use positive language, then that is what will show up for you externally.

Conversely, if you use negative language to describe your situation and convey hopelessness, then those words are likely to shape your outcome. When the language you use is incorrect, you may appear to lack knowledge or credibility, which can diminish how your co-workers and patients perceive and relate to you. Whether you are talking to patients about the best treatment for their illness or discussing performance issues with your supervisor, it is important that you speak effectively and choose the correct words to ensure the greatest outcome and best result.

An important aspect of choosing your words is knowing the meaning of the word and expanding your vocabulary. Vocabulary development is about exposure and our ability to use language. The more we engage with language, the more we learn and develop our vocabulary. When we know more words, we are able to express our thoughts more accurately. Moreover, a more diverse, colorful vocabulary commands attention and makes you more interesting. Instead of concentrating on big words that others may not know, use smaller words that are heard less often but convey the same meaning.

Reading is the single best way to improve your vocabulary. To expand your vocabulary, it is good to read content outside of your interest area. For example, if you enjoy reading about technology, consider reading science fiction or health care news. Expanding your vocabulary means reading more challenging material, which can be difficult. If you are having trouble comprehending the message, examine the context. The words used around an unfamiliar word or concept will usually give you clues to the meaning of the new word. Bookmark a dictionary website on your computer and stick it on your toolbar so you will always have immediate access to it. You may also want to keep a print dictionary nearby while you are reading to reduce frustration when you encounter new words.

Consider using a "word a day" app. These apps provide you with a new word each day, along with the definition and context. Many apps include audio support to ensure you know how to pronounce the word correctly.

Research shows that reading as little as 20 minutes a day will have a positive effect on growing your vocabulary. Keep a list of the new words you learn. In your spare time, review them, pronounce them, and use them in a sentence. Research shows if you use the word seven times, it will become part of your vocabulary. Additional tips for building your vocabulary are listed in Box 4.1.

If you wish to converse with me, define your terms.

—Voltaire

Voice and Tone

An important component of verbal communication is our tone and pitch. Although what you say is important, the way we say it and how we say it communicates a great deal. The tone of your voice affects how

---

BOX 4.1

Tips on Vocabulary Building

- Choose words deliberately based on your professional or personal need. You will be more successful when your motivation is clear.
- Collect new words as you read the newspaper.
- Establish a place to collect words you want to add to your vocabulary and adopt a methodology for learning them, such as writing sentences with them or working them into conversations.
- Learn how to correctly pronounce and spell each new word as you learn it. You never want to mispronounce or misspell a word you are trying to learn.
- Look for prefixes, suffixes, and root words you already know. Try to understand how they contribute to the meaning of the new word.
- Use a thesaurus as well as a dictionary. Every word carries its own unique meaning. Understand the essential differences between words and their synonyms.
- Be aware of words that present usage problems. For example, "enervated" and "energized" are opposites, not synonyms. Study the differences between "affect" and "effect" and use them correctly.

---

people perceive you, although there is a limit to what you can do to change the sound of your voice. If you have a high-pitched voice or a low-pitched, gravelly voice, try to develop a pleasing tone somewhere between the two extremes.

When we are angry, frustrated, or upset, our pitch may raise, which is communicated to the listener. This might be necessary at times. When it is not, being able to control your tone and pitch is helpful in effectively communicating and ensuring that only the appropriate emotion is conveyed.

The manner of your speech is important as well. Speaking too fast or too slow, too loud or too soft, can be off-putting to your audience. It is worth taking time to improve your command over your voice, especially if you find it challenging to speak in public.

When interacting with patients, you want to instill confidence by sounding confident and speaking with authority, both in what you say and how you say it. Your voice should be strong and delivered with a confident smile. Pronounce words correctly, starting with the patient's name. If you do not know how to pronounce the patient's name correctly, simply ask. In most cases, patients will be happy to tell you and are pleased that you care enough to ask.

You can still command attention by speaking slowly and pausing frequently. It is better for you to speak accurately and thoughtfully than fast and being haphazard. To build positive interpersonal relationships in an office environment, we should all endeavor to speak in a professional and respectful tone.

Nonverbal Communication

Nonverbal communication is a form of communication where we send and receive messages without using our verbal communication skills. Research has shown speech only makes up about 20% to 30% of communication. The rest of communication is conveyed through our nonverbal communication skills or body languages, such as facial expressions, eye contact, gestures, and posture.

* **Facial expression.** Our face is incredibly expressive and often conveys our feelings of happiness, frustration, or confusion. It is important to be aware of the impression we are creating by using our eyes, eyebrows, mouth, and other facial features. For example, we often use facial expressions to communicate that we are listening and engaged with the person speaking. A smile, furrowed eyebrows, or an inquisitive expression all convey information

to the speaker about how you are responding to their conversation.

* **Eye contact.** We make eye contact to tell someone we are interested and paying attention to what they have to say. In contrast, if we frequently look away or refuse to make eye contact, we are sending a message that we are not interested. Maintaining good eye contact is an easy way to build rapport and trust when you communicate.

* **Gestures.** A gesture is any physical movement that helps you express an idea or opinion. It is important to try and coordinate your physical gestures to match your speech as a way to naturally reinforce your message.

* **Posture.** The way we carry ourselves, sit, stand, and move our body can be used to reinforce our verbal communication. How you position yourself during a conversation is important. For example, slouching, leaning back, crossing arms, or turning away from the speaker shows that you are not interested in the other person, and tapping your hand or fingers on a table may demonstrate you are bored or disinterested. If you angle yourself toward the person, with a relaxed and open posture, you invite them to engage with you more fully.

Part of catering to your listeners involves taking cues from their behavior. If they speak softly, lower your volume as well. If they are embarrassed, move to a private place. If they are emotional, be calm, make eye contact, nod affirmatively, and listen. Avoid interruptions, which may suggest that you are not listening.

As we learn more about how to effectively use our body language, we can improve our overall interpersonal communication and minimize misunderstandings. The good news is that we can all improve our nonverbal communication skills with practice. By learning more about how we use nonverbal communication, you will be better able to master yours and ensure that you are conveying your message exactly the way you wish to.

? WHAT IF?

What if a co-worker was describing the busy morning schedule to the office manager and you overheard her say, "Then, I had four stupid calls in a row!" What is your impression of your co-worker? What is she communicating to you and your office manager? How would you explain to your co-worker that her words may have been offensive to the office manager? What might she have said instead?

Aspects of Professional Speech

Consider Your Environment

It is always important to consider your audience when speaking. Think about conversations that you have with family and friends throughout the day. These conversations are likely to be casual and contain familiar language that you use when speaking to people who already know you. Do you use certain popular words, such as "whatever"? Do you find yourself using a lot of slang terms and even including some profanity? Using slang is generally inappropriate in the workplace, so be prepared to change some of your more common phrases. Of course, profanity is never acceptable at work.

➔ JOURNALING 4.1

Make a list of common phrases you say when you are not at work, and state their meaning. Which ones would be inappropriate for work? Write out substitutions using more professional language for those that are considered inappropriate.

When health care team members speak to one another, many levels of communication occur. Some experts believe that what you say is less important than your tone of voice, your word choice, and your body language. In addition, your audience, location, and comfort level will affect the quality of your communication. You can see these differences for yourself if you pause to notice that your breakroom conversations are casual in contrast with discussions in front of patients. Speaking professionally requires you to stop and think before you speak. You will have to rephrase what you might be thinking to express only those thoughts that are acceptable in professional situations. The first rule of all communication is to always identify your audience, so you may speak appropriately in all situations.

One of the best ways to set yourself apart from the crowd is to be gracious and display good manners. Saying "please," "thank you," and "you're welcome" is an easy way to ensure that people will remember you in a positive light. Many patients will be unfamiliar with your facility, and your welcoming demeanor will make them feel at ease.

Oversharing

Conversations with supervisors, co-workers, and patients may include many topics, both personal and professional. It is acceptable to share small details of your life with those you see every day. In fact, it is sometimes a good way to build a positive rapport with your co-workers.

However, do not share too much personal information. A detailed conversation about last night's escapades is never appropriate at work. Likewise, discussions about your health, salary, or relationships should be reserved for friends and family and should occur outside the workplace.

> *The game of life is a game of boomerangs. Our thoughts, deeds and words return to us sooner or later with astounding accuracy.*
>
> —Florence Scovel Shinn

Using Professional Language

Different professions have different languages and terms. This is true for the health care profession with the language of medicine or medical terminology. While you are learning about your chosen field, practice your medical terminology as much as possible. Educators will tell you that these words are the new language you need to use in the workplace, but you may not fully realize the importance of pronunciation and usage until you are in clinical situations.

Learn all the words you can and the proper way to say them. Play vocabulary games with a group or read health care journals to immerse yourself in the language. Using medical terminology correctly marks you as a professional and instills confidence in the patients you are speaking with and the co-workers you will be working with (Figure. 4.2).

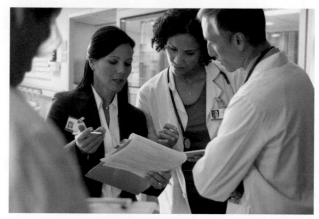

Figure 4.2 Hospital staff members discuss patient charts. (Copyright © istock.com.)

CASE STUDY 4.1
The Best People in the World

Dr. Avila was nervous about introducing his new office manager to the medical assistants and the support staff. As the managing partner of a large practice of over 75 physicians, Dr. Avila was acutely aware of the importance of this position and the success of the person he selected. He had passed on several senior staff members who had long been trusted employees of the practice, because they just were not quite what he felt the practice needed. He wanted an experienced professional, an excellent communicator, and a warm individual to fill the position.

He was about to introduce his choice, Roberta Candalaria, to the group of almost 200 staff members. Although Dr. Avila was uncomfortable in front of large audiences, he mumbled his way through an unremarkable introduction. He felt relieved to walk away to the sound of applause, shaking Roberta's hand as they passed from the center of the conference room.

Roberta stepped quickly to the podium. "You know, the best thing that any of us can do is give our very best to care for the people we actually come into personal contact with.

This includes not just the patients, but the family members. Those are the people we are in the best position to help, the ones who come to this practice seeking help from us. They are our customers. We are here to serve them."

"I'm a Certified Medical Assistant and have been for more than 20 years," she said. "How many of you are certified in your profession?" Most of the hands went up. "That's great," she said, "I think we owe it to our patients to give them the best our profession offers, don't you?"

"As you know, this practice already sponsors many CMA continuing education programs. In addition, if you are an AAMA member, the practice will pay your recertification fee. If you're not an AAMA member, we'll pay the portion we would pay if you were. We will reimburse you for any preapproved continuing education. If you're not certified, we will work with you to get you certified, including offering tutorials for the CMA examination. I want our patients to know that they are being cared for by some of the best professionals available."

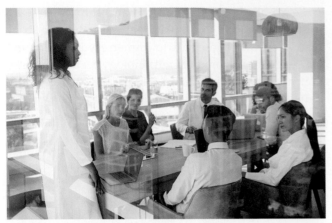

istock.com/monkeybusinessimages/677892282

Once the meeting was over, Dr. Avila watched Roberta walk up the aisle and stop next to a middle-aged man whom Dr. Avila said was one of the people who had applied for the job that went to her instead. "I'm Roberta," she said, extending her hand. "LeRoy," said the man, surprised and annoyed.

"LeRoy Walker?" asked Roberta. The man nodded. "LeRoy, haven't you been managing things on an interim basis since my predecessor left?"

LeRoy nodded again, a little less annoyed. "I have been."

"Thank you, LeRoy, for your service and leadership," said Roberta. "I already know you've made the transition much easier. I certainly know who to go to when I have questions."

By now, Dr. Avila was feeling a lot better.

QUESTIONS FOR THOUGHT AND REFLECTION

1. What was Roberta's challenge in making this speech?
2. Do you think Roberta had given thought to the needs of the audience in planning her speech? Why or why not?
3. What was Roberta's purpose in talking with LeRoy?
4. Why was Dr. Avila apprehensive at first? How do you think he feels now after the meeting? Why?

A Different Path

Kristen and Erika, both medical assistants and mutual friends outside of work, were huddled at the front desk on Monday at about 7:30 a.m. No patients were expected for 30 minutes and they were ready for the day, so they began catching up on the social events of their weekends.

"Where'ya go last night?" asked Erika.

Kristen whispered, then Erika squealed, "Seriously?"

Erika leaned in for more details, and soon the women were engrossed in their conversation. They did not hear Mrs. Long, the 8:00 a.m. patient, enter the reception area, and they had just about finished their conversation when Mrs. Long cleared her throat.

Mrs. Long, unfortunately, overheard Kristen share with Erika the club she went to last Saturday night, how much she drank, and the guys she met.

"I'm Bethany Long and I have an 8 o'clock appointment with Dr. Wen." Mrs. Long looks both uneasy and annoyed. "I hope I'm not interrupting anything."

Kristen and Erika scuttled to get Mrs. Long checked in.

During their break, Ellie, the office manager, asked to meet with them. She told them that Mrs. Long mentioned overhearing their conversation, and she thought it was inappropriate. She and Dr. Wen had to apologize to Mrs. Long.

"Not only did you keep her waiting, but your conversation was inappropriate for the office. I understand casual conversation is normal. But please keep the topics to more G-rated content, okay?"

QUESTIONS FOR THOUGHT AND REFLECTION

1. What do you think Kristen and Erika were talking about that offended Mrs. Long?
2. How should the office manager and physician handle this problem?
3. When is it appropriate to talk about your social life in the workplace?

⊛ EXPERIENTIAL EXERCISES

1. Spend a half-hour in the lobby of a hospital or medical office. Observe the language used between the medical staff. Note words or conversations you feel are professional and ones that are not. Can you spot patients and staff as being different by the way they speak?

2. Review your medical terminology textbook. Write down all the terms you forget. Ensure that you know what they mean and how to pronounce and spell them correctly.
3. Read a health care–related article. Write down at least five words you are not familiar with. Write a sentence with clear meaning for each word, and practice using it.

4. Play a word or vocabulary game with a group of friends. Playing games is a valuable way to increase your vocabulary, and the more diverse the people you play with, the more exposure to new words you will have.

🌐 **CROSS CURRENTS WITH OTHER SOFT SKILLS**

LISTENING ACTIVELY: To speak effectively, you should be listening more than speaking (Chapter 6).

READING AND SPEAKING BODY LANGUAGE: Sometimes the key to communicating is the things we do not say (Chapter 6).

SHOWING EMPATHY, SENSITIVITY, AND CARING: You can demonstrate empathy and caring to others professionally. Professionalism can be warm and comforting (Chapter 5).

COMMITTING TO YOUR PROFESSION: Good, knowledgeable speakers will always be in demand in your profession (Chapter 8).

EXUDING OPTIMISM, ENTHUSIASM, AND POSITIVITY: Smiles can be heard in all languages, and it is amazing what a positive attitude will do for your communication skills (Chapter 2).

Writing, Grammar, and Spelling

A synonym is a word you use when you can't spell the other one.

—Baltasar Gracián

LEARNING OBJECTIVE 2:
WRITING, GRAMMAR, AND SPELLING

- Think about your audience before you write anything.
- Learn to communicate concisely in your writing, respecting your reader's time.
- Use correct grammar and spell every word correctly.
- Understand how to adjust your tone so you convey the attitude you intend.
- Arm yourself with email best practices.
- Gain familiarity with writing for social media and digital environments.

Good writing skills enable you to communicate your messages clearly and concisely to your intended audience. Did you know that writing is not really about writing? Writing is all about your reader. You are writing to communicate. If you make one change now in how you write, it should be to remember that you are writing for your reader, no matter how easy or difficult writing is for you. Constantly ask yourself, "What does the reader want to know? Will this be clear to the reader? What are the different ways that the reader can interpret this?"

Reflect on what you want from someone's writing when you are the reader. Writing should be clear, interesting, informative, and concise.

You don't start out writing good stuff. You start out writing crap and thinking it's good stuff, and then gradually you get better at it. That's why I say one of the most valuable traits is persistence.

—Octavia E. Butler

Basic Aspects of Good Writing

Whether you are writing patient notes, problem-oriented notes, general documentation, thank you notes, or a referral, you are leaving behind a permanent record that will always reflect on you. If the grammar and spelling are correct, the tone appropriate, and the words concise and well chosen, you will be seen as a person of competence and professionalism.

Grammar

Using correct grammar together with a good vocabulary will ensure your message is delivered effectively. Grammar inconsistencies and mistakes in grammar usage can create confusion for readers and hinder your intended message. You put a lot of thought into what you want to write, and grammar and punctuation let you express your ideas and more easily communicate with your reader.

One of the easiest and most enjoyable ways to improve your use of grammar and punctuation is to read. Every time you read, pay attention to grammar usage. Where is the writer using punctuation to separate sentences, phrases, or ideas? How are they formatting lists, quotations, or long sentences? Use the structures you see in your reading as models when you write. The more you read, the more you will be able to recognize and adopt effective uses of grammar and punctuation.

There are also a number of free online resources and computer applications that can be helpful in monitoring and using proper grammar:
* **Grammarly.** This is a free, online writing assistance that lets you copy and paste text into Grammarly's editor. The tools flag potential issues in the copy

and suggest context-specific corrections for grammar, spelling, and punctuation. It can also be downloaded as an application and can grammar and spell check documents, emails, and even texts.

* **The Purdue Online Writing Lab.** The site offers free resources on grammar, writing business communications, and other tools.
* **GrammarBook.** This site offers detailed rules and examples on various areas of grammar.

Reviewing grammar is beyond the scope of this book. However, you can improve your skills by taking classes or reading books on the topic. In the meantime, write simple sentences that have a clear subject and an active verb. Short, simple, direct sentences minimize errors and increase understanding.

? WHAT IF?

What if you received a note from a co-worker that used incorrect grammar, run-on sentences, and so many typos that you could not even figure out what the person was trying to say? What impression would you have of the writer?

Spelling

In health care, you are writing to an audience who knows correct word spelling, especially if it is medical terminology. Therefore, when you misspell a word, it distracts from the message you are trying to communicate. Plus, misspelled medical terms can result in incorrect dosages, treatments, or insurance billing.

Recognize that spelling is something you can master with simple analysis, repetition, and attention to detail. When you first encounter a new word, take a few seconds to examine it carefully. What are its syllables? Is there anything unusual about the word, such as surprising combinations of letters, letters that do not match how they are pronounced, double letters, or letters that are not doubled when you would expect them to be?

For example, if we apply this process to the word *parallel*, the first half, para, is easy. It is just like all the other instances of para you know: parasympathetic, paranormal. The last four letters might trip you up if you do not learn them now. There is no particular rule that justifies the double "L," so just remember it: *llel*. In fact, when you think of these four letters standing alone, they may look so peculiar to you that they just might stick in your memory.

Although spelling is usually considered either correct or incorrect, it is important to keep in mind that the spelling of some medical terms may be different in America compared to other countries, for example, anemia versus anaemia, dyspnea versus dyspnoaea, or tumor versus tumour. They all have the same meaning, and you may see them in medical journals. These spellings are all acceptable, but it will be important to use the American version while working in the United States.

Tone

Although we discussed tone in verbal communication, tone can also be conveyed in written communication. For example, does the sentence include please or thank you? Is it written in capital letters? Are you intentionally using complex terms to overcompensate or intimidate the reader?

The tone we use in writing should reflect the writer's attitude toward the audience and the content that is being written about. The tone of our written messages affects readers in the same way that our tone of voice affects our conversations. Think of your writing tone as your manners. How do you come across to your reader? Polite? Respectful? Sarcastic? Hostile?

Your tone reflects your attitude. The nuances of tone can be subtle. Word choice can also affect your tone. For example, do you see problems or disasters? The way you frame ideas and experiences can affect the outcomes. Box 4.2 explains methods to manage tone.

Additionally, here are a few questions to help you discern the correct tone to use:

* **Why am I writing this document?** Always take time to consider the purpose of your messages. This

BOX 4.2

Elements to Manage Tone

- Short sentences suggest simple, often powerful ideas.
- Long sentences suggest complicated, nuanced ideas.
- Is the vocabulary appropriate for the audience?
- Active voice seems personal: "I thank you."
- Passive voice seems impersonal: "You are to be thanked."
- To increase formality, eliminate contractions.
- To decrease formality, use slang and lingo.
- Avoid overuse of the exclamation point, and never use emoticons as substitutes for tone.

process will help shape how you should express the message to reach your intended audience.

* **To whom am I writing?** When you take time to consider to whom you are writing specifically, your tone will adjust to ensure it is more effective.

* **What do I want them to understand?** It is important to emphasize the benefits for the reader and to use emphasis to highlight key information in your writing. When writing for business, we generally strive for a tone that is confident, sincere, and polite.

Be Concise

I didn't have time to write a short letter, so I wrote a long one instead.

—Mark Twain

Some people think that lengthy discourses, complicated sentences, and fancy words equal good writing. Nothing could be farther from the truth. It takes time and thought to craft your message down to its final length. An important skill in writing is being concise and succinct. This is expressing or stating ideas using only enough words as necessary.

It is likely that your readers may be busy or may have a short attention span. It is important to get to the point and communicate the most important information as soon as you can before your message is lost. State what you are trying to convey in as few words as possible. This requires some effort and thoughtfulness on the writer's part. For some writers, it is easier to get all the information down on paper quickly and then review it to tighten the piece. For others, it can be more helpful to begin by thinking instead of writing. If you are one of these writers, Box 4.3 contains questions to consider before beginning to write.

However, there may be times when you must over-explain or provide a lot of detail, such as in the case of describing instructions to a patient for a procedure or training a new employee on the electronic health records software. Thus, it is important to understand the situation and the audience when writing.

Advanced Elements of Good Writing

Powerful Verbs and Punchy Words

Along with adjectives, verbs add emotion to a sentence. They are the action words that drive your thoughts forward. Writers who make an effort to

BOX 4.3

Questions to Ponder Before Writing

- Who is my reader? Who will read this?
- What does my reader need to know about this subject?
- How can I put the essential information in the first sentence?
- What tone or attitude should I adopt?
- How can I create that tone?
- What is my intention: to inform, persuade, amuse, applaud?
- Am I making a request or call to action?
- How can I keep this as short as possible?
- How can I end on a strong note?

choose interesting verbs will develop an engaging writing style. Instead of writing, "He sat up straight," you might consider, "He sprang to attention." Strong verbs can improve your writing and help you:

* **Eliminate wordiness.** Strong verbs can help you eliminate different forms of the verb "to be" and eliminate using words such as "is," "was," "are," and "were." For example, instead of saying, "He was the owner of a fleet of trucks," you can say, "He owned a fleet of trucks."

* **Use active voice.** When writing in active voice, the subject (noun) of a sentence performs an action (verb) on an object. For example, Jaime kicked the ball. Avoid passive voice writing where possible, as you want to engage the reader and add more impact to your content.

* **Reduce adverbs.** When you choose strong verbs, you can be more specific and descriptive in your writing. Ask yourself if the adverb tells the reader something you can convey to them through a better description.

Modification

Modifiers add details. Not surprisingly, modifiers modify the meaning. It was not just a shirt, it was a yellow shirt. The patient did not just shuffle, they shuffled precariously. These are examples of adjectives and adverbs, respectively—adjectives modifying nouns, adverbs modifying verbs. If you do not overuse adjectives and adverbs, they can add personality to your writing.

Phrases or clauses can also be used to modify and add meaning, color, and precision. You can modify phrases and clauses in three places in a sentence:

before the subject, between the subject and the verb, and after the verb. Here are some examples:

* "Before surgery, the patient signed the consent form."
* "The patient, with little hesitation, signed the consent form."
* "The patient signed the consent form, after consulting his wife."

You can improve your style by placing modification phrases throughout your sentences to achieve variety and interest. The great thing about modification is that there is no limit to the kind of variety possible and the ways it can contribute to your style. When you ask yourself how you might modify a word or a sentence, you are actually asking yourself for additional observations, important details, and vivid language to help achieve the purpose of your writing assignment.

Transitional Words

Transitional words help the reader follow your thoughts and logic. For example, to remind your reader that you are making the second of three points, start your second point with "second" or "secondly." To announce a conclusion, write "Therefore." To move on to your next point, write "Next." To show that you are wrapping up a list of steps, write "Finally." To introduce an exception or a contrasting view, write "However." Transitions keep the reader on track to grasp your message and keep them engaged.

This is the sort of bloody nonsense up with which I will not put.

—Sir Winston Churchill

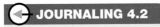 **JOURNALING 4.2**

Describe what is unique about your particular writing style. Do you tend to write lengthy paragraphs and documents?

Electronic Communication

Although you may still need to write on paper to complete some documents and forms, most of your writing and documentation will likely be done electronically. Electronic communication is any form of communication that's broadcast, transmitted, stored, or viewed using electronic media, such as computers, phones, email, and video. The most common types of electronic communications are:

* Email
* Instant messaging and live chat
* Websites and blogs

* SMS and text messaging
* Phone and voicemail
* Video

In the health care setting, you may use some or all these types of electronic communications. Additionally, they all may be used in appointment reminders, patient portals, and telemedicine. Electronic communication can be a useful tool in the practice of patient care and can facilitate communication with a patient.

Email communication can raise special concerns about privacy and confidentiality, particularly when sensitive information is to be communicated. When health care professionals and providers engage in electronic communication, they hold the same ethical responsibilities to patients as they do during any other clinical encounters. Any method of communication, virtual, telephonic, or in person, should be appropriate to the patient's clinical need and to the information being conveyed.

Emails

Every email is an opportunity for you to present yourself in a positive light. However, email requires special attention and involves additional constraints.

First, when you write a professional email, ensure that your message is concise and free of emoticons, garish colors, and backgrounds. Your recipients may receive at least 50 emails each day, so consider if this email is truly necessary or not. Begin your emails with the most important details and information and follow up with any necessary information. Make any requests early in the email so they will not be overlooked. If possible, state your key message in the subject line. "Carefully monitor Mr. Souza today" immediately conveys the most urgent part of the message, but the reader can open the message for additional information.

Second, use email for its intended purpose of instant communication and not as a substitute for face-to-face communication. Remember to keep your audience in mind and write accordingly.

Acronyms like "lol" or "smh" should not be used in professional emails. Even common business acronyms are out of place if your audience does not know them. Use work-related acronyms only if they hold meaning for everyone who may be reading your email.

Do not write anything in an email that you would not say to someone in person. Further, do not write anything you may regret later. Do not write emails when you are emotional. Take advantage of the time that electronic communication allows. Remember,

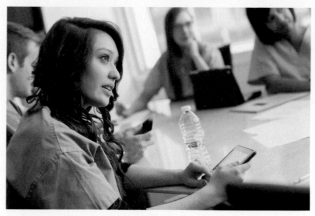

Figure 4.3 A health care team member uses her personal mobile device during a staff meeting. (Copyright © istock.com.)

emails last forever. They can be used as legal documents and as evidence in court or a complaint to human resources. It is always helpful to pause before hitting the Send button during these situations. Box 4.4 suggests additional email practices to avoid.

Blogs, Twitter, and Digital Communication

If you are a good writer and have something important to say, you may want to expand your writing to the web. In no way, however, can you appear to represent your employer unless your employer explicitly authorizes you to do so. Nevertheless, social media are here to stay, and it is likely that health care facilities will increasingly use Facebook, blogs, Twitter, TikTok, or LinkedIn to market themselves and interact with their customers or patients.

Of course, you can make personal use of social media, but you should still be cautious to not do or post anything that would embarrass your employer or raise concerns with your supervisor. For example, avoid venting or complaining about your co-workers, supervisors, or employers. The advent of social media calls for incredible professionalism, restraint, and social intelligence (Figure. 4.3).

The key to writing online is having something of value to say or to share. If you consistently offer information and views that are helpful to others, you will attract an audience and be in a position of influence.

The First Draft

Over the course of your career, you may be asked to write longer and more extensive documents, such as a report or an important letter. How would you start? Each writer must experiment and find the style that works best for them. Try one of the following methods to see which approach fits you best.

The Color Code Approach

Some writers must write fast to catch their thoughts as they get them. Then, once captured, the writer follows these steps:
* Highlight the various thoughts in different colors, according to their focus, to form connections.
* Group like colors together.
* Number thoughts within each color section.
* Determine the order in which to present each section.
* Organize each thought to achieve a unified flow.
* Create an opening and ending.
* Edit the final read-through.

Mapping and Webbing

Does forming a sentence onscreen or on paper just feel totally paralyzing? If so, mapping might work best for you. Forget the computer screen or lined paper at first; instead, make a "thoughts web" or "mind map" to act as your first draft before you write. To try your hand at mapping or webbing, start with a blank sheet of paper:

* In the center of a sheet of paper, write down a single word or phrase that is central to what you want to say. Then circle it.
* Next, as other thoughts about your message come into your head, jot these down at random around your central word, making a spider web of words. Include phrases that occur to you or words you want to use as well. Take your time. The more thoughts you can capture in these circles, the better.
* Now draw lines between all of them that connect.
* Look for meaningful links. Do you see connections and patterns that you want to talk about?
* Later, you can link these connections to make larger webs until you have cohesive paragraphs. This usually frees you to connect and construct a solid first draft.

* Once you are satisfied that you have covered everything, make a short outline.

Mind mapping is a valuable technique because it uses the spatial, creative, and imaginative parts of your brain and enables you to make more connections. Figure. 4.4 is an example of a mind map.

The Diving Board Approach

Many people simply plunge into writing. They may think about their audience and start "talking" to them on paper. They may like starting with an interesting first sentence that will grab the attention of the reader. Others know right away how they want their document to end and write from there. Later, after this "diving-in" approach, they find it easier to go back, fill in the blanks, rearrange things, choose words thoughtfully, and edit.

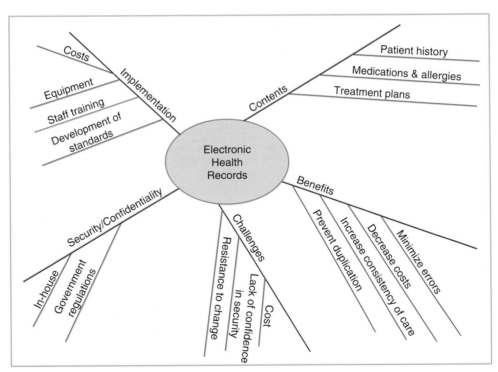

Figure 4.4 Mind map. (From Haroun L: *Career development for health professionals: success in school and on the job,* ed 4, St Louis, 2016, Saunders.)

CASE STUDY **4.2**
Donna Wong, PhD, RN, PNP, CPN, FAAN

Dr. Donna Wong wrote the best-selling nursing textbook of all time, *Nursing Care of Infants and Children.* Like you, she started out as a health care professional and only later came to see writing as a way to contribute to her profession.

When Dr. Wong met someone for the first time, she would often say, "Were you expecting a little Chinese lady?" In fact, born in 1948, Donna looked a lot like her Italian American mother. She was raised in New Jersey and became a nurse after attending Rutgers University. In 1971, she married Dr. Ting Wong, a Chinese immigrant who became an officer in the Air Force and whose last name she took.

Dr. Wong started out as a young nurse working with children. She was dismayed to encounter children with serious illnesses who were not being treated effectively for their pain. In fact, in those days, it was not widely recognized that infants even experienced pain because it was believed their nervous systems were not fully developed. Moreover, young children could not effectively communicate the level of pain they were experiencing, and thus they were usually undermedicated.

Even though this was one issue that concerned the young nurse, there were many others, and she often thought how poorly student nurses had been served by the pediatric nursing textbooks that were available at the time. After earning her master's degree in nursing from the University of California at Los Angeles, she began thinking seriously about what could be done to better educate student nurses in the field of pediatric nursing. Through a series of fortunate coincidences, she teamed up with Lucille Whaley and wrote the now-famous textbook *Whaley & Wong: Nursing Care of Infants and Children*, first published in 1979 and now in its ninth edition.

Dr. Wong went on to earn a doctorate degree in child development from Oklahoma State University. She was a professor at the University of Oklahoma Medical Center, Oral Roberts University, and the University of Oklahoma School of Nursing. For many years, Dr. Wong was a nurse consultant at the Children's Hospital of the St. Francis Medical Center in Tulsa.

Dr. Wong had an amazing ability to synthesize new knowledge reported in the literature and translate it to nursing practice in her books. These assimilations went into her files, one for each chapter in the forthcoming edition. Dr. Wong published extensively in journals and peer-reviewed articles for publication. She formed an organization called Pediatric Nursing Consultants, teaching some of the most talented pediatric nursing researchers about writing and publishing. She also became a popular speaker at conferences and conventions. She started an ongoing conference on pediatric pain.

Additionally, Dr. Wong developed the Wong-Baker FACES Pain Rating Scale (Figure. 4.5), which is now used worldwide to assess children's pain. Recognizing that children were inconsistent in how they reported their pain, resulting in inconsistent treatment for pain, Dr. Wong and her colleague Connie Baker extensively researched graphic representations of faces expressing comfort and pain.

Dr. Wong encouraged friends and colleagues to research issues that needed answers. She talked to kids about what it felt like to have a cast removed, get blood drawn, or experience chemotherapy. Moreover, her book reflects the very latest in the pathophysiology of disease, explaining the mechanisms of disease, and what that means for treatment and nursing care.

QUESTIONS FOR THOUGHT AND REFLECTION

1. What role did writing play in Dr. Wong's life?
2. What effect did her writing have on others and her profession?
3. What inspires you about the life of Dr. Wong?
4. How might you use writing to improve and expand your job? How can writing advance your career and promotability?

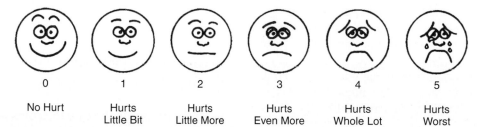

0	1	2	3	4	5
No Hurt	Hurts Little Bit	Hurts Little More	Hurts Even More	Hurts Whole Lot	Hurts Worst

Figure 4.5 Wong-Baker FACES Pain Rating Scale. (From Hockenberry MJ, Wilson D: *Wong's nursing care of infants and children*, ed 10, St Louis, 2015, Elsevier.)

The hospital's general counsel, Arthur Adams, was reviewing a patient's chart, which had been subpoenaed by the patient's attorney in connection with a lawsuit that the patient had filed. The patient, Mrs. Roberta DeMasi, alleged that she received substandard care at Buchanan Hospital, which led to the amputation of her left foot. Mr. Adams was dumbfounded by what he saw. In particular, there were four progress notes by a "M. O'Brien, PCT," or patient care technician.

The first one, dated April 2, read: "The patient has a sticky wound on the bottom of her foot with this black stuff oozing out. Charlie, one of the dietary aides, helped me take off the bandage for changing. Had a terrible smell. I squirted some cream on it and covered it up as fast as possible. M. O'Brien, PCT."

The next one was worse. "April 4. Roberta was in a bad mood tonight. Constantly complained about pain in her foot. RN gave her PRN pain medication. Patient still complained. M. O'Brien, PCT."

The next note was the biggest liability: "April 7. Patient's foot worse than ever. I had RN take a look, and she called DOC. MD arrived and said it was the worst he's ever seen. He said she had "green." He had to debride the wound. MD put on cream, rewrapped bandage. Patient's temperature elevated. M. O'Brien, PCT."

"Elevated?" thought Mr. Adams. "Elevated to what?" The last note did not help.

"April 8. Somebody said they might have to amputate. MD changes bandage now. Roberta in a nasty mood. Medical students observed wound. Patient complained she didn't give consent for this. M. O'Brien, PCT."

Mr. Adams met with the president of the hospital, his legal team, and the vice president of human resources.

"We have no choice but to settle this case. Once the plaintiff's attorney sees the patient's medical records, it will be obvious that we have some liability here," Mr. Adams said.

QUESTIONS FOR THOUGHT AND REFLECTION

1. What are some of the mistakes M. O'Brien made in the documentation?
2. In your opinion, what was more damaging—the patient's medical care or the way she was characterized in the chart?
3. What was the liability Mr. Adams is referring to?

⭐ EXPERIENTIAL EXERCISES

1. Determine whether your employer or externship site has any written policies on documentation. Ask your co-workers or supervisors for an example of what they consider good documentation.
2. Explore mind mapping online using the Internet.
3. Read a short story. Observe the use of language, word choice, attention to details, and how the details contribute to the tone and meaning of the story.
4. Read a journal related to your field. What kind of observations can you make about the writing style you encountered there?
5. Ask a friend to critique an email you wrote. Did it seem to address its intended audience? Was it clear and concise? How was the tone?

CROSS CURRENTS WITH OTHER SOFT SKILLS

THINKING CRITICALLY: Thinking is a prerequisite for writing (Chapter 6).
COMMITTING TO YOUR PROFESSION: Writing and researching are key components to advancing knowledge in your profession (Chapter 8).

Professional Phone Etiquette

Tomorrow you might get a phone call about something wonderful, and you might get a phone call about something terrible.

—Regina Spektor

LEARNING OBJECTIVE 3: PROFESSIONAL PHONE ETIQUETTE

- Know proper technique to professionally answer the phone.
- Convey emotions through tone, pitch, and volume.
- Know what kinds of calls to expect and how to triage them.
- Defuse emotional callers.
- Commit to learning the technology associated with the telephone.

Preparing to Answer the Phone

When you answer the phone, it is a mistake to think that your voice is doing all the work. Your posture, breath, smile, tone, and attitude are, in fact, conveyed through your voice.

Who are you when you answer the phone? You get to choose. It is almost as if you choose a persona, like an actor in a play. Make sure your phone persona is the best "you" it can be, and then use that version of you every single time.

Your professionalism is challenged every time you answer the phone at work. Every caller will judge you and form an opinion of your employer based on their interaction with you. Plan your phone presence. At health care facilities, callers may be anxious or ill. Be sensitive to their needs.

The Greeting

You should have a well-rehearsed greeting when you answer the phone. Of course, you will want to follow any policies and practices in place at your place of employment, but you will probably want to identify the facility, followed by your name: "Hello, Riverside Labs. This is Lori." You want to speak slowly and clearly, so the caller knows immediately that he has reached the right place.

Prepare your telephone voice ahead of time. You will want to speak in a moderately loud voice in case the caller has a hearing deficit or a poor connection. Plan to enunciate and speak directly into the phone. You can train your voice to sound clear and professional by humming for a minute at the lowest register of your voice. That is also an effective way to clear your voice after you have consumed dairy products or other foods that can produce mucous around your vocal folds.

Keep a notepad near the phone and plan to take messages or notes (Figure. 4.6). Write the caller's name, affiliation, and the time on the notepad. That way, you can clarify the caller's name right away if you need to, and you will have it to refer to later in the call without forgetting it. Write down any important information.

Answering the Phone

Just before you answer the phone, sit up straight to open the full capacity of your lungs. You want to have your whole lung capacity available to you. Smiling, with your posture and body language in ready position, state your rehearsed greeting directly into the receiver. The greeting and introduction should be

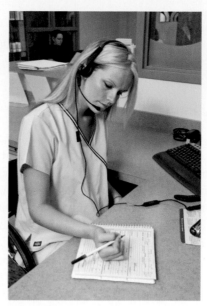

Figure 4.6 A health care professional on the phone, taking notes. (From Proctor DB, Adams AP: *Kinn's the medical assistant: an applied learning approach*, ed 12, St Louis, 2014, Elsevier.)

consistent every time. You will have practiced it to get as much inflection, warmth, and enthusiasm into your voice as possible.

Your main job as the recipient of a phone call at your health care facility is to listen. You should verify the caller and listen for the purpose of the call. Try not to interrupt. Take a breath before you speak to ensure that the caller has provided all the information. Obviously, your caller will be seeking information, but very often your answer will be in the form of a question because you want to clarify the caller's need and get as much information as you can.

Quite often, you are going to take a message, transfer the call, or arrange for a callback from one of your colleagues. It is your job to anticipate the questions your colleague will have and record that information.

Telephone Triage

You should answer the phone as quickly as possible. The general rule is you should answer the phone by the third ring. You never know which calls will be an emergency.

An important aspect of answering the telephone in a health care setting is knowing how to triage. Telephone triage is the process of managing a patient's call to the office to determine the urgency of the medical issue, the level of staff or provider response required, the appropriate location if the patient needs to be seen, and the timing of appointment scheduling.

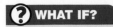

Routine Calls

Most calls will be of the routine nature. Box 4.5 lists the different types of common telephone calls that you may experience in a health care setting. The telephone is still a common form of exchanging information, and the need for information in health care is fast-paced. You are likely to spend a significant amount of time on the phone every day, depending on your job and duties. Be prepared to make this time as economical as possible.

For many health care professionals, a flurry of information is exchanged over the phone every day. Many times, callers will miss you, or you will be unable to reach your parties, and follow-up calls are needed, adding to the confusion. You will need a system if there is not one already. Regardless of whether you have to create your own system or whether your office has an established system or policy, it will only be successful if you use it every single time. It must be consistent and a habit. You cannot suspend the phone record or

BOX 4.5

Common Types of Phone Calls in the Health Care Setting

- New patients
- Appointments and cancellations
- Insurance and billing inquiries
- Fee queries
- Questions about whether your providers are in or out of a network
- Laboratory reports and results
- Patient documentation (e.g., workers' compensation)
- Medical records
- Office administration
- Vendors
- Referrals and referral requests
- Prescription refills
- Sales and vendors
- Complaints
- Calls from family members or caretakers of patients
- Calls from other doctors and health providers
- Social calls
- Return calls from previous information requests

phone log system just because it gets busy. It is precisely at these times that the system is most needed.

Emergency Calls

Emergencies demand special skills. You should always be prepared to respond effectively and efficiently to an emergency call. As soon as you realize you are dealing with an emergency, ask, "Please state the nature of your emergency." Emergency callers are often quite emotional, so you should use some of the techniques you use with any other emotional caller.

Concentrate on getting the facts. If possible, get the person's name and location or the exact location of the emergency. The caller's number should be recorded on your telephone equipment but try to obtain it anyway. Ask the person to tell you what you can do to effectively respond to the situation. Identify the severity of the situation and identify others who may be in the best position to help, whether it is the police, an ambulance service, the poison control center, or the attention of a physician or other emergency professional. In almost all cases of an emergency call, you should be instructing the caller to dial 911.

Other Types of Calls

Follow-up calls are not difficult, unless they are not made. When you need to or promise to follow up, something is at stake. Information must be obtained or clarified to ensure the smooth operation of the enterprise. Somebody is waiting to hear back from you, and their impression of your employer depends on whether you follow through and meet this obligation.

Confidential calls also require special attention. When what you say should not be overheard, try to move away from others or lower your voice or avoid using identifying patient information (Figure. 4.7). If the situation is confidential, arrange to return the call in a private setting. Care should be taken that any notes are conveyed verbally or transcribed to the appropriate record and the notes destroyed.

Complaints are part of any enterprise. Mistakes will be made. Misunderstandings will occur. And when they do, you will receive a complaint. Health care professionals deal effectively with problems all day long. Develop solutions by examining the problem itself rather than its delivery.

Patients may call in a very angry mood. Try to defuse the emotion surrounding the problem. Speak in a calm voice and indicate a willingness to assist. Usually, you are not the reason the person is angry; you have simply answered the phone. However, you are your employer's representative, and so it is your job to manage the

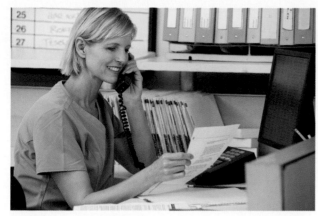

Figure 4.7 A nurse calls a patient with confidential information. (Copyright © istock.com.)

angry caller. Say something empathetic, such as, "I can understand your frustration. Let me see what I can do to help you." Listen actively and ask good questions so you have a good grasp of the caller's problem.

If the anger persists, you should deal directly with it. "I'm having a hard time trying to help you. So, I do need you to lower your voice." If this does not help, you may need to escalate it to a co-worker or supervisor. You can arrange a callback, either from yourself or from someone who can address the problem effectively.

Of course, if the angry caller is abusive, uses coarse or offensive language, or is completely consumed with rage, you are not required to continue the conversation. Use the following explanation to communicate with the caller: "Unfortunately, I am not able to assist you when you're speaking to me this way. Please call back when you're ready to focus on a solution." Your duty is to follow procedures and protocols, while doing your best to meet the caller's needs. Firmly repeat the policy and offer to do what you can do. "Sir, I cannot put you through to the doctor. However, I would be happy to take a message for her."

JOURNALING 4.3

Think about telemarketing calls you have received at home or at work. Write down the kinds of techniques the more aggressive callers use. How have you responded? Think about how you might respond even more effectively.

Making Calls and Leaving Messages

When placing calls, clearly identify yourself, your role, your employer, and the person on whose behalf you are calling. Make an effort to engage with the person you are calling and smile while you are talking; often people can "hear" that you are smiling and

BOX 4.6

Tips for Leaving a Message

- State your name, role, affiliation, and the time of your call, including the date.
- Name the person or the role of the person you are leaving the message for.
- State your message concisely. If your message is complicated, give an idea of what it is about and state that you will provide details when the call is returned.
- If the message is urgent, make that clear.
- State when you can be reached.
- State your name again. You are reinforcing the memory of your call to the recipient.
- State your telephone number slowly. Repeat your number, so the recipient can record it correctly.
- Thank the recipient for the requested action in advance.

this encourages their cooperation. Be precise about the information you are seeking or the request you are making. Write down any information you receive. Arrange any follow-up that may be needed. Thank the person for their help or kindness.

Frequently, you will have to leave a message to achieve the purpose of your call. Box 4.6 offers suggestions for making your messages more effective.

Phone Technology

In this age of global telecommunication and technological advances, all of us are challenged to master existing technologies and learn new ones. Functions you will have to learn include transfers, holds, call waiting, conferencing, voicemail, answering services, caller ID, call forwarding, pagers, faxes, international calling, and operating headsets.

Reliable communication is essential to the safe and efficient delivery of health care. Therefore, technological skills are required of you. You must take this training seriously and practice it. Identify more than one mentor or resource you can consult until you are comfortable with the technology used at your facility. Finally, keep frequently called numbers on hand so you can access them easily and quickly, whether your calls are routine or emergencies.

The telephone is an amazing invention, but who would ever want to use one?

—Rutherford B. Hayes

CASE STUDY 4.3
Angry Husband

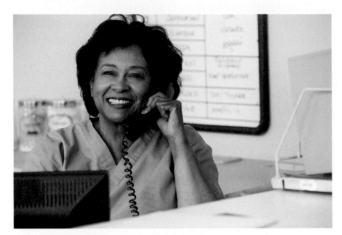

iStock.com/monkeybusinessimages/161824863

Charlissa had just arrived for her night shift in the Emergency Department when the phone rang. She took a deep breath, put a smile on her face, and said "Community General Hospital. This is Charlissa speaking. How may I help you?"

"I'll tell you how you can help me, Charlissa," said the caller, an agitated male. "You can put me on the phone with Dr. Horace Skinner … right now!"

Charlissa took a deep breath before she replied. "Sir, could you give me your name?"

"Tell him it's Jerry Pacheco, and I need to speak with him right now."

She wrote his name down on her pad. "Mr. Pacheco, Dr. Skinner is unavailable just now. Could I help you or take a message for him?"

"Is he there?"

"I believe so, however …."

"Then put him on!"

"Unfortunately, sir, he's unable to come to the phone. Can I help you or take a message?"

"Put Skinner on this phone. Right now!"

"Mr. Pacheco, again, Dr. Skinner cannot come to the phone right now. But let me see if I can help you. Please give me some information about your situation."

She heard a deep sigh on the phone. Then the male voice, softer, more controlled, between gritted teeth, continued. "I am out of town. I got a call that my wife was taken to your emergency room. Dr. Skinner spoke to me and told me she was stable. He said he would call me back. I have not heard from him!" he finished, returning to his original state of agitation.

"I can certainly understand why you're concerned, sir. Could you tell me your wife's name?"

"Lisa," he said.

"Sir, can you hold? I'll see what I can find out."

"Of course, put me on hold!" he almost shouted.

Charlissa pressed the "Hold" button. Despite being calm during the call, her heart was racing, and she had to take a moment to close her eyes and take a deep breath.

She checked her procedures and Ms. Pacheco's privacy statement. "Does anybody know where Dr. Skinner is?"

"In surgery," somebody said.

"Does anyone have a condition report on a Lisa Pacheco?"

"In surgery with Dr. Skinner."

Charlissa pressed the "Hold" button again. She was able to relay an update to Mr. Pacheco. "Mr. Pacheco. Your wife is currently in surgery with Dr. Skinner."

"Oh God, oh God."

"Mr. Pacheco, I know you are very anxious. I am going to find out what is going on in surgery and call you back. Will that be all right?"

"Oh, God, yes. Call me back. Please call me back."

She took down his cell phone number, which matched the number on her display. "I will call you as soon as I speak with Dr. Skinner, Mr. Pacheco."

After Dr. Skinner came out of surgery, Charlissa updated him on her phone call with Mr. Pacheco. Once Dr. Skinner gave her an update on Mrs. Pacheco's condition, Charlissa dialed Mr. Pacheco's number.

"Mr. Pacheco, your wife is out of surgery and is stable. Dr. Skinner will call you as soon as he is out of the surgical unit. That's why he didn't call you before. I gave him your cell number."

"Thank you, Charlissa," he said, barely audible. "Thank you so much."

QUESTIONS FOR THOUGHT AND REFLECTION

1. How did Charlissa prepare for this call?
2. What did Charlissa do when she realized the caller was agitated?
3. What steps and actions did Charlissa do make sure the interaction was successful and professional?

A Different Path

Brittany was chatting with the other medical assistants when the phone rang. She picked it up before she really finished talking. "Tell him to buzz off," she said, laughing. "Hello."

"Hello?" said a male voice.

"Hello? This is Brittany."

"Is this Dr. Lorris' office?"

"Yup. What can I do for you?"

"Well, actually, I have terrible pain in my hip joint. I know I have to have a hip replacement eventually, but right now, I'm in a lot of pain. Do you think Dr. Lorris could help me?"

"I don't know. He's a GP, you know, not a bone and joint doctor."

"That's OK," said the voice. "I just need help with the pain, until I can get the hip taken care of. I'm in a lot of discomfort. Do you think he can see me?"

"Sure, I guess so. Do you want an appointment?"

"No, I'll just stop by."

"Ok. He's not that busy today."

"Does it matter which pharmacy I use?"

"Not that I know of. It depends on your insurance."

"I'll be right over."

QUESTIONS FOR THOUGHT AND REFLECTION

1. What information did Brittany get from the caller? What information was missing?
2. What mistakes did Brittany make in this interaction?
3. Based on Brittany's behavior, how would you describe the kind of clinic she works at?

⭐ EXPERIENTIAL EXERCISES

1. Watch a local newscaster. Notice the animation in their voice and how that is achieved with facial expressions.
2. Put a mirror across from you the next time you answer the phone or talk on the phone. See if the way you speak on the phone is influenced by your facial expressions.
3. Record yourself taking a phone call. Play back the recording. What observations can you make about your voice and the messages carried along with it? How could you improve your phone voice?
4. Familiarize yourself with office policy regarding phone calls, including answering protocols, screening procedures, emergencies, and complaints.

🔄 CROSS CURRENTS WITH OTHER SOFT SKILLS

LISTENING ACTIVELY: Your main function on the phone is to listen (Chapter 8).

ADOPTING A POSITIVE MENTAL ATTITUDE: Your attitude is the foundation of your voice and your message (Chapter 2).

MODELING PROFESSIONAL BEHAVIOR: The principles of courtesy and professionalism should guide your phone presence (Chapter 13).

SPEAKING PROFESSIONALLY IN YOUR WORKPLACE: Speaking on the phone is an important part of your workplace speech. You want to convey warmth, caring, and helpfulness (Chapter 6).

Building Relationships

- Understand the Importance of Trust to Your Success in the Health Professions
- Develop a Strategy to Earn and Keep Trust in Your New Job
- Understand Why Empathy Is a Critical Trait in the Health Professions
- Describe an Empathic Organization
- Explain the Importance of Diversity in Health Care
- Understand the Differences Between Stereotypes, Prejudice, and Bias
- Understand and Practice Cultural Competence

Building Trust

The best way to find out if you can trust somebody is to trust them.

—Ernest Hemingway

LEARNING OBJECTIVE 1: BUILDING TRUST

- Understand how people learn to trust others.
- Know how to build trust among your co-workers.
- State the benefits of a trusting organization.
- Consider the advantages of forgiveness.
- Gain insight into how broken trust can be rebuilt.

Trust is important in any workplace, but especially in the health care field. Building trust involves respect, empathy, and listening skills, which require time and practice. In the following sections, we will discuss the building blocks of trust, how to instill trust in others, understand the nature of organizational trust, and know what to do when trust is broken.

JOURNALING 5.1

Because likability facilitates building trust, list the characteristics that make you likable. Explain how you can make these traits more obvious to people you meet.

The Building Blocks of Trust

Most people do not listen with the intent to understand; they listen with the intent to reply.

—Stephen R. Covey

Listening

Listening is a key skill in establishing trust and building relationships. It fosters rapport and mutual respect. When people can express their thoughts fully, they feel valued, respected, and empowered. They know they will be able to get their views across without being interrupted. Feeling heard and understood, they will likely be more willing to listen to others, as well.

At work, listening to your supervisor, co-workers, and staff will also help you gather feedback and understand others' ideas and opinions about an issue. It will help you build trust in your work relationships as you learn more about the people you work with through meaningful dialogue. If you do not understand someone's comment, ask clarifying questions. If you would like to learn more about someone's idea, ask a question about it. Questions serve to draw out information, create mutual understanding, and help drive a conversation forward.

When conversing with your co-workers, avoid interrupting or talking over them. Listen fully to what each person says, considering the meaning of the words, rather than simply thinking about what you will say when your turn comes. To know when it is your turn to speak in a conversation, wait for breaks or pauses. However, try to gauge whether a pause indicates that a person is done speaking or simply taking a rest while they try to find the right words or take a breath. If the person is done speaking, the person most likely will make eye contact with you to indicate it is your turn to speak.

Practice active listening. Try to listen without interpreting. Let your body language communicate your engagement in the conversation by making eye contact, nodding, smiling, and maintaining open posture. If you become distracted or feel your mind wandering, try to direct your attention back to the speaker by taking notes or mentally (and silently) summarizing what the speaker said in your own words. You can use the latter to provide feedback to the speaker once the person is done.

As soon as you trust yourself, you will know how to live.

—Goethe

Respect

Another building block of trust is respect. As discussed, listening is one way to demonstrate respect. In addition, take an interest in the experience and well-being of others. Remember that small efforts make a big difference: greet people and use their names, ask about family they have mentioned before, offer to help, say "thank you" when others offer you help, pay sincere compliments. Be considerate of your co-workers by keeping your workspace neat and watching the volume of your conversations. When you demonstrate this kind of interest, openness, and consideration, people will perceive you as accepting, reasonable, and kind.

Show your respect for your co-workers in the way you interact and collaborate with them to complete your work. Recognize others' contributions, respond in a timely manner, do your fair share, participate, and follow through on your commitments. In addition, honor differences and diversity. We will discuss multicultural competence and the benefits of diversity more later, but part of respecting your co-workers is treating them fairly and without bias while valuing their uniqueness.

Showing respect is particularly important to maintaining positive relationships in the workplace, as there is likely a greater degree of hierarchy than in other areas of life and less freedom to make decisions for oneself. In this context, allowing people to express their thoughts, taking their ideas seriously, and incorporating their feedback and ideas when possible can contribute to a greater sense of agency and autonomy for workers and increase job satisfaction.

As a manager, you can demonstrate respect by ensuring that co-workers and direct reports understand new policies or procedures, allowing them time to ask questions. In any role, avoid insulting people or talking behind their backs, dismissing others' views, nitpicking, demeaning, or micromanaging. Showing people that you value their input and regard their work highly enough to give them freedom to make decisions on their own is a form of respect.

Respect in the workplace should always extend to your patients (Figure. 5.1). As a health care professional, you should try to express genuine interest in your patients. This interaction displays the trust that you should work to achieve with every patient.

R-E-S-P-E-C-T. Find out what it means to me.

—Aretha Franklin

Empathy

The final building block of trust is empathy, which we will explore in greater depth later in this chapter. Empathy is the capacity to recognize and understand another's situation or feelings as if they were our own.

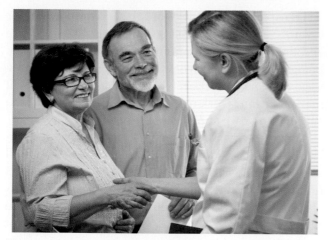

Figure 5.1 Health care professionals should always show respect to patients. (Copyright © istock.com.)

That is, it refers to the ability to put yourself in someone else's shoes, so to speak. When we empathize with another person's situation, we often rely on our experience with a similar situation, which enables us to relate to what that person is feeling or dealing with.

Empathy differs from sympathy. Whereas the former denotes an ability to imagine the other person's feelings based on your experiences or what you know about that person, the latter describes sharing a person's feelings. Sympathy refers to the ability to take part in someone else's feelings; for instance, if a childhood friend's mother passes away, you would likely share in their sorrow. It can also be an emotional or intellectual agreement with people's tastes, opinions, or attitudes. Empathy concerns the ability to identify with or understand another's feelings or experiences.

As a health care professional, you will need both sympathy and empathy to succeed in your work. For example, you may offer your sympathy to a patient who receives a terminal diagnosis or to the family of a critically injured patient. Empathy will enable you to understand what your patients and their loved ones experience and provide them with the quality care they need.

JOURNALING 5.2

Consider the idiom "to put oneself in another's shoes." Reflect on a time in your life when you did that, and record the example in your journal. How do you think your ability to understand another person's feelings affected your relationship with that person? If you have never done so, try to do it now. How does it change your perspective about that person?

Being honest may not get you a lot of friends, but it'll always get you the right ones.

—John Lennon

BOX 5.1

Behaviors That Build Trust

- Be on time all the time. No exceptions!
- Be friendly. Greet people you encounter. Make eye contact.
- Remember the names of the people you are introduced to.
- Ask for help and advice.
- Keep your elevator speech—a standard, short, and interesting introduction—at the tip of your tongue.
- Dress professionally and be well groomed at all times.
- Observe business etiquette and culture so that you will be in sync at your workplace.
- Complete all your tasks professionally.
- Pitch in when there is work to be done.
- Show kindness toward patients and clients in all your interactions with them.
- Display a positive attitude.

Developing Trust in Others

Earning trust takes a long time. Trust is a founding principle that shapes a relationship between two people. It builds the foundation for a better working relationship and directly affects things like productivity, communication, job performance, and the overall outlook a person has toward the employer and profession.

To build trust, it requires honesty, competence, transparency, and good communication. You will have to demonstrate all these qualities and behaviors consistently to build trust with your co-workers, employer, and patients. Follow the tips in Box 5.1 to start building trust.

Communicate

Communicate clearly, ask and answer questions honestly, and seek help when you need it. Asking for help can function as a strong relationship builder (Figure. 5.2). In fact, research suggests that people tend to like those for whom they have done a favor, a phenomenon known as the Ben Franklin effect.[1]

---

[1] While serving in the Pennsylvania legislature, Franklin asked a rival legislator if he could borrow a rare book from his personal library. The man agreed. Franklin returned the book to him about a week later, along with a thank you note, and thereafter observed a shift in the man's demeanor toward him. His former rival now approached and spoke to him for the first time, and the two men remained friends for the remainder of his life.

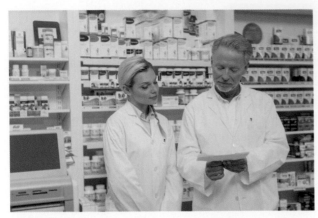

Figure 5.2 New employees can learn about job duties and build positive work relationships by communicating with co-workers. (Copyright © istock.com.)

Asking for help is not a sign of weakness or lack of intelligence. When you ask for help, you receive assistance for your immediate problem but also strengthen your relationship with your co-workers. Health care professionals are usually eager to share their expertise when asked, and the time you spend with your new co-workers may help you build trust and rapport.

As a new team member and beginning to comprehend your new role and interact with a lot of new people, focus first on observing, helping, and executing your job correctly. Always clarify expectations. Never make assumptions or walk away from a conversation with only a vague understanding of what your supervisor or co-workers expect you to do. Communicate clearly to avoid misunderstanding and refrain from offering strong opinions until you have formed relationships with your new co-workers. Do not be afraid to ask questions. Otherwise, you may be bound to make an error.

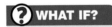 **WHAT IF?**

What if someone does not remember your name? How will you be able to tell? How can you tactfully remind them of your name?

Being Transparent

Transparency is the practice of being open and honest with others, no matter how challenging it might be. Being transparent in the workplace simply means operating in a way that creates openness and develops trust between people. Being transparent should not just be between co-workers but also between supervisors and employees and the facility and patients.

Transparency in the workplace is important for several reasons. Transparency means that you are encouraging clear communication and collaboration. Being transparent at work allows you to get to know your co-workers better, which creates trust and will make the team work more efficient knowing that you support and care about one another.

Transparency allows people to better communicate their ideas and opinions more freely. They will feel more open to discussing their strengths and areas of improvement. When your employer and co-workers know they can trust you, you will be given more responsibility and be seen as an integral member of the health care team.

Consistently using and improving your skills will demonstrate your reliability. As you gain proficiency, remaining open and transparent about your challenges and weaknesses will foster trust with your co-workers and supervisor.

Over time, as you become more familiar with routines and procedures, you will overcome the "learning curve" that accompanies new jobs. You will find yourself improving and developing a sense of where your skills are most needed. As your performance naturally evolves, you can start to contribute your ideas and experiences. Your transparency about benefiting from your co-workers' help may also encourage your co-workers to trust and depend on you as your skills continue to grow.

Strive for transparency in your actions, as well. Say what you mean, and ensure that whatever you say about someone when they are not there is the same as what you would say to their face. If you speak negatively about someone, your co-workers may wonder what you say about *them* when they are not around. The best course of action is to try to say only positive things about your co-workers, knowing that your comments could get back to them.

Accountability

Accountability at work is accomplishing your goals and responsibilities and taking responsibility for your actions. Set goals for yourself that are clear and measurable so everyone, including you, knows what you are trying to achieve. Once you understand your goals and expectations, you can bridge the gap between what you are actually doing and what you are supposed to be doing.

Patients and co-workers alike award their trust to employees who tackle problems and address difficult issues when they arise. Strive to do what you say you will do. Hold yourself accountable when you fail. Accountability establishes expectations, boundaries, safety, and trust. Finally, demonstrate your own accountability by making commitments and consistently keeping them. Over time, your impeccable track record will inspire trust.

Organizational Trust

Few things help an individual more than to place responsibility upon him and to let him know that you trust him.

—Booker T. Washington

Trust is all about relationships. Each role is interrelated, and co-workers must be able to trust each other to get their jobs done. In a workplace setting, organizational trust is essential. Organizational trust is employees' belief in the company's conduct. This can involve faith in management or team members, and it may include the company's goal, vision, culture, ethics, equality, diversity, and inclusion.

While interpersonal trust is important, or trust between individuals or teams, the importance of organizational trust should not be overlooked. Employers cannot achieve their mission and goals without establishing a foundation of trust. For example, employers must have trust that employees will do their work and meet their responsibilities based on the deadline.

In an atmosphere of trust, people share information and accept mistakes, because they acknowledge that mistakes are necessary steps on the path to learning and for professional and personal development. People are loyal and support one another. The environment fosters creativity, innovation, and workflow improvements. Co-workers, who are able to trust one another, regularly demonstrate a high degree of productivity and good morale (Figure. 5.3).

In contrast, a low-trust environment can breed divisiveness, poor morale, and increased turnover. Further, patients may leave after experiencing that kind of

TABLE 5.1

Characteristics of Organizations That Trust and Those That Do Not Trust

Trusting Organizations	Organizations Without Trust
Information is shared	Information is withheld
People support one another	People look out for themselves
Teams	Cliques
Communication	Gossip
Autonomy	Micromanagement
Innovation	Bureaucracy
Fun place to work	Low morale
Longevity, experience	Turnover
Satisfied customers	Customer turnover

environment. After all, why would patients trust health care workers if those workers do not trust each other? Table 5.1 compares the characteristics of trusting organizations and organizations where trust is lacking.

Trust is the lubrication that makes it possible for organizations to work.

—Warren Bennis

When Trust Is Broken

Our distrust is very expensive.

—Ralph Waldo Emerson

Trust is fragile. It takes a long time to build it, but it can be broken in seconds. Once broken, trust can take even longer to rebuild.

If you break someone's trust, two things can help you repair the damage. First, apologize. You must genuinely acknowledge your offending behavior or action and understand the effect it had on the other person. Second, commit to a new course of action. You will have to start all over to rebuild trust slowly, but with effort and consistency, you should be able to redeem yourself in time.

What if a co-worker betrays your trust? Though it may be tempting to lash out emotionally, it is best to control this urge. Saying nothing is sometimes the wisest course. After all, everyone slips up now and then, and we usually feel bad enough without being reminded of our errors. However, if the error is significant, and you feel it is more constructive to say something, it might be appropriate to calmly address your co-worker. Make your feedback easier to deliver by first calling attention to your co-worker's strengths.

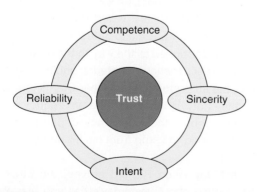

Figure 5.3 Important aspects of trust.

For example, you might say, "You are usually such a great team player, Anna. I was just really surprised by the way you acted."

Whether you address the situation or not, give yourself a little time to heal before attempting to mend the relationship. It is best to forgive a co-worker even if they do not ask for your forgiveness. We all make mistakes. Forgiveness means letting go of resentment and bitterness, not forgetting. Although you may remember the incident, you are no longer emotionally affected by it. Forgive, move on, and leave the door open to repair the relationship. After all, you likely must continue working with this person.

Like a broken bone, broken trust will take time to heal. Even after everyone involved forgives, the relationship may be irrevocably changed. For this reason, you should do your best to respect and protect the trust that grows between you and your co-workers. However, if something does happen to threaten that delicate trust, aim to understand how the incident happened in the first place, so you can learn how to address the issue and avoid similar instances in the future.

The weak can never forgive.

Forgiveness is the attribute of the strong.

—Mahatma Gandhi

 JOURNALING 5.3

Reflect on a time when you betrayed someone's trust. Imagine how the other person felt. Did they forgive you? Did you redeem yourself? Where does the relationship stand today, and why is it the way it is?

CASE STUDY 5.1
Trust Me

Richard Brecht was not a typical student. He had struggled through high school and worked a series of odd jobs since graduating. After several years stuck in a rut, Richard decided he needed to start over. He packed up his Jeep and drove to Flagstaff, because he had heard the area had a shortage of EMTs. The training was even subsidized by the county. Richard signed up for an EMT program and worked at a nursing home to support himself while attending school.

Richard's EMT-Basic class was a diverse group. At 40 years old, Richard was among the oldest in his class. Richard felt out of place at first, but once the training began, he started to think that being an EMT was going to be a great fit for him. He felt a sense of direction for the first time in his career.

A local company hired Richard once he completed his training. The company put Richard with a different crew every few days, so he could get to know the other employees. He asked everyone he met the same questions. How long did it take them to feel comfortable with the job? What did they like about the company? What was their background? His co-workers were generally very open and willing to answer his questions. Richard heard many stories about memorable runs and imagined what he might have done if he were faced with the same situations, so he could try to learn from their experience. He kept a notebook to write down everything he learned.

One day, the company installed new HeartStart defibrillators on each unit. Everybody received training on the new defibrillators, but some of the EMTs complained about always having to get used to new equipment. Rather than complaining, Richard picked up a copy of the training manual and watched several training videos to familiarize himself with all the defibrillator's functions.

A few days later, Richard's efforts paid off. His unit got a call from a woman whose infant son was not breathing and was turning blue. His crew started performing heart compressions as they carried the infant to the ambulance. The team was unable to find a heartbeat, so Richard prepared the defibrillator. "Here," said Richard. "We need to turn the infant key."

"Are we ready?" one of Richard's teammates, Rachel, asked as she grabbed the paddles.

Richard nodded. "Clear!" yelled Rachel. She shocked the infant twice and was able to detect a feeble heartbeat. The heartbeat continued all the way to the medical center, but it was erratic. Richard located a cable to attach his iPhone to the strip stored in the HeartStart's memory. As soon as they got the infant into the emergency room, he worked with one of the emergency department technicians to download the strip from his iPhone to their main system.

The next day when Richard arrived, the other EMTs were all chatting about yesterday's call and his excellent

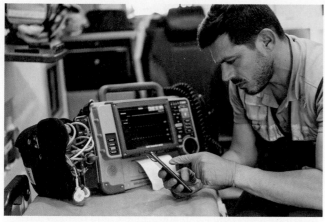
iStock.com/Raul Navarro/1394594870

downloaded the sinus rhythm strip. He was happy to be able to answer their questions for a change.

"Lucky to have you aboard," said Art, the crew chief.

Ms. Carmichael, the vice president of operations, asked Richard to develop a more in-depth training course for the defibrillator.

QUESTIONS FOR THOUGHT AND REFLECTION

1. What listening skills did Richard demonstrate?
2. List the trust-building efforts that Richard made throughout this story.
3. How did Richard manage to demonstrate his clinical skills, even though he was new to the profession and the company?

performance and teamwork. Richard explained the infant key to the rest of his team and explained how he

A Different Path

Will Davis had been working at the Arcadia State Hospital for more than 40 years. He had seen huge changes in the care of the mentally ill, but he thought his job as a mental health worker was more dangerous now than it had ever been. Long ago, patients had few rights. Many were committed by courts. Restraints and seclusion rooms were common responses to patients who were aggressive or suicidal.

Now, the least dangerous patients have been moved out of the state hospitals and into the community in halfway houses and group homes. Many are cared for by their families, but a large percentage of mentally ill people who used to receive treatment in state-supported psychiatric hospitals ended up being homeless. It seemed to Will that only the most dangerous patients remained. Mental health workers have to think on their feet to manage patients, and assaults are common. "A lot of people I've worked with over the years live on disability," he told a group of new employees. He was teaching a class on restraints and self-defense, and he wanted them to understand how important these skills would be to them.

One of the six new employees, Keith Cummings, was assigned to the unit where Will worked. Will was paying special attention to him, because he had a few concerns about Keith. For one thing, Keith did not maintain eye contact with Will.

"You have to be on the same team as your fellow staff members and have good communication at all times," Will said to the new employees. Will demonstrated all the physical techniques. Having the new staff members stand in as patients, Will taught them how to protect themselves and other patients against assaults. They learned how to safely restrain a patient, getting the patient to the floor and immobilizing all the limbs. "It takes four people to carry a patient, so nobody gets hurt," he explained. "You carry the patient face down," he said as he demonstrated the skill. "The patient won't be as strong that way and won't feel as panicked."

Keith seemed tentative, even when Will showed him the techniques. "Grab the wrist and put your other hand on their shoulder. If the patient is still fighting with you, twist the wrist a little." Will told them that if they worked as a team, built their skills, and learned to trust one another, they could minimize the chances of getting hurt or injuring a patient. "Everything we do here," he declared, "is in the interest of the patient."

One week after orientation, Keith showed up for his first shift with Will. Fortunately, the unit was going through a quiet time. The mix of patients did not appear too volatile, and the staff seem to have developed strong relationships even with the more dangerous patients. Keith had majored in psychology at Bates College, and he eventually hoped to become a psychologist. This looked like a difficult job, but he wanted to get some exposure to people who had severe mental illnesses; he hoped the experience would help him get accepted to graduate school in a year or two.

Keith introduced himself to the psychiatrists and residents and would try to discuss the patients. He wanted to understand the etiology of their illnesses, the dysfunctional parts of their brains, the treatment, and the prognosis.

At the end of the first week, there was a minor scuffle involving a new patient, Larry, which was quickly resolved. Will, Keith, and two other experienced staff members were on the scene. They lowered the patient to the carpet, keeping his arms and legs immobilized until he calmed down. Keith was confused about his responsibility as he moved around the patient nervous and unsure how to assist his co-workers. By the time Keith composed himself and felt ready to help, the patient was ready to be escorted to the day room.

Keith's poor performance confirmed Will's initial concerns. He took Keith out to the side yard to practice some of the moves. He was trying to be patient but got frustrated as he saw how little effort Keith put forward. "I don't think I like this part of the job," Keith told Will. "Nobody does," said Will, "but it's not optional. It's a critical skill for this work."

Everything stayed quiet for the next few weeks until a serious incident occurred. Will and Keith were by themselves with Lou, a burly patient with a persecution complex. Without warning, Lou attacked Will. Will shouted for help as the two crashed to the floor, Will covering himself against Lou's blows. He thought he saw Keith run to get help. After a few tense seconds, several staff members arrived to help Will, but Keith was not among them.

"Where'd that kid go?" said one of them, after Lou had been subdued.

"He called us for help, but that's the last we saw of him."

QUESTIONS FOR THOUGHT AND REFLECTION

1. Why did Will have little confidence or trust in Keith?
2. What interest did Keith show in learning his new job?
3. What do you think Keith should have done after the incident with Lou?
4. How do you think Keith could repair the damaged trust between himself and Will?

⭐ EXPERIENTIAL EXERCISES

1. Ask an acquaintance to do a favor for you. Note any changes you observe in your relationship after that.
2. The next time a friend talks to you about a problem they are having, think about ways to show sympathy or empathy. Note which seems like the better response in that instance. Why?
3. Make a trust chart. Using graph paper, list the important people in your life across the top. Color in the squares of the graph paper below each name to show your level of trust in each of the people. Consider how these levels of trust affect your relationships with these people.

CROSS CURRENTS WITH OTHER SOFT SKILLS

ADOPTING A POSITIVE ATTITUDE: A positive attitude is fundamental to forming trust (Chapter 3).
ACHIEVING HONESTY AND INTEGRITY: Consistently honest behavior helps build trust (Chapter 1).
STRIVING FOR TOLERANCE: Building trust means requires open-mindedness, which enables you to accept and respect others and learn from them (Chapter 7).
LISTENING ACTIVELY: Active listening is a key skill for building trust (Chapter 6).
CONTRIBUTING AS A MEMBER OF THE TEAM: Trust is a social enterprise (Chapter 13).

Demonstrating Empathy and Sensitivity

How far you go in life depends on your being tender with the young, compassionate with the aged, sympathetic with the striving and tolerant of the weak and the strong. Because someday in life you will have been all of these.

—George Washington Carver

LEARNING OBJECTIVE 2: SHOWING EMPATHY, CARING, AND COMPASSION

- Identify multiple ways of increasing and deepening your empathy.
- Understand the role of social intelligence in relationships.
- Explain mirroring and its effect on empathy.
- Describe the empathic organization.

When you start to develop your powers of empathy and imagination, the whole world opens up to you.

—Susan Sarandon

Empathy is the ability to recognize, understand, and share the thoughts and feelings of others. Developing empathy is crucial for establishing relationships and behaving compassionately. It involves experiencing another person's point of view, rather than just one's own. Empathy helps us cooperate with others, build friendships, make moral decisions, and intervene when we see others being bullied. In health care, we are in the business of alleviating worry and suffering, helping people to heal, and maximizing their wellness. Without empathy, these outcomes would be difficult to achieve.

Empathy enables us to establish rapport with another person, make them feel that they are being heard, and, through words and body language, mimic their emotions. Perspective-taking, or the empathic ability to assume the cognitive state of another person and see a problem through their eyes, can further cement a connection.

Developing Empathy

Health care professionals must have empathy. Fortunately, most people seeking careers in the health care field have a strong sense of empathy, but there is always room for improvement. Even though you may believe that empathy is an innate quality, whether you are born with it or not, it can be developed and increased in all of us.

We begin to show signs of empathy in infancy and the trait develops steadily through childhood and adolescence. Most people generally are likely to feel greater empathy for people like themselves and may feel less empathy for those outside their family, community, ethnicity, or race. However, people who spend more time with individuals different from themselves tend to adopt a more empathic outlook toward others. Other research finds that reading novels can help foster the ability to put ourselves in the minds of others.

As you recognize and increase your empathy, your work and your relationships will likely improve as a result. By understanding how empathy combines with other elements of emotional and social intelligence, you can pursue a number of strategies to become even more empathetic (Box 5.2).

Emotional intelligence and social intelligence are both important competencies for working in health care facilities. We defined and discussed emotional intelligence in Chapter 2. In the following sections, we will examine the related concept of social intelligence.

Social Intelligence

Social intelligence is a measure of interpersonal skill that describes the ability to have successful social interactions and build relationships. It is the capacity

---

BOX 5.2

Strategies for Becoming More Emotionally Aware

- Develop a plan to improve your active listening skills and practice this plan.
- Consciously search for the emotional content expressed by others.
- Reflect upon your own emotions in a quiet place.
- Observe body language and try to interpret nonverbal cues.
- Make eye contact and provide nonverbal feedback, such as smiling or nodding.
- Allow pauses and silences in conversations.
- Confirm your observation of others' emotions by using statements such as, "You seem disappointed" and "How did that make you feel?"
- Maintain a healthy sense of curiosity about other people.

BOX 5.3

Social Intelligence Skills

- Conversation skills, including verbal and nonverbal
- Knowledge of social rules and etiquette
- Listening skills
- Understanding how other people's emotions work
- Adapting to different social roles and environments
- Self-image and impression management

---

to know yourself and others and exercise appropriate emotional management. As we have learned, emotional intelligence comes from introspection and emotional awareness and the role of emotions in the problem-solving process. It has more to do with how people manage themselves before they make contact with another person. In contrast, social intelligence is something that develops once we start interacting with people and includes skills, such as expression, dialogue, listening, and learning through communication with others (Box 5.3).

There are five components in social intelligence, sometimes referred to as SPACE: Situational awareness, Presence, Authenticity, Clarity, and Empathy (Figure. 5.4). Situational awareness involves understanding the context of a situation and knowing how to act appropriately. People who lack situational

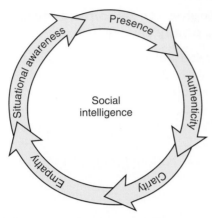

Figure 5.4 Components of social intelligence.

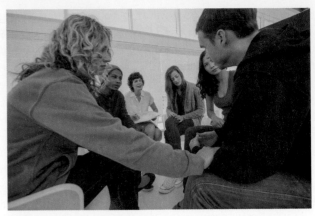

Figure 5.5 A therapist and group members console a distraught man. (Copyright © istock.com.)

awareness might have poor manners, for example. Presence describes your overall "bearing" or total impression you make on people through your behavior, body language, and charisma. Authenticity refers to how much others perceive that you act in accordance with your ethics and values. It involves the honesty of your behavior. Clarity represents the ability to express ideas clearly, effectively, and impactfully. Moreover, people who possess clarity will use a range of communication skills to convey their message, including listening, feedback, and metaphor. Finally, empathy, as we have seen, is more than just identifying with others. It involves building connections with people so that you understand how they feel.

Social intelligence is essential for unlocking the skills of effective communication, dialogue, and teamwork to create an optimal and productive work environment.

Developing a sense of empathy will help create a smooth work environment and ensure that patients feel cared for.

Active Listening

Listening actively involves a lot more than hearing and understanding words. It includes asking perceptive questions and then listening actively. While you are listening, notice the nonverbal communication that accompanies the speaker's words, such as their gestures, facial expressions, pauses, and tone. What can you tell about their emotions? How do they *feel* about what they are saying? What are they conveying that you want to ask about next? Showing interest in people is the first step in forming an empathetic relationship, followed up by your genuine curiosity about them as individuals. Withhold judgment; just

learn. Listening is one of the simplest and most effective ways to build empathy.

Compassion begins with attention.

—Daniel Goleman

Imagining Others

Have you ever identified with a character in a movie or a book? Of course, films and novels are constructed to maximize the audience's emotional response as they imagine what it must be like to be in a character's shoes. Use your empathetic skills to try to relate to a patient or a co-worker as if they were a character you are curious about, reflecting on what they say and paying attention to their emotional content (Figure. 5.5).

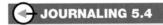
JOURNALING 5.4

List three of your behaviors you would like to change. Record when these negative behaviors occur, and consider how you can become more aware of them so you can change them more effectively.

Mirroring

One way we can connect and build rapport with others is to mirror their behavior. Mirroring is used to improve rapport with another person by imitating their nonverbal mannerisms and by reflecting their verbal style. Sometimes called *blending*, mirroring is not mimicking every movement or expression the other person makes but taking a clue from the person's communication style to bring yours into accordance with that person's to build rapport.

All of us can practice empathy by picking up on facial expressions, tone, gestures, or posture. We even have mirror neurons in the premotor cortex of our brains, the area responsible for planning actions. These cells fire automatically, helping us mirror each other's actions. We see this when babies mimic their parents' facial expressions, for example, or when we feel like yawning after seeing another person yawn. They help us "read" each other, laughing when others laugh, and wincing when we see violence. These neurons also help us learn by watching someone perform a skill. The existence and role of mirror neurons suggest that human beings are wired for social interaction and that empathy is a natural human response to that interaction.

Mirroring often communicates empathy, particularly with your patients. When you are in sync with their tone, gestures, and expressions, your patients will feel that you understand them better, and you will. For example, if a patient is expressive, animated, and uses the hands often to gesture, you may want to express the same behavior. Otherwise, the patient may find you cold, distant, and uninterested. Patients are looking for acceptance and comfort in an unfamiliar setting, where they may feel anxious and vulnerable. If you can successfully mirror a patient's body language, you will receive the patient's cooperation.

Organizational Empathy

Similar to organizational trust, organizational empathy is empathy embedded throughout an organization and a commitment to understanding and meeting customers' needs. In a health care organization, the customers are the patients or clients, and every one of them is looking for empathy, as a large part of their experience when they come to your facility. Knowing that, you should regard each interaction as an opportunity to gain insight into a patient's needs and deliver compassionate, effective service.

Put yourself in your patient's shoes. Try to figure out what is worrying them, whether they are feeling any pain or anxiety, or what kind of care the patient's family members expect from you. You will become a better health care professional when you can understand where your patients are coming from, what the health care experience is like for them, and what they most need from an interaction with you.

Keep in mind that you are likely not the only person at your facility or organization with whom the patient has interacted or will interact with. Understanding what each role or department does and how they interact with patients will help you not only meet patients' needs but also effectively collaborate with and support your co-workers. For instance, try to understand what your co-workers need from you in order to provide excellent care to patients. Different disciplines speak different languages or lingo, require different types of information, and have different ideas about how best to do things and what success looks like. Use empathy in all your interactions, and you will help your patients and contribute to the organization's mission.

Valuing Cultural Competence

It is not our differences that divide us. It is our inability to recognize, accept, and celebrate those differences.

—Audre Lorde

LEARNING OBJECTIVE 3: VALUING MULTICULTURAL COMPETENCE

- Define diversity and culture.
- Understand how culture affects your role in providing patient care.
- Explain the differences between stereotyping, prejudice, and bias.
- Identify the cultural competence needs of health care professionals.
- List several ways you can enhance your own cultural competence.

Diversity and Culture in the United States

The United States comprises many different cultures, and many Americans identify closely with their cultural backgrounds. Although it is a very broad concept, culture can be defined as the act of belonging to a designated group or community which shares common experiences that shape the way its members understand the world. Cultural practice and norms are often learned, shared, and passed on through generations. It may include groups that a person is born into, such as race, national origin, gender, class, or religion. It may also include groups the person joins or becomes part of, such as acquiring a new culture by moving to a new country or changes in their economic status. As a result, every person belongs to and is influenced by and is a part of many types of cultures.

Culture is a strong part of people's lives. It influences our views, our values, our humor, our hopes, our loyalties, and our fears. Culture helps guide our thinking, decision-making, and actions. Culture provides security and reassurance. All humans have a great need to feel connected and bonded with other people. When bonds are weak and we do not feel connected or safe, it affects our health and wellness.

Culture also affects our interpersonal relationships, including marriages, communication patterns, and sexual habits. Even the concept of time, display of emotion, and speech patterns such as loudness and

BOX 5.4

Examples of Cultural Influences

- Eating habits
- Language
- Dress
- Hobbies
- Living patterns
- Occupation choices
- Education
- Religious affiliations
- Political view

speed of delivery are influenced by culture. No aspect of our lives is free from cultural influence. As a result, our culture is expressed daily in many different ways (Box 5.4).

The United States is rich in cultures that include ethnic customs, traditions, languages, and religions. No matter where you live or who you are, every person you will be working with and establishing relationships with will be from many different cultures. It will be important to remember that many people may view the world differently than you do because of their culture.

In order to build communities that are successful at improving conditions and resolving problems, we need to understand and appreciate many cultures, establish relationships with people from cultures other than our own, and build strong alliances with different cultural groups. This is particularly true in health care since you will need to successfully interact with patients, family members, and co-workers from many different cultures.

JOURNALING 5.6

Describe your heritage. What do you know about it? How can an understanding of your cultural identity help you gain perspective and acceptance from people of different cultures?

Benefits of Diversity

With increased diversity comes increased opportunity. In a shrinking world, where transportation is fast and communication is instantaneous, exposure to diverse cultures helps make us better world citizens and better workers. For instance, research has demonstrated that diverse groups tend to be more creative and innovative than homogenous ones. Having a more diverse talent pool also increases productivity and the value of goods and services produced, helping fuel overall economic growth.

Perspective and Experiences

Having co-workers who represent many different cultures and backgrounds gives us much more experience to draw from in solving problems or coming up with innovative solutions. We will make better decisions and be more inclusive in our thinking. In fact, researchers have found that when we hear ideas or perspectives from people who are different from us, we tend to perceive them as more novel and give them greater consideration than we would if someone more similar to us had expressed them.

One reason for this is that we tend to believe that people who are similar share the same information and hold the same views as we do. Working with people from a variety of cultures exposes us to diverse perspectives and views and helps build empathy, making us more effective as health care professionals.

Performance and Innovation

As noted previously, when groups are more diverse, they often outperform groups made up of people who are more similar. In organizations focused on innovation, for instance, female representation in top management positions is often associated with increased financial gains.

Similarly, racial diversity contributes to greater financial performance in innovation-focused companies. When greater social and cultural diversity exists in an organization or group, individuals are more likely to anticipate differences of opinion and perspective, which makes people work harder to express their views clearly, remain open-minded, and come to a consensus. Overall, diversity contributes to enhanced performance and innovation.

Pluralism

Pluralism describes a system in which different races, ethnicities, religions, and social groups maintain and develop their respective cultures within a common society, and diversity is regarded as a social good. In the workplace, pluralism can mean not only respect for diverse employees but also active engagement with and inclusion of a range of work styles, perspectives, and ideas. These diverse interests may be represented through collective bargaining, trade unions, and public policies, or less formally through responsive management practices that incorporate employees' perspectives in their decision-making.

In health care settings, pluralism can be defined as the use of both conventional medical practices and complementary or alternative medicine, health services, and practices. Most facilities in the United States practice conventional, Western medicine, and there are standard practices that must be followed in hospitals and health facilities, such as sterilization procedures and protocols for infection control. However, alternative medicine and traditional healing practices are becoming more widely accepted. For instance, acupuncture has increased in popularity in the United States in recent years. Whether or not you work in a facility with a variety of treatment modalities, the patients you care for may seek various types of health services beyond those provided by your facility. Additionally, patients' religious beliefs and cultural practices may affect their preferences regarding health services and treatments, and as a health care practitioner, you must respect their views and wishes.

Diversity is about all of us, and about us having to figure out how to walk through this world together.
—Jacqueline Woodson

Understanding Intolerance and Discrimination

Although culture influences a large part of our lives, its effects are often unconscious. As a result, perceptions of culture can be based on past experiences and ideas passed from generations and family structures. This can result in some people's difficulty in embracing diversity and other people's culture, potentially resulting in issues in the workplace and when interacting with other people.

Stereotyping

A stereotype is a preconceived notion or oversimplified opinion about a group of people. Stereotyping often serves as a mental shortcut that enables people to classify others. One advantage of stereotypes is that they simplify our social world, enabling us to respond quickly to situations that we have experienced or heard of before (Griffin et al. 2007). Stereotypes categorize certain attributes, characteristics, and behaviors as typical for members of a particular group of people. This is usually done by categorizing social groups based on visible features,

such as ethnicity, gender, age, and religion. In an evo-
lutionary sense, the ability to stereotype could have
life-or-death consequences: If you saw a lion attack
your cousin, for example, you would likely keep
your distance from lions and potentially save yourself from a future attack, or you may have learned
to identify which plants are poisonous based on
the shape or color of their leaves. However, stereotyping has serious disadvantages in modern society. Stereotypes may make us overlook distinctions
between individuals or make false generalizations
about people based on their group membership.

Although members of a group may share traits or
characteristics with other members of a group, it does
not mean that any given individual will have any or
all those traits. Even stereotypes that seem positive on
the surface can nevertheless have negative effects on
individuals. For instance, the stereotype that Asians
are good at math can place undue pressure on Asian
Americans, pigeonhole them into certain academic
subjects or career fields, and make them feel deper-
sonalized and devalued as individuals. In health care,
studies have shown that racial stereotyping may exist
in assessing pain in Black Americans versus White
patients, which may affect the kind of treatment each
group receives.

As stereotypes are based on impressions, opinions,
misconceptions, myths, rumors, prejudices, and fears,
they can be inaccurate or limiting at best and prejudicial or damaging at worst. Although members of a
group may share traits or characteristics with other
members of a group, it does not mean that any given
individual will have any or all of those traits. Overall,
stereotypes do little good in a modern, information-
age society. You will be a better health care professional if you learn to combat any stereotypes you have
and greet each person you meet as an individual, not
merely a representative of a social group.

*It is never too late to give up our prejudices. No way
of thinking or doing, however ancient, can be trusted
without proof.*

—Henry David Thoreau

Prejudice and Bias

While a stereotype is a thought about a person or group
of people, a prejudice relates to feelings and attitudes
about that person or group of people. Prejudices are
opinions, feelings, or ideas that are based on personal
perception and not on reason or facts. It can be based
on a number of factors, including age, race, sex, sexu-
ality, gender expression, nationality, religion, socioeconomic status, or even appearance. Prejudices are

often rooted in the idea that certain types of people are
worth less or are less capable than others.

While prejudice is not necessarily specific to race,
racism is a stronger type of prejudice used to justify
the belief that one racial category is somehow superior
or inferior to others; it is also a set of practices used by
a racial majority to disadvantage a racial minority.

Similar to prejudice, a bias denotes a preference for
a certain group, concept, or set of things. Biases may
be held by an individual, group, or institution and can
have negative or positive consequences. However,
even seemingly positive or neutral biases often have
negative consequences and can lead to inequality and
discrimination.

The key distinction between bias and prejudice is
that bias denotes a preference for a certain group, concept, or set of things, whereas prejudice is more about
judging individuals based on their group membership. For instance, our society has a *bias* toward right-
handed people and against left-handed people; most
desks, spiral notebooks, and tools are designed with
right-handed people in mind. In contrast, an example
of *prejudice* against left-handed people would be judging an individual as more likely to engage in crimi-
nality simply because they are left-handed, based on
the belief that left-handed people are more prone to
criminal behavior.

As an example of how stereotypes, bias, prejudice,
and discrimination can work together in a negative
feedback loop, consider gender roles and gendered
characteristics. Our society holds certain ideas about
what constitutes appropriate behavior for men and
women, such as the stereotype that women are more
nurturing and supportive than men and that men
are more assertive and dominant, and thus are more
natural leaders. This stereotype can lead to bias. For
instance, based on these gendered ideas, people may
show a preference for men who demonstrate stereo-
typically male traits and women who embody ste-
reotypically female characteristics. In an often cited
Harvard Business School experiment, a professor
gave one half of his class a case study about a successful entrepreneur and venture capitalist named Heidi
Roizen, who is outgoing and maintains an extensive
personal and professional network, which she lever-
ages to benefit both herself and others. He gave the
other half of the class an identical case study but
changed the name from Heidi to Howard. The students rated Howard as a more appealing colleague,
whereas they viewed Heidi as selfish and not the kind
of person they would want to hire or work for. The
only difference between Heidi and Howard in this
experiment was gender. This example illustrates how

gender stereotypes can lead to bias and prejudice and even discrimination.

While prejudice refers to biased thinking, discrimination consists of actions against a group of people. Discrimination can be based on age, religion, health, and other indicators. Discrimination based on race or ethnicity can take many forms, from unfair housing practices to biased hiring systems.

Conscious and Unconscious Bias

The two main types of biases are conscious bias (also known as explicit bias) and unconscious bias (also known as implicit bias). In the case of an explicit or conscious bias, the person is very clear about their feelings and attitudes, and related behaviors are conducted with intent. We know we are being biased toward a particular person or group.

Conscious bias in its extreme is characterized by overt negative behavior that can be expressed through physical and verbal harassment or through more subtle means such as exclusion. For example, an employer only wants to hire men and not women or only people under 40 years of age. These are all dangerous biases. Most people understand that there is no place for this in the modern workplace. In fact, there are many laws and policies that exist to prevent prejudice based on race, age, gender, gender identity, physical abilities, religion, sexual orientation, and many other characteristics. Violations of these laws and policies may result in disciplinary action, termination of employment, and even being charged with a criminal offense.

Unconscious biases are social stereotypes about certain groups of people that individuals form outside their own conscious awareness. Everyone holds unconscious beliefs about various social and identity groups, and these biases stem from one's tendency to organize social worlds by categorizing.

Unconscious bias can occur when we need to make decisions and judgments. We are not always making conscious decisions which are well thought through, taking all factors into account. Our brains work quickly so they access information which is known and familiar to us first. This information is based on our personal experiences, meaning there is a natural bias toward views and opinions which fit with the worldview we are most familiar and comfortable with. By doing this unconsciously, there is no malicious intent; we are often unaware that we have done it, and of its impact and implications. Unconscious bias clouds and undermines decisions. Unconscious bias holds on to stereotypes and will disregard anyone who fits into these groups.

Unconscious bias is far more prevalent than conscious prejudice and often incompatible with one's conscious values. Certain scenarios can activate unconscious attitudes and beliefs. For example, biases may be more prevalent when multitasking or working under time pressure.

It is important to note that biases, conscious or unconscious, are not limited to ethnicity and race. Though racial bias and discrimination are well documented, biases may exist toward any social group. One's age, gender, gender identity, physical abilities, religion, sexual orientation, weight, and many other characteristics are subject to bias.

Whether recognized or not, bias and prejudice can substantially undermine multicultural acceptance and tolerance in the workplace. Confronting our own biases and prejudice is a great first step toward building multicultural competence. Box 5.5 lists important strategies for addressing unconscious biases.

← JOURNALING 5.7

What cultural groups are predominant in your community? What do you know about these groups? What would you like to learn?

Workplace Diversity

Workplace diversity refers to the differences among people who interact with one another at work or in an organization. As the United States becomes more diverse, this will impact how employers address diversity in the workplace, including recruiting and hiring new employees.

Workplace diversity not only includes how individuals identify themselves but also how others perceive them. Diversity within a workplace encompasses race, gender, ethnic groups, age, religion,

BOX 5.5

Strategies to Address Unconscious Bias

- Promote self-awareness by first recognizing one's own biases.
- Understand the nature of bias.
- Take opportunities to have discussions about bias in a safe space with others, especially from different cultural groups.
- Attend facilitated discussions and training sessions on recognizing and unlearning unconscious biases.

BOX 5.6

Benefits of Workplace Diversity

- Improves creativity with new ideas and innovation
- Improves productivity and profits by increasing local knowledge
- Improves employee engagement and employee retention
- Increases the range of skills and knowledge
- Expands the talent pool and attracts more candidates

sexual orientation, citizenship status, military service, and mental and physical conditions, as well as other distinct differences between people.

There are many benefits to having a diverse workplace (Box 5.6). Employers that commit to recruiting a diverse workforce have a larger pool of applicants to choose from, which can lead to finding more qualified candidates and reducing the time it takes to fill vacant positions. Employers who do not recruit from diverse talent pools run the risk of missing out on qualified candidates and may have a more difficult time filling key roles, which increases recruitment costs.

? WHAT IF?

What if you felt pressure from a group you identify with to share the group's bias against another group? What could you do to resist?

Cultural Competence in Health Care

Each interaction with a patient will have cultural implications. As a result, it is important for all health care professionals to have a cultural awareness and awareness of their own unconscious bias, and how it impacts patients. For example, many health care professionals were taught that their personal backgrounds and the characteristics of their patients should be excluded from clinical decisions and that the type of patient care should not be different. But health care professionals are just as susceptible to unconscious bias as workers in any industry. Many non-health factors influence medical decisions and patient care, including a patient's style of dress, race, ethnicity, gender, insurance status, employment status, and the

clinical setting. Evidence shows that medical conclusions can be based just as much on who a person is as on the symptoms they present.

When health care professionals ignore or deny cultural differences, patient care suffers, resulting in the loss of trust and respect. Patients and family members who lack a sense of trust or respect from their health care professionals will not follow treatment regimens, resulting in poor health outcomes.

To prevent discrimination and unconscious biases in health care, it is important to build skills to ensure the quality and equality of patient care and patient interactions. These skills are often called cultural competence, which is the ability to meet the health care needs of patients while meeting and adhering to their cultural values, beliefs, and practices. It requires sensitivity to the patient's needs and wants and a deep understanding of their views and values. For health care professionals, it involves respecting patients' health beliefs and practices and accommodating their cultural and linguistic needs in the services provided. Every future and current health care professional should be able to interact effectively with people from a wide range of cultures while recognizing the cultural context of the community in which you are working.

You can increase your cultural competence by learning about cultural groups different from your own. Read books, ask questions, and attend diversity and tolerance workshops to raise your cultural intelligence. Take care, however, not to place the burden of your multicultural learning on cultural minorities. It is not others' responsibility to teach you about their culture. Thus, when asking questions, remember to be respectful and not overwhelm people with too many questions, especially those that could be answered by a little research on your own. Box 5.7 lists some helpful skills-building strategies for cultural competency.

For a health care organization to create truly welcoming and accepting environments for all cultures and people, everyone must embrace cultural diversity as core to the mission of the organization (Figure. 5.6).

← JOURNALING 5.8

Think about a co-worker who you had a bad first impression of but now get along with. What did you not like about them? Was it based on any biases? If so, how did you overcome it to now become good colleagues?

Skills Building for Cultural Competency

- Learn to correctly pronounce the names of co-workers and patients from other cultures.
- Introduce yourself and explain your role.
- Explain what patients can expect, because they are likely to be uncertain about what to do.
- Recognize that direct and prolonged eye contact may be offensive in some cultures.
- Be sensitive to personal space and touching, which varies by culture.
- Teach important American cultural concepts, like punctuality, directness, informality, and equality of gender, age, and social class.
- Pay more respect than usual to older people, who are highly valued in many cultures.
- Define medical terms, which may be a mystery to patients whose first language is not English.
- Learn to say "hello" and "thank you" in the languages of the people you serve.
- Be careful of gestures; they can mean different things in different cultures.
- Smiles are universal.

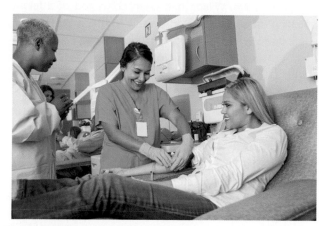

Figure 5.6 A young phlebotomy student draws blood. (Copyright © istock.com.)

CASE STUDY 5.2
Second Chances

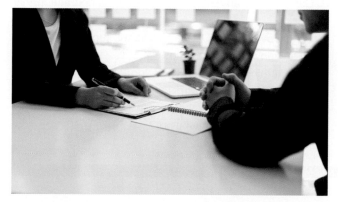

iStock.com/Wasan Tita/1359838986

Bill Wilson warned the hospital that his criminal background check would come back with bad news. He had served 8 years in state prison for drug trafficking. He had checked the box on the application that said, "Have you ever been convicted of a felony?" He had written in, "May I explain?"

"I did a stupid thing when I was a teenager," he told Georgia James, the Human Resources Director. "The strict Rockefeller drug laws were in effect then. I got caught with too much marijuana, but I never sold any. I have not taken any drugs now for over 10 years. I go to Narcotics Anonymous meetings, and I have a sponsor. I also sponsor others, and I volunteer in drug treatment centers. I paid for what I did and I'm still paying every day. Most people won't hire me because I have a felony conviction. I always wanted to be a lawyer, but my conviction made it unlikely that I would ever be allowed to sit for the bar examination. When I was in prison, I learned how to be a medic, and, when I got out, I got my degree in Respiratory Therapy. I understand how people feel, but I'm a good person and I'm good at my job. Will you give me a chance?"

Georgia said, "Let's see what the background report shows, and I'll get back to you."

Bill nodded, rose, and shook her hand. "Thank you for your consideration."

Outside, he sighed. This has been the story of his life. The only jobs he could get were manual labor jobs. Maybe he should have learned one of the construction trades or how to drive a rig or heavy equipment.

Inside, Georgia arranged a meeting with the hiring manager, Philip Acosta, the Head of Respiratory Therapy, and Jim Mandeville, Chief of Pulmonary Medicine. The feedback they gave on their interviews with Bill was positive, and she needed to facilitate a hiring decision made with the full disclosure of Wilson's background.

At the meeting, Georgia disclosed what Bill had said and that his criminal background check would likely come back as positive. Wilson had been convicted of a felony, trafficking drugs, and served 8 years in Attica State Prison in upstate New York.

"Wow," said Philip. "Huh. Well, I guess that's it. Too bad. I kind of liked him."

"Well, I should point out that, although we are required to perform a criminal background check before we make an offer to new employees, there is nothing that says we can't hire the person, if we feel the circumstances warrant it."

"No, no. We can't have a drug trafficker working in a hospital. I think we all understand that," Dr. Mandeville replied.

Georgia proceeded carefully. "Let's just take a quick look at the report before we move forward," she said. "He said he had almost 6 ounces of marijuana in his possession. By law, that amount was automatically considered trafficking at the time. Mr. Wilson claims he never sold any drugs, but he has accepted his punishment and paid his debt to society."

"Well, that's most unfortunate for poor Mr. Wilson," said Dr. Mandeville, with a smile and wink at Philip. "But I don't think we should hire a marijuana smoker as a Respiratory Therapist. Do you, Philip?"

"That wouldn't seem to make a lot of sense, Jim. Is there anything else we should know, though, Georgia?"

Georgia then explained the circumstances as Bill Wilson related them. Georgia had also called the drug treatment center where Bill volunteered, and they offered a glowing recommendation for him.

"Look, Georgia," said Dr. Mandeville. "I'm sure we would all like to help Mr. Wilson. He seemed like a fine man before all this came up. But really, Georgia, a drug user? Have you ever known a *former* drug user? I mean, come on."

"Actually, there are millions."

Dr. Mandeville rolled his eyes.

"Like your friend, Dr. Barton," Georgia offered.

"Let's not get personal," said Dr. Mandeville, losing whatever good humor he was still trying to show. "Dr. Barton was under a lot of stress. His wife divorced him. He's an extraordinary man, one in a million. Do you know what he had to go through to get off the stuff? It cost him over $200,000 out of his own pocket." His voice was rising now. But then Philip spoke up. "I'm willing to give Wilson a chance, but under only one condition," he said.

"What, drug testing around the clock?" exclaimed Dr. Mandeville.

"No. I'll hire him if you agree to give him a chance to show that he can change like Dave Barton did."

That silenced Dr. Mandeville for a moment. "Barton didn't go to prison," he muttered, but he said nothing more because he knew that not everyone had David Barton's resources. Dr. Mandeville rose and went over to the window overlooking the river below. He said nothing for long enough that everyone was experiencing some discomfort. Georgia knew that the decision would now be based on the next words out of Dr. Mandeville's mouth.

"Yes," said Dr. Mandeville. "We should hire this man." He turned toward Philip. "He has my support."

"I'll let Mr. Wilson know that," Georgia replied.

QUESTIONS FOR THOUGHT AND REFLECTION

1. Do you think people with positive criminal backgrounds should be allowed to work in hospitals?
2. How did bias factor into this story?
3. Can you find any instances of personal courage in this story?
4. Do you believe that Dr. Mandeville will support Bill Wilson on the job? Why or why not?
5. Do you think that the HR department, Philip Acosta, or even Bill Wilson should disclose his past felony conviction to the staff members in the Respiratory Therapy Department? Why or why not?

A Different Path

Brent had been a laboratory technician for a few years before he got a new job at the state university's student health center. The first thing that surprised Brent was the diversity of students who sought health care at his new job. He was from a small farming town and went to school with very few African American and Hispanic people. He also previously worked in a suburban laboratory and rarely was exposed to such a diverse patient population. In addition to the patient population, the staff at the student health center was also very diverse, with different racial and ethnic backgrounds, such as Dr. Yee, one of the physicians, and Mr. Jayakumar, the pharmacist.

Brent was doing well with working with all of his co-workers, but he was having a harder time dealing with student patients. As a phlebotomist, he had to get very close to patients in order to find their arteries to get blood. Some patients were particularly difficult for Brent. For example, Africans and African Americans with very dark skin were hard, as he often had trouble finding their arteries. He learned to take some deep breaths and remain as patient as possible. He did not know why but he often found himself uncomfortable around African American men, and he hoped he could find their vessels quickly and get them out of a laboratory room as soon as possible. But he would be gentler and take his time with Asian women.

One day, a Muslim woman in a hijab arrived to have her blood drawn. Brent was apprehensive about taking blood from her. Was it okay to be touching this woman and asking her to reveal the lower half of her arm? Before he could speak, the patient asks, "Is it possible to have my blood drawn by a woman?"

"No," said Brent. "I'm the only tech here. You can come back on Monday, but I think your doctor wants these results before then."

"Yes, he does. It's all right. I have my husband's permission."

"Permission?" said Brent. That didn't sit well with him. "Well, I never had anyone dressed like you before. What do you want to do?"

"I can pull back the sleeve on my abaya," she said, "but I would like you to sterilize the site with one of these," she said, pulling a jar of damp pads from somewhere within her gown. "They don't have alcohol."

Brent rolled his eyes but used the nonalcoholic pad she offered once he got approval from the doctor.

Later that afternoon, Brent had a young Middle Eastern man as a patient. Just the appearance of this patient put Brent in a surly mood.

"You Muslim?" said Brent, startling the man, who nodded. "Any special procedures or rituals?" said Brent.

"No," said the man, confused, not sure if Brent was being hostile or sarcastic. Soon he knew.

"Do you have your wife's permission?" said Brent.

"I'm not married, and why do I need to get my wife's permission even if I was?

"Isn't that the way it works for you guys?" Brent replied.

"Is there anyone else who can do this?" asked the man.

"Nope, you're stuck with me." He grabbed the man's wrist harshly and started rubbing the site with an alcohol pad. "Don't worry about the alcohol," he said. He jabbed the man's arm coarsely with the needle, not really seeking an artery. He wiggled the needle around, making the man wince in pain. "Don't worry," said Brent. "I'll find one eventually."

Brent heard a noise behind him and noticed Dr. Yee was at the door. He had a stern look on his face and said, "Please finish with this patient and then meet me in my office."

QUESTIONS FOR THOUGHT AND REFLECTION

1. Brent felt he tried to act professionally in the face of uncomfortable situations. What strategies did Brent use to deal with his discomfort? How successful were his strategies?
2. What could Brent have done to deal better with his cultural biases?
3. In your opinion, did Brent have good clinical skills?
4. How do you think Dr. Yee should manage Brent and this situation? Should he be fired?
5. What kind of training opportunities are there for Brent?

⭐ EXPERIENTIAL EXERCISES

1. Think back on a time in your life when you did not fit in or experienced prejudice. Recall how you felt. Think of how you can use this memory to foster empathy for others who may feel out of place.
2. How many cultural groups do you belong to? Think broadly and write a list. Include beliefs, activities, affiliations, habits, preferences—everything you can think of.
3. Explore a world map to refresh your memory of world geography.
4. What is your place of employment doing to welcome a diverse patient population? What else do you think they could do?

CROSS CURRENTS WITH OTHER SOFT SKILLS

VALUING MULTICULTURAL COMPETENCE: This will help you regard working with people of different backgrounds as an asset rather than a challenge (Chapter 6).
STRIVING FOR TOLERANCE: Tolerance is the prerequisite for multicultural competence (Chapter 7).
TAKING ACCOUNTABILITY: Only you can increase your multicultural competence (Chapter 3).

References

Griffin RA, Polit DF, Byrne MW. Stereotyping and nurses' recommendations for treating pain in hospitalized children. *Res Nurs Health.* 2007;30(6):655–666.

Communicating in Health Care

- Develop Professional Skills to Improve Work Relationships
- Understand the Benefits of Taking Accountability and Ownership
- Effectively Use Critical Thinking Skills in Your Profession
- Develop a Process to Improve Your Problem-Solving Skills
- Recognize Challenges Related to People With Communication Barriers
- Take Responsibility for the Success of Your Interactions With Co-Workers and Patients
- Use Communication Strategies to Support Diversity in the Workplace

Developing Professional Skills

The most precious gift we can offer anyone is our attention.
—Thich Nhat Hanh

LEARNING OBJECTIVE 1: DEVELOPING AND IMPROVING YOUR PERSONAL SKILLS

- Demonstrate how to use critical thinking skills in a workplace setting.
- Learn how to problem-solve by identifying issues and evaluating solutions.
- Understand accountability and its importance in the workplace.
- Define ownership and how to take it.
- Know how to build trust as an employee and co-worker.

In previous chapters, you learned about different interpersonal skills, such as time management, integrity, and adaptability, and how to more effectively communicate. In addition to these, there are a number of professional skills that are critical to ensuring your success as a health care professional.

Teamwork

Teamwork is when team or staff members interact interdependently with one another for a common purpose or working toward a goal, such as ensuring or improving patient care and safety. Teamwork may minimize issues caused by miscommunication with co-workers and misunderstandings of roles and responsibilities.

Working well in groups requires some understanding of how teams function and the way that relationship can change group dynamics. It is important to understand that challenging team behaviors may occur. Knowing how to manage difficult behaviors is an important skill to learn in any organization. The most effective teams are those that can see what skills are available in the group and use their own skill set to fill any gaps. Good team workers strive hard to ensure that the group communicates well, helping to make sure there are no misunderstandings or conflicts between team members.

In addition to leveraging your new communication skills, it is important to learn techniques around building rapport, allowing for different perspectives, which improves productivity and conflict management. Process-focused skills tend to be about people, and about building rapport within the group and making sure the group works effectively together (Figure. 6.1).

* **Building rapport.** Rapport is based on building an emotional connection with another person. Employers look to hire people they feel will get along with their co-workers or other team members and be able to connect with patients. It is easier to build rapport with someone who shares your interests or, in this case, profession. When you lack common interests, you need to work harder to build rapport and find common ground.

* **Use positive communication skills.** We often create and maintain rapport subconsciously through nonverbal communication, including body positioning, eye contact, and tone of voice. For example, behaviors that build rapport are leaning toward the person you are talking to using open body language, making eye contact, using encouraging gestures, smiling, and asking questions to demonstrate you are interested in what they have to say.

* **Creating unity.** Teamwork promotes an atmosphere that fosters friendship and loyalty. These relationships motivate employees in parallel and align them to work harder, cooperate, and be supportive of one another. When an environment of teamwork exists, the whole team is motivated and working toward the same goal.

* **Allowing feedback.** Individuals possess diverse talents, weaknesses, communication skills, strengths, and habits. Good teamwork provides the facility with a diversity of thought, creativity, perspectives, opportunities, and problem-solving approaches. A team environment allows individuals to brainstorm collectively, which in turn increases their success in problem-solving and arriving at solutions more efficiently and effectively. Sharing differing opinions and experiences strengthens accountability and can help make effective decisions faster than when done alone.

* **Improves productivity.** With effective teamwork, you and other team members become more efficient and productive. This is because it allows the workload to be shared, reducing the pressure on individuals, and ensuring tasks are completed within a set time frame. Ultimately, when a group of individuals works together, compared with one person working alone, they promote a more efficient work output and are able to complete tasks faster due to many minds intertwined on the same goals and objectives of the business.

Problem-Solving

Another key professional skill involves working with others to identify, define, and solve problems. Everyone can benefit from developing good problem-solving skills, as we encounter problems every day. Large problems can often overwhelm us and leave us with self-doubt. The first stage in solving any problem is to try and break the problem into smaller components. Once we clearly define the problem and break it into smaller, manageable parts, we can begin to methodically tackle each part.

Planning and structuring will help make the problem-solving process more successful and less difficult. A lot of the work in problem-solving involves understanding what the underlying issues of the problem really are, not necessarily the results. Effective problem-solving usually involves working through several steps, including:

* **Problem identification.** The first phase of problem-solving requires identifying a problem, recognizing the source of the problem, and defining the problem. By spending some time defining the problem, you will not only understand it more clearly yourself but also be able to communicate it better to others.

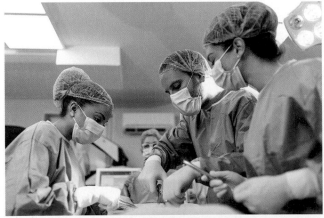

Figure 6.1 A surgical team must effectively work together as a team. (iStock.com/stefanamer/1408931473.)

* **Structuring the problem.** This phase focuses on gaining more information about the problem and growing your understanding; it is all about fact-finding and analysis. Building a more comprehensive picture of the problem and the barrier to implementation is essential to resolve more complex issues.
* **Identifying possible solutions.** This stage lets you identify a range of possible solutions to the identified problem. In a group situation, this stage is often carried out as a brainstorming session, letting every person in the group express their views on possible solutions. In the workplace, different people will have different expertise in different areas, and it is helpful to hear the views of each concerned party.
* **Making a decision.** This is the stage where you will do an analysis of the different possible solutions and then select the best possible solution to implement. The information-gathering phase should have provided sufficient data to base a decision on, and you now know the advantages and disadvantages of each option. For important decisions, it is worth keeping a record of the steps you followed in the decision-making process. That way, if you are ever criticized for making a bad decision, you can justify your thoughts based on the information and processes you used at the time. By keeping a record and engaging with the decision-making process, you will be strengthening your understanding of how it works, which can make future decisions easier to manage.
* **Implementation.** This is the phase where you will implement the decision you have made. It is important to remember that obstacles typically surface during the implementation phase, so it is important to build in extra time to test and fix issues. During this phase, you will want to solicit feedback from people affected by the new solution. It is good practice to keep a record of outcomes and any additional problems that occurred.

Critical Thinking

Similar yet different from problem-solving, critical thinking is the ability to think clearly and rationally, understanding the logical connection between ideas. Critical thinking and problem-solving can both help you resolve challenges, but the two practices have distinct purposes and strategies. As we just learned, problem-solving is a set of techniques you specifically use to find effective solutions. Critical thinking is a lifelong practice to improve your overall thinking process. In fact, critical thinking is an important part of

problem-solving. Once you identify the problem and collect all the information, you can use critical thinking to guide you to the best solution.

Critical thinking is our ability to engage in reflective and independent thinking. Critical thinking requires you to use your ability to reason. It is about being an active learner rather than a passive recipient of information. By analyzing your thoughts, you can improve how efficiently you think, how intuitively you organize your thoughts, and how often you recognize your biases. When you think critically, you can study arguments, analyze what evidence supports them, and make a reasoned decision about whether the arguments are correct. Adopting critical thinking as a long-term practice can help you consider the perspectives of co-workers more often, become more honest about your mistakes, and commit to the process of lifelong learning.

Critical thinkers rigorously question ideas and assumptions rather than accepting them at face value. They will always seek to determine whether the ideas, arguments, and findings represent the entire picture and are open to finding that they do not. Critical thinkers will identify, analyze, and solve problems systematically and logically rather than by intuition or instinct. Box 6.1 lists common critical thinking skills.

In addition to clinical skills, employers are looking for employees and job candidates who are able to think critically, analyze a situation, and problem-solve. Critical thinkers are able to bring creative ideas and solutions to a problem. Developing your critical thinking skills will make you a better candidate for that new job or promotion.

As a health care professional, critical thinking skills are essential and common skills employers are looking for. Poor judgment and being unable to logically problem-solve with the facts at hand may lead to

---

BOX 6.1

Critical Thinking Skills

- Understand the links between ideas.
- Determine the importance and relevance of arguments and ideas.
- Recognize, build, and appraise arguments.
- Identify inconsistencies and errors in reasoning.
- Approach problems in a consistent and systematic way.
- Reflect on the justification of their own assumptions, beliefs, and values.

BOX 6.2

Steps to Improving Critical Thinking

- **Define your question.** Know what you are trying to achieve, and then figure out how to best get there.
- **Gather reliable information.** Make sure that you are using sources you can trust—that they are factual and without biases.
- **Ask the right questions.** Asking the right questions that are going to get you to your answer.
- **Look for short- and long-term consequences.** Both are important when considering solutions.
- **Explore all sides.** There is rarely just one simple answer. Explore all options and think outside of the box before you come to any conclusions.

errors and poor patient care and outcomes. A critical thinker understands the connections between ideas and is able to construct arguments based on facts, as well as find mistakes in reasoning. Box 6.2 lists ways to improve critical thinking skills.

Power of Observation

In the fields of observation, chance favors only the prepared mind.

—Louis Pasteur

An important part of critical thinking is being a good observer. Observation is the action or process of observing something or someone in order to gain information. Our observation skills inform us about events, attitudes, and experiences, using one or more senses. Being able to observe and gather information will also improve your ability to communicate well. Improving your observation skills allows you to "listen" with more than just your ears and make better decisions. It also enhances your ability to interact with others and to respond in an appropriate manner. Both are keys to success personally and professionally. In the workplace, a good employee not only listens well but also is aware of what is happening around them.

Develop the skill of observation by testing yourself each day. Practice the following skills: focusing, noticing, and remembering. Observe someone around you, inspect a photo, or listen to an overheard conversation. *Focus* on details that stand out for some reason or another, and then *notice* why the details are interesting or strange. Take your time with each section of this activity to ensure you do not stop observing too soon. When you are training your brain to observe, speed is not a factor. You are more likely to make a good observation and *remember* as you concentrate more thoroughly on the object of your examination.

Learning to focus on the matter at hand requires good observational, concentration, and communication skills. You may have to become skilled at silent signals to keep others from interrupting your concentration. Try avoiding eye contact with others outside of your focus until you have completed the task at hand. Avoid interrupting others and observe how successful co-workers keep their focus. After an issue has been identified and the key features noted, your focus may then be diverted. Thus, your focus of attention can zoom in and zoom out, depending on where you need to place your attention at any given moment.

The power of observation is used by employees to develop effective relationships with their co-workers. You are likely to emulate others in the same position in the work environment to find the appropriate level of assertiveness, humor, and familiarity with others in the work environment. Choose people in your work environment that you respect. Observe their qualities and how they deal with different patients and professional situations. Watching others who are successful is a key step toward developing your own critical thinking.

Being observant is a habit that can be developed with practice and mindfulness. In the workplace, employees who are observant are more easily trained, perform their jobs better, and are more productive while working. It is easy to see why employers value the observant employee.

JOURNALING 6.1

Write in your journal the ways you show attention to a person who is speaking to you. How do you listen to friends? Is this different from how you listen to teachers or a supervisor at work? Do people often tell you to pay attention, or are they trying to get your attention? Do you find yourself having to ask people to repeat themselves, or are you missing information when in a conversation? How can you improve your focus and concentration?

Logical and Reasoned Thinking

As a health care professional, you have been trained in reasoning and the scientific method of inquiry. Although intuition will develop with experience in the field, the conclusions and decisions you make must be based on logic and sound thinking.

Maintaining Objectivity

Education, reading, and exposure to different people and experiences are the best tools to open up your mind to possibilities beyond those you have already encountered in your own life. Think about all the people and situations you have experienced while in school and how these different scenarios and experiences have helped to broaden the way you think. How do you use this broader thinking to keep your main objective in mind?

First, identify facts and do not rely on subjective impressions. Avoid allowing personal biases to influence decisions before all the facts are known. Practice not jumping to conclusions or making quick decisions. Instead, let your mind be free of stereotyping and preconceived ideas at work. Only in that way will you be able to become more selective before reaching a conclusion.

Inference

Inference is the ability to draw on past experiences to guide you through current issues and situations. In contrast with biased thinking, inference draws on successful resolutions to past problems and does not rely on only one incident. It may combine many past events to help solve today's issue. Using a prior situation and its outcome is helpful to problem-solving. It will give you a basis for what to do and what not to do in the health care setting.

As a new employee, you may find it difficult to focus and be overwhelmed by the many inputs and trivial details you encounter at work. As your experience grows, so will your confidence, objectivity, and organizational skills. Employers value inference because the employee will be able to have a greater understanding of situations and be able to better communicate with patients and co-workers.

However, developing inference skills takes time and experience. One effective method is the reverse engineering process, which helps improve your inference skills by considering or asking yourself the following in future situations:

* Are your answers or conclusions supported by any evidence or information?
* Does the evidence or information add to what you already know?
* Can more than one answer be possible?

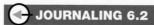 **JOURNALING 6.2**

Consider a recent debate or argument you were involved in. What did you and the other person believe to be true? Using critical thinking, outline the facts that support your argument. Then outline the facts that support the other person's argument. What do you conclude?

Taking Accountability

I've missed more than 9,000 shots in my career. I've lost almost 300 games. Twenty-six times, I've been trusted to take the game-winning shot and missed. I've failed over and over and over again in my life. And that is why I succeed.

—Michael Jordan

Accountability is a choice. Accountability is accepting responsibility for your activities, behaviors, and the outcomes of your actions. Sometimes, it means admitting that you made a mistake. There are plenty of people to blame when things go wrong. But to be fully accountable means taking initiative and performing your job well because your employer, co-workers, and patients depend on it. It also means taking responsibility for results and not assuming it is someone else's responsibility.

Taking Responsibility

When something goes wrong, what does true accountability and responsibility look like?

* Being annoyed with yourself for not taking ownership earlier.
* Regretting not admitting up front that you needed more training before taking on a task.
* Being annoyed with yourself because you depended on someone who was not dependable.
* Recognizing the benefit of an event turning out a certain way and using it as an opportunity to practice your accountability skills.

If you experience any of these feelings or have asked yourself any of these questions, you are taking ownership and are learning to take accountability. Taking accountability is not an easy thing. Behaving and acting with accountability is a heavy responsibility that involves difficult decisions and extra effort.

When you and your co-workers demonstrate accountability, trust is formed. Knowing that your co-workers are doing what they said they were going to do and when they said they were going to do it results in a high-performing team. But accountability starts with you. You need to model the behaviors you want to see in your workplace. Certainly, there will be times when a task is not your job. But instead of refusing to help, ask, "How can I help?"

Taking Ownership

Whereas accountability is taking responsibility for completing a task as assigned, ownership is the initiative of standing up and saying, "I will do it." Sometimes, taking ownership is taking action and believing it is your responsibility to do so, even when it may not be. For example, your supervisor assigns you a task and you successfully complete it—that is accountability. However, if you volunteer to take on this task before your supervisor assigns it, that is ownership.

However, ownership is difficult because it puts you at the very center of the outcome. If you make a mistake, you will need to admit it. If you fail, you will need to take responsibility for it. But this is the risk you must take to advance personally and professionally. This is when you must decide what you are made of. Taking ownership means focusing on solutions rather than problems. The focus is always on what's next. "What about this?" "Let's try this." Ownership means devising solutions, and owners who create solutions are known as leaders.

Ownership is an important quality to have in an employee, even more than accountability. Ownership puts you in charge, which gives you a sense of being part of the team and organization. When you feel you are a part of the bigger picture and that you are an integral part of a team, you will feel more confident and ready to take on more responsibility. Employees who take ownership are often more driven, are more motivated, and seek creative and innovative ways to improve and develop what they are doing, rather than going through the motions and fulfilling the minimum of their jobs.

Trust and Be Worthy of Trust

Accountability and ownership can only be successful if trust exists between you, your co-workers, and supervisor. All relationships at work must be built on a sense of trust. An employee who is worthy of trust should not be micromanaged. Employees should not be suspicious of one another's motives.

The first step is to always try to tell the truth, even when it is difficult, embarrassing, or may jeopardize your job. Being polite or wanting to spare someone's feelings are not excuses for avoiding the truth. Truth takes courage, but the benefit is that others will trust you even if you make a mistake. When there is a high level of trust, there is a higher level of productivity. If your supervisors do not trust you, they will spend too much time and energy following up on you and managing details of your job. Further, if you do not feel trusted, you are less likely to take initiative or ownership.

The next step to being trusted is to avoid talking about people behind their backs, especially if you have criticism to offer. Instead, always bring concerns directly to that individual. Talking poorly about someone never solves problems, and it marks you as untrustworthy. For example, if you have concerns about someone else's ability, should you stand on the sidelines and let the disaster unfold? Instead, you can be honest but supportive at the same time. Volunteer to help or suggest other resources to assist your co-worker. Collaborating with a co-worker to arrive at the right solution is a great opportunity to build trust.

Similarly, when someone complains to you about a co-worker behind their back, direct that person to the third party. Say you are uncomfortable with the conversation and feel the issue should be discussed with the person being talked about so something can be done about it. Gossip can be highly destructive to the process of building trust. Box 6.3 suggests some ways you can respond to avoid gossip.

BOX 6.3

How to Avoid Getting Involved With Gossip

- Assume that everything you say about a co-worker will be repeated.
- When gossip starts, and you are there:
    - Say something positive about the person being gossiped about.
    - Change the subject.
    - Leave.
- Remember: You want to create positive relationships, not negative ones.
- Just because others gossip doesn't mean you have to.
- If you have a concern about a co-worker, address it directly with them.
- When you gossip, you open a process that can spin out of control.
- People who gossip become the topic of gossip.

Back to Basics

Direct Conversations and Interactions

We have learned a lot about the role of verbal, nonverbal, and listening communication skills, along with other key skills to improve your interpersonal relationships. However, to successfully execute these skills, we must engage in conversations and effectively interact with different people. Advances in technology enable us to have a lot of our conversations via text, email, tweets, and other social platforms. In many ways, we are communicating more than we use to, but we are doing it without using certain communication skills while using many others and in different ways.

Direct conversations, or face-to-face communications, are declining, and many experts feel we are losing our ability to have deep, personal interactions. Direct conversation is a form of social communication between two or more people without any form of mediating technology, such as a phone or computer. With technology and more jobs being remote or working from home, including some in health care, direct conversations may include virtual meetings. Electronic communications, such as texting, messaging, and emailing, are typically shorter than verbal communications, and important nonverbal signals, such as body language, tone of voice, and facial expressions, are lost.

Having direct conversations encourages engagement, rapport, and participation in meetings, even if they are informal, and builds a company culture of trust. In fact, direct communication is often more effective than written or audio-only conversations. This is because seeing one another allows us to pick up on nonverbal cues and body language. Because a lot of communication is nonverbal, being able to see each other helps us understand each other better.

Although digital communication teaches critical skills, it should not replace face-to-face conversations. Verbal communication teaches other skills and is important for our overall well-being. When you are having a bad day or struggling with difficult work conflicts, a real-life conversation can boost your morale and help you manage and work through problems more effectively (Figure. 6.2).

Introductions

One of the best ways to make a good first impression is to properly introduce yourself. Meeting someone in our personal life or in business can be the beginning of something great. We meet new patients, patients, friends, and co-workers daily. However, we often miss an opportunity to make a great first impression. For example, you should have a specific short introduction ready to use every time you greet a new patient, focusing right away on your name and your role (Figure. 6.3). Plan what to say in advance, so it comes naturally. On the other hand, introducing yourself to a co-worker or prospective employer requires a more detailed approach. For example, when you meet people at a new job, you might use a longer introduction because your new co-workers want to get to know you and what your role will be at work.

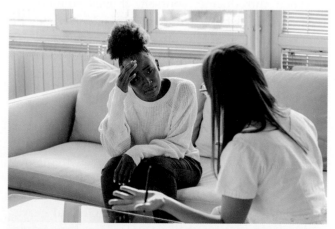

Figure 6.2 Direct communication is important in observing nonverbal signals, such as body language, tone of voice, and facial expressions. (iStock.com/stefanamer/1182390029.)

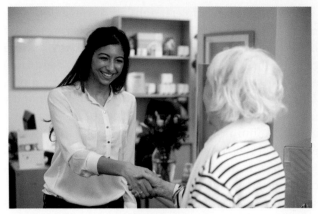

Figure 6.3 A medical office manager introduces herself to a patient. (Copyright © istock.com.)

Introduce yourself with "Hi, I'm Sandra. It's a pleasure to meet you." In some instances, it will be appropriate to include a few more details about what you do, such as, "Hi, I'm Sandra and I'm a medical assistant. I'll will be working with Dr. Archer." This stage will establish the flow for the rest of the conversation. Remember to wait for the other person to respond and make introductions, too, before continuing.

To develop the introduction into a conversation, simply ask a question about the other person. This will allow the patient to feel like you are interested in learning more about them. Many good conversations begin with a question. You might ask for information, such as directions, advice, or guidance. This stimulates conversation by focusing the conversation on the other person, which gives you an opportunity to listen actively and learn more about them. It also pays the other person a compliment because you are seeking and valuing the other person's experience and thoughts.

When introducing yourself, it was common to include a handshake. Although a handshake may be common outside of a health care setting, more health care professionals and settings are opting to avoid shaking hands with patients to prevent the transmission of pathogens. Despite strict hand-washing policies in virtually all health care facilities, studies have found that a significant portion of health care providers and professionals are poor at complying with these policies. Health care professionals frequently wash their hands, but often do not wash as long as they should or use the proper techniques. Further, bacterial live on computers, phones, medical charts, and uniforms. As a result, many facilities have implemented "handshake-free zones" to help reduce the transmission of pathogens and diseases.

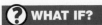

? WHAT IF?

What if you encounter a co-worker at your new place of employment and they do not introduce themself? What steps would you take to handle the situation?

Listening

Why is it so easy to get lost in your own thoughts when you are supposed to be listening to someone? Distraction has a lot to do with the difference between the speed of speech and the speed of thought. We usually think at a rate of about 500 words per minute, while most of us speak at about 130 words per minute. Someone who speaks at 150 words per minute is considered a fast talker, and someone who speaks at 200 words per minute would not be intelligible or understandable to most people.

Because we think faster than we speak, we must make a concerted effort to concentrate to actively listen to someone speaking at a much slower pace than our thoughts. Teach yourself powerful concentration skills and consider the three phases of a productive conversation: active listening, reflecting, and asking questions (Figure. 6.4).

There's a lot of difference between listening and hearing.
—G. K. Chesterton

Active Listening

Listening is an active process in which you make a conscious decision to listen and understand the message of the speaker. Active listening involves using all your senses and giving full attention to the speaker. You should remain neutral and nonjudgmental, which includes not taking sides or forming opinions early in the conversation. Active listening also involves patience. You should anticipate pauses and short periods of silence and avoid jumping in with questions when there is silence. Remember to leverage your nonverbal skills and use your body language

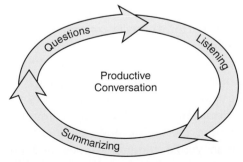

Figure 6.4 The listening process will repeat itself several times in a conversation.

to communicate your interest in the conversation by making eye contact, nodding, smiling, and maintaining an open posture.

Listening to your colleagues helps you gather feedback and understand their ideas and opinions about an issue. It will help you build trust in your work relationships as you learn more about the people you work with through meaningful conversations. Remember to try not to interrupt or talk over others. Listen fully to what each person says, considering the meaning of the words, rather than simply thinking about what you want to say next.

To know when it is your turn to speak in a conversation, wait for breaks or pauses. The listener propels the conversation forward by making gestures and interjecting to encourage the speaker to continue. Typical expressions for encouraging a speaker are listed in Box 6.4. Give speakers sufficient time to express themselves. You want them to say as much as possible to share as much information as possible. As you listen, observe body language and assess the speaker's emotions.

Reflecting

As an extension of good listening skills, it is important to develop the ability to reflect words and feelings to ensure you have understood the message correctly.

Reflecting is the process of paraphrasing and restating both the words and the feelings of the speaker. After the speaker has expressed themself, clarify what you heard with statements, such as, "If I understand you correctly," followed by key phrases or ideas you have heard.

The purposes of reflecting include:

* Showing the speakers that you are listening and trying to understand the messages they communicate.
* Encouraging the speakers to continue talking.
* Allowing the speakers to hear their own thoughts and giving them the opportunity to focus their ideas.

Another benefit of repeating the speaker's ideas is that it helps you avoid misinterpreting the speaker by making assumptions that may or may not be true. A skilled listener will be able to reflect feelings from nonverbal body cues as well as verbal messages. Reflecting combines content and feelings to mirror what the speaker has said. For example, the speaker says, "I don't understand my boss. He says one thing and then does another." The listener conveys, "You feel confused by him." You can see that the listener has linked the speaker's words and emotional response.

Questioning

The listener can demonstrate that they have been paying attention by asking relevant questions or making statements that build on or help to clarify what the speaker has said. Questions used as clarification are important to minimize misunderstanding and to improve communication. By asking relevant questions, the listener also helps to reinforce that they have a genuine interest in what the speaker has been saying. Questioning lets you learn more about the speaker, which can be helpful when you begin to build rapport and get to know the other person better. It can also be used to understand problems that another person may be experiencing, for example, when a physician is trying to diagnose a patient.

Being an effective communicator has a lot to do with how questions are asked. When you are sure that you understand the speaker, ask open-ended questions beginning with who, what, where, when, how, and why. However, ask one question at a time. Every time you ask an open-ended question, or one that cannot be answered with a simple "yes" or "no" answer, you repeat the listening process.

Knowing when to begin asking questions is important. As discussed earlier, the pause, or a natural break in the conversation, is a signal to change speakers and listeners. Try to avoid interrupting and wait for that

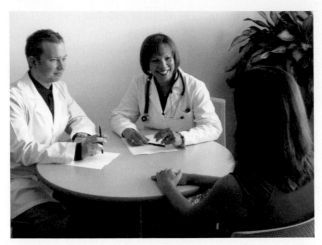
Figure 6.5 Two health care professionals listen to a patient.

pause. People who interrupt have already stopped listening. They have already decided what they want to say in response, even before the other person has completed their thought. If you speak after a pause, it shows that you were listening actively, especially if you make a logical comment, make an observation, or ask a relevant question. Then, once you pause, you have invited your partner to respond, and you can again encourage them to continue (Figure. 6.5).

Two monologues don't make a dialogue.

—Jeff Daly

Listening Empathetically

Listening is the best approach to resolving conflict or responding to strong emotions. When a patient or co-worker is angry or emotional, your job is not to solve their problem or even agree with the person but to first simply listen and support the person who is experiencing these feelings. Their feelings are real and a part of their current experience. At this point, they are most likely not looking for advice, answers, or an easy dismissal of their feelings or problems. They want their feelings to be recognized, accepted, and understood. Encourage them to express their feelings first, then ask thoughtful questions when they are done talking.

Health care professionals may need to share bad or unexpected news with patients and relations of patients, such as diagnosis and prognosis. It is important that you give patients as much time as they need to speak and ask questions. Once you have finished listening and eliciting all the information you can, summarize what you have heard. Summarizing

clarifies issues, validates the speaker, and calms emotions by remaining neutral. Start by saying, "If I understand you correctly ..." followed by your paraphrased summary.

? WHAT IF?

What if you do not understand what someone is saying? Or, what if you strongly do not agree with what someone is saying? What strategies could you use to get the conversation back on track?

Your real objective is not to solve the person's problem or stop any irrational emotions but to help the person do that for themselves. Solving someone else's problem can foster a dependent relationship in which the other person approaches you to resolve every problem he or she encounters. By simply listening and questioning, you empower them to solve their own problems. Besides, if you are tempted to give the person advice and your advice does not work, that person may resent or blame you.

It can be difficult reasoning with a person who is emotional. Listening patiently will help people talk themselves into a calmer state, especially if you are modeling as you listen and staying calm with a level tone. In many instances, by staying calm, the person may be better at assessing the situation and coming up with a solution. Once you practice and master this skill, your co-workers will observe your behavior, which may help them in future similar situations.

Prioritize Listening

Health care settings can be chaotic, and we will sometimes find it difficult to listen. According to studies, the average length of time for a medical visit is less than 18 minutes. The median talk time by the patient was 5.3 minutes, and the physician was 5.2 minutes. The median time during which neither part spoke was 55 seconds.

In one study (Beckman and Frankel, 1984), the listening behaviors of physicians in a health clinic were examined by measuring and recording the time patients were permitted to speak at the beginning of their appointment. The study found that physicians only let patients speak for an average of 18 seconds before interrupting them. When informed of the findings, the physicians responded by denying that they interrupted their patients that quickly. They also explained that they were busy and that patients would talk endlessly about their problems if they were not interrupted.

The researchers repeated the study but instructed the physicians to let patients speak without interruption, no matter how long the patients took. The average patient only spoke for 30 seconds, and the longest amount of time only lasted 90 seconds. Are we really too busy to listen? What can we learn from patients and their health status if we allowed them to speak for an additional 12 seconds?

The time and capacity to truly listen to patients, hear their stories, and learn not only what the matter is with them but also what matters to them. Some health care providers and professionals claim that workload and other factors have compressed medical encounters to a point that genuine conversation with patients is no longer possible or practical. In fact, the opposite may be true. By not fully understanding the patients' concerns and what they are experiencing, health care providers may miss pertinent information, which may lead to a misdiagnosis and ineffective or incorrect treatments. These consequences have clear human and financial costs.

CASE STUDY 6.1
A Deep Discovery

Alicia was dreading her 3:00 p.m. appointment with Mr. Cruz. Her employer, Dr. Lin, charged a $75 fee when a patient missed a dental appointment without 24 hours' notice. Mr. Cruz had missed an appointment several months ago and exploded at Alicia when she told him about the fee. She could not get him to calm down long enough to explain that the fee was waived the first time it happened. But, unfortunately, Mr. Cruz also missed his next appointment. Alicia thought they had seen the last of Mr. Cruz, but then his wife called and rescheduled.

Mr. Cruz seemed to be in a good mood when he arrived. He even waved at Alicia. Alicia thought he might not even be aware he had missed his last appointment, even though she called him the day before to remind him.

Mr. Cruz was still smiling as he approached her counter. "Good afternoon, Mr. Cruz. How are you?"

"Better than you might think for somebody who has to see the dentist."

"That's great," said Alicia. "Now, when was your last appointment?"

"I was here in September or October, I think. I'm not quite sure."

"Hmmm," said Alicia, looking at his chart. "It says here that you had an appointment in December, but it looks like you didn't make it to the appointment. So, unfortunately, there is a $75 penalty for missed appointments."

"I don't see why I have to pay this $75 penalty," he said as he recalled his missed appointment. "Things come up, you know. Nobody's perfect. I'm an insurance adjuster, and my schedule is very unpredictable," he continued. "When there is a claim, I have to be there. I try to keep these appointments, but my job is a higher priority."

Alicia noticed that he was talking faster now and more color rose in his face. But she made a point of just nodding and occasionally saying, "I understand."

"I guess I could have called, but would that have helped? I mean, if I called, and it wasn't the day before, would you still charge me?" he said.

At this point he paused, and Alicia knew she had to choose her reply carefully. She saw that he was trying to contain his emotions, but she knew that he had a short fuse.

"Yes, calling and letting us know always helps," she said. "We understand that your job is important, and we try our best to accommodate every patient. But we only have so much availability. So, when an appointment is scheduled and it's a no-show, it's one less patient for the doctor to see and an appointment another patient would have appreciated having."

"We want to make sure everyone is aware of the policy, so that's why it's clearly stated here. We never want to surprise anyone," Alicia lowering her voice a bit and pointing to the sign taped to the window that stated the policy. "We understand that things come up and that's why we do waive the penalty for the first time. After that, we must follow the policy."

"Well, I understand," Mr. Cruz said begrudgingly.

"Thank you for understanding," said Alicia. "I think the doctor is ready to see you now. We can make payment arrangements when you are through."

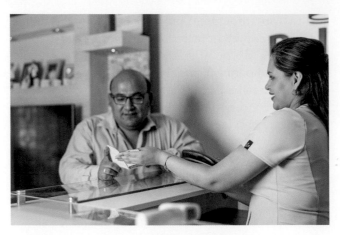
iStock.com/Guillermo Spelucin Runcimn/1395391606

QUESTIONS FOR THOUGHT AND
REFLECTION

1. What tactics did Alicia use to avoid getting into an argument with Mr. Cruz over the penalty fee?
2. What communication skills did Alicia use in this exchange?
3. Why did Alicia enforce the penalty fee? Would you have enforced the penalty? Why or why not?

A Different Path

Prima finally got a job as a sonography technician at the obstetrical practice of Drs. O'Malley, Kendrick, and Anselmo. She had done very well in her program, but she knew she had a lot to learn on the job. She had already learned how to use a more advanced sonography imaging machine than the ones she had used at school and during her clinical externships. She had encountered some anomalies—that was what Dr. Anselmo called them—in some of the sonograms she had taken. She was not sure Dr. Anselmo was using that term correctly.

Prima pursued sonography because she liked babies, and she thought it would be a very positive profession, with a lot of happy moms, as well as opportunities to learn and advance. She had not seen a miscarriage yet, but she dreaded the day when that would come. She told her boyfriend that the job was a lot more complicated than she thought. Some of the patients had to have amniocentesis, and it struck her that there were many more complications than she had originally anticipated.

At the end of her third week, Prima did a sonogram for a woman whose name showed up as Dr. Alison DeMoure in the medical record.

"I noticed doctor on your chart. Are you a medical doctor?" she asked when Dr. DeMoure arrived.

"No, I teach engineering at the University. You can call me Alison." She pointed in the direction of the man who was with her. "That's Mitch, my husband." She was soft-spoken, and she seemed to lower her voice even more as she shared that this was their first child.

"Wow, that's great," said Prima. "Let's see, your birth date is April 2, 1985. Is that right?"

"Yes."

"Wow, and this is your first baby? You're getting a late start."

Alison exchanged a glance with Mitch, who stepped forward. "The baby will be fine," he said to both of them as he took Alison's hand.

"Sure, she will," said Prima with sudden enthusiasm. "What are you guys hoping for—a boy or a girl?"

"A healthy baby," Alison said, laughing.

"We don't care about the sex," said Mitch. "We want to be surprised." He nodded at Alison, as if to reassure her.

"Well, you are far enough along that we can probably tell," said Prima.

"Well, we prefer not to know. We don't care one way or the other," said Alison.

"Sure, you want to have a healthy baby. Let's get started then."

Pretty soon, they all heard a healthy heartbeat. "He's got a great heartbeat," said Prima. Alison and Mitch glanced at each other.

"Oh my God, look at him!" Prima felt happy that the baby seemed healthy. "Do you want to take a print of this, so you can put the little guy on your refrigerator?"

Alison and Mitch seemed relieved that the baby seemed healthy.

Later that day, Dr. O'Malley came out and asked to speak to Prima in his office. "Did you tell the DeMoures that they are having a boy?"

"No, I mean, they were so happy about the heartbeat. I hope the little guy is going to be OK."

"The little guy?"

"The baby. You know."

"Didn't they tell you they didn't want to know what the sex was?"

"Well, I'm not sure … I don't think I heard that."

"They told me they did tell you. You really need to work on listening and paying a lot more attention when patients are communicating with you."

EXPERIENTIAL EXERCISES

1. Listen to your friends or patients talk without interrupting them. How long do they talk before they pause?
2. Write two introductions for yourself—one introducing yourself to a patient and one introducing yourself to a new co-worker. Memorize them and say them out loud until they sound natural.
3. Use your "co-worker" introduction on a partner. Observe where the conversation goes from there.
4. Compliment a friend or family member. Observe where the conversation goes from there.
5. Watch the news or a late-night talk show. Pay close attention to the questions the reporters ask. Are they open-ended questions? How effective are they in encouraging conversation and dialogue?

CROSS CURRENTS WITH OTHER SOFT SKILLS

MODELING PROFESSIONAL BEHAVIOR: What is the connection between listening and etiquette? (Chapter 13)

MANAGING YOUR MANAGER: This is when listening can really pay off for your career (Chapters 13 and 14).

GAINING ENERGY, PERSISTENCE, AND PERSEVERANCE: Learn how listening fuels your energy (Chapter 3).

MANAGING ANGER AND STRONG EMOTIONS: Why is listening a good strategy here? (Chapter 5)

Communicating With Special Groups of Patients

Anything that's human is mentionable, and anything that is mentionable can be more manageable. When we can talk about our feelings, they become less overwhelming, less upsetting, and less scary. The people we trust with that important talk can help us know that we are not alone.

—Fred Rogers

QUESTIONS FOR THOUGHT AND REFLECTION

1. What mistakes did Prima make during this patient visit?
2. Why did Dr. O'Malley express concern about Prima disclosing the baby's sex?
3. What communication skills should Prima work on improving?

LEARNING OBJECTIVE 3: COMMUNICATING WITH SPECIAL GROUPS OF PATIENTS

- Assess special communication challenges in the health care setting.
- Have strategies at hand to communicate effectively with patients who are deaf or hard of hearing.
- Understand the needs of disabled people and learn to anticipate their needs.
- Know how to guide and seat a visually impaired person.
- Help people with speech impairments to express their needs and thoughts.
- Use an interpreter correctly.

Effective communication is critical when caring for patients; it is also the health care provider's primary tool for showing respect, empathy, and compassion to patients and their families. In the health care industry, we need to adapt our own communication skills to help others, including those with disabilities and other challenges.

Patients With Hearing Loss

The terms "deaf" or "hard of hearing" usually refer to individuals with very little, impaired, or no functional hearing. The deaf and hard-of-hearing community is diverse, and individuals have different levels of hearing, age of onset, and methods to communicate. Although there are many ways that individuals may identify themselves, the terms "deaf," "hard of hearing," or "people with hearing loss" are considered the most inclusive and accepted, according to the National Association of the Deaf.

Generally, hearing loss is categorized as mild, moderate, severe, or profound. An individual with moderate hearing loss may be able to hear sounds but has difficulty distinguishing specific speech patterns in conversation. Those with profound hearing loss may not be able to hear sounds at all.

The many different ways under which individuals develop hearing loss can affect the way they experience sound, communicate with others, and view their hearing loss. For example, some may use American Sign Language (ASL), others read lips, and some people use their voices. People with hearing loss have made many adjustments that make it easier for them to function in society. Nevertheless, they frequently encounter communication challenges that may create feelings of helplessness. Be empathetic to these challenges.

Conversations require a lot of focus, energy, and patience, so keep this in mind when communicating with people with hearing loss. Focusing on hearing can be tiring, and people have an even more difficult time when they are tired, sick, anxious, or in a bad mood. Some people are very open about their hearing loss, and they will ask you to make adjustments to help during a conversation. However, some people may not realize they have hearing loss, are not ready to address it yet, or may have hearing loss but do not wear hearing aids.

Patients Who Are Deaf or Hard of Hearing

Successful communications require the efforts of all people involved in a conversation. Even when the person with hearing loss utilizes hearing aids and active listening strategies, it is crucial that others involved in the communication process consistently use good communication practices. As health care professionals, it is our responsibility to actively identify patients who have hearing impairments.

A person who is deaf or hard of hearing who visits a health care facility usually informs you about the hearing loss. Some patients who are deaf or hard of hearing may also have speech difficulties. It is important for you to understand that the impairment is the result of hearing loss and not an intellectual disability or an impairment of their voice or vocal cords. You also cannot tell by speech quality alone that a person is hard of hearing. For example, if a person loses hearing after about age 12 years old, the person's speech is likely to be unimpaired. If a person loses hearing before the ages of 5 and 12 years old, the person will have some noticeable speech impairment but will likely be easy to understand. People who are born deaf or lose their hearing early in life will have a significant speech impairment, and you may have greater difficulty in understanding them.

Communicating With Patients Who Are Deaf or Hard of Hearing

Once you realize that you are communicating with a person who is deaf or hard of hearing, adopt a strategy to communicate effectively (Figure. 6.6). Deaf individuals typically use sign language to communicate. Hard of hearing refers to individuals who have mild-to-moderate hearing loss. Hard-of-hearing individuals may use sign language, spoken language, or a combination of both. Some hard-of-hearing people rely on their lipreading abilities. This form of communication is helpful, but medical terminology can be confusing. It is, therefore, important that you confirm comprehension. If you ask, "Are you having a hard time understanding me?" and your patient continues to smile and nod, you should be concerned about the quality of communication taking place. The best approach is to simply ask each patient how they prefer to communicate.

Use these strategies to improve your communication with patients who are deaf or hard of hearing:

* **Face the patient directly.** Position yourself on the same level and in good light whenever possible.
* **Speak clearly, slowly, and without shouting.** Shouting distorts the sound of speech and can make speech reading more difficult.
* **Say the patient's name before starting a conversation.** This gives the listener a chance to focus their attention and minimizes the chance of missing words at the beginning of the conversation.
* **Avoid talking too fast or using long, complex sentences.** Remember to slow down a little, pause

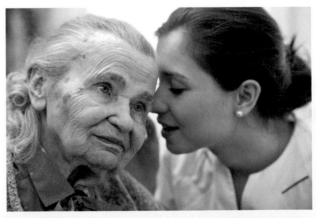

Figure 6.6 A nursing assistant speaks to a hard-of-hearing nursing home resident. (Copyright © istock.com.)

between sentences, and wait to make sure you have been understood.

* **Keep your hands away from your face.** If you are talking or using hand gestures near your face, your speech will be more difficult to understand. Beards and mustaches can also interfere with the ability to read lips.
* **Minimize background noise from music or TV.** Many people who are deaf or hard of hearing have difficulty understanding speech when there is background noise, as it can distort sound and affect their ability to hear.
* **Provide critical information in writing.** Whenever possible, write down information such as medications, directions, and phone numbers.
* **Pay attention to the listener.** A puzzled look could indicate a misunderstanding or hearing difficulty.
* **Take advantage of technology.** Use computer screens, texting, or email to communicate with your patient.

The problem with communication is the illusion that it has taken place.

—George Bernard Shaw

JOURNALING 6.5

Think about your senses: sight, smell, taste, hearing, and touch. Which sense would be the hardest for you to lose? Describe how you would adapt to this loss.

Writing is one way to avoid confusion. You can supplement written communication with signage or objects that will clarify the message you are trying to communicate. In your clinic or health care facility, suggest installing a series of helpful signs created specifically to enhance communication with the hearing impaired.

As discussed in earlier chapters, body language and gestures are great tools for communicating with patients who are deaf or hard of hearing. Even with people who are not impaired, body language can convey as much as 70% of the communication. Use body language to aid your communication with patients who are hard of hearing, especially in adding the nuances that words and voices usually carry, such as warmth, urgency, or seriousness. Exaggerate gestures to help your words carry more meaning. Finally, remain alert to your patient's use of body language. Additional suggestions to facilitate communication with people who are hard of hearing are listed in Box 6.5.

BOX 6.5

Improving Communication With Patients Who Are Hard of Hearing

- Smile and offer positive and welcoming body language.
- Indicate your willingness to stop if the patient does not understand you.
- Frequently assess whether or not you are being understood.
- Never cover your mouth or do anything to interfere with lipreading.
- Maintain eye contact to indicate attention and interest.
- Use your eyes to direct your patient's attention to another object, such as a sign or a hallway.
- When the patient is looking away, stop speaking.
- Get the patient's attention by placing yourself in their visual field or gently tapping their shoulder.

Deafness has left me acutely aware of both the duplicity that language is capable of and the many expressions the body cannot hide.

—Terry Galloway

Using Interpreters

Many people who are deaf or hard of hearing know American Sign Language (ASL). Many health care facilities employ professional interpreters or offer interpreter services, including those fluent in ASL. These expert interpreters not only translate between languages but also "interpret" language for patients by explaining medical terminology, answering simple questions, and clarifying any confusion between the patient and the health care professional. Additionally, interpreters used in the health care setting have an understanding of local knowledge and cultural beliefs and practices that will help in the communication exchange between the health care provider and the patient.

When you are using an interpreter, remember to talk directly to the patient and not to the interpreter. Use the interpreter to convey what is being spoken or signed. The interpreter should not be an active participant in the conversation or give opinions. It is important to position the interpreter close to the patient, ensuring the patient can easily see both you and the interpreter at the same time. If no professional interpreter is available, determine whether there is someone in your office who may know some sign language.

Using Others As Interpreters

Many patients who are deaf and hard of hearing—as well as people with speech impairments and language deficits—may bring along friends, family members, or caregivers who may serve as interpreters. Although it is thoughtful for them to offer support, be careful of relying on them as an interpreter. As a health care professional, you must protect the privacy of the patient's confidential medical information. Having a friend or family member act as the interpreter might also result in misinterpretation, especially if they have to explain information rather than just translate it. Moreover, this dynamic presents a conflict of interest because the friend or family member may have an agenda or may not be objective. Sometimes, sensitive information, perhaps involving contraception, domestic abuse, or a poor prognosis, is information that a family member serving as a translator might be hesitant to share with you or the patient.

Before using a family member or friend as an interpreter, you need to gain approval directly from the patient. You must do everything you can to support the confidentiality and best interests of your patients. Finally, you should document in the medical record that an interpreter was used, any information you received from the patient that was provided by an interpreter, and any concerns you may have about the accuracy of the information.

Patients With Visual Impairment

Legal blindness refers to vision that is no better than 20/20 with correction or to a restricted visual field of 20 degrees in diameter or less. Legal blindness presents obvious challenges to health care professionals who need to communicate with patients about their health. The visual difficulties of your patients do not have to be a barrier to effective communication, however. Do not assume people who are visually impaired also have other impairments, such as hearing. There is no need to raise your voice for them to understand you. They, in fact, may find it offensive and embarrassing.

There are many degrees of visual impairment. Many individuals are able to discern movement, shapes, and contrasting colors. Take as much advantage as you can of whatever abilities the person may have, but also be prepared to interact with a person who is totally blind.

As with any patient interaction, introduce yourself and describe your role. Address the visually impaired patient, so they know you are speaking to them. People who are visually impaired do not have access to nonverbal cues, such as facial expressions and body language, that aid in comprehension. Thus you have to recognize this and be able to put yourself in your patient's shoes. Ask yourself what you need to do to be considerate. For instance, explain any sudden loud noises. Do not be afraid to use subtle touch, such as a pat on the hand, because it indicates that you are listening and paying attention.

When escorting the visually impaired patient to an examination room, for instance, allow the patient to take your arm (Figure. 6.7). Give verbal directions as you move together. Describe any obstacles. When you arrive, explain the layout of the room, if necessary. When you offer a seat, place the visually impaired patient's hand on the back of the chair, which enables the patient to navigate the seating. When you leave, tell the patient you are leaving the room, and then introduce the patient to any staff member.

Some people with severe visual impairments will have professionally trained service dogs. Remember, the dog is "on the job" and do not pet or engage the dog without asking the patient's permission first.

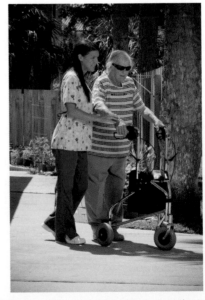

Figure 6.7 A nursing assistant directs a patient with a visual impairment. (Copyright © istock.com.)

Patients With Speech Impairments

A speech impairment is a condition in which the ability to pronounce sounds necessary to communicate with others is impaired. Speech impairment can be mild, such as slurring of words or stuttering, to severe, such as not being able to produce speech at all.

There are many reasons why people are speech impaired. They may have been born deaf or lost their hearing, which affects their ability to develop proper speech patterns. They may have uncorrected or untreated speech impediments. They may have disfiguring injuries affecting their tongue, mouth, teeth, or jaw. They may be recovering from a stroke and have trouble recalling or forming words. They may be suffering from a neurodegenerative disease, such as cerebral palsy or Parkinson's disease.

Remember that speech impairment and hearing impairment do not necessarily go hand-in-hand, so resist the temptation to speak louder than normal. Some people are offended by this unnecessary gesture.

Communicating With Patients With Speech Impairments

Do not pretend to understand something the patient says when you do not. Ask the patient to repeat what was said, and then repeat it to confirm your understanding. Be patient and take as much time as necessary. Concentrate on what the patient is saying, moving closer or to a quieter location if necessary. Resist the temptation to speak for the patient or attempt to finish the patient's sentences. Some people with speech impairments may have to exert tremendous effort to speak and be understood. It is important to give patients as much time as they need to complete their thoughts and express their feelings.

Ask questions that require only short answers. Consider writing as an alternative means of communication if you are having difficulty understanding the patient; first ask the patient if this is acceptable and if the patient is comfortable doing this.

Use strategies to improve your communication with speech-impaired patients.

When you are the talker:

* Speak at a normal volume.
* Do not assume you have to speak slowly or use simple language.

* Check with the patient to make sure they have understood each point before continuing.

When you are the listener:

* Do not hurry the patient. Patience is the key when communicating with someone with a speech impairment.
* Always let the patient finish their sentence. It is discouraging to interrupt a patient or complete their sentence.
* Let the patient know if you do not understand them; simply ask the patient to repeat what they said.

? WHAT IF?

What if, despite your best efforts, you simply cannot understand what a patient with a speech impairment is saying? What should you do?

Patients With Limited English Proficiency

The complex mosaic of the cultural and linguistic patterns in US society places new demands on health care professionals, who must effectively communicate complex medical information to patients with limited English proficiency. Effective patient-provider communication is essential to providing good patient care.

Language barriers can hinder care and affect communications with health care providers and professionals, such as calling for an appointment, describing symptoms to a paramedic, or discussing treatment risks. The consequences of not communicating effectively due to language barriers can be dire.

← JOURNALING 6.6

Think about an interaction you have had with someone who spoke little or no English. How did you communicate with this person? Describe this experience, your communication strategies, and any emotions or frustrations you or the other person experienced.

Communicating With Patients With Limited English Proficiency

As you can imagine, it is extremely difficult to communicate with someone when you do not share the same language (Figure. 6.8). Accurate communication is essential in a health care setting, where many words and concepts are unfamiliar to the patient.

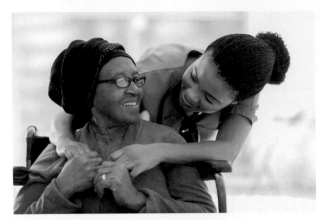

Figure 6.8 A nurse comforts a non-English–speaking patient. (Copyright © istock.com.)

Communicating With Patients With Limited English Proficiency

- Learn a few polite expressions. Learning "thank you" or "good morning" will go a long way toward improving rapport and building trust.
- Draw an object on paper, or write things down. Many foreign speakers of English have larger vocabularies of written words than spoken words.
- Use simple language free of metaphors, slang, or colloquialisms.
- Make simple and direct requests, saying "please" and "thank you," which are universally recognized for their politeness. Aim for words and phrases that are simple to understand and easily translated.
- Speak a little slower than normal and articulate clearly, although not in an exaggerated fashion.
- Speak in full sentences. This keeps information in the proper context and minimizes inaccurate translation.
- Make many more gestures than normal when speaking.
- If another language is prevalent in your area, your clinic might make a small electronic translation device available to the staff.
- As long as you understand your patient, do not correct their English.

One solution is the utilization of a professional interpreter. If a friend or family member accompanying the patient serves as a translator, you must consider the concerns discussed earlier in this chapter. Box 6.6 lists suggestions on how to communicate with patients with limited English proficiency.

In the absence of an interpreter and in the case of complete inability to communicate in any common language, it is best to try to reschedule the appointment until suitable communication arrangements can be made. Measures might include arranging for a dial-up interpreter service. In an emergency, however, you will have to communicate as much as possible, using body language to reassure the patient. In some cases, health care professionals have used translator applications on their smartphones to aid in communication.

Communicating With Pediatric Patients

Most health care professionals have an affinity for small children (Figure. 6.9). However, communicating with them may not always be so easy. Children may be shy, fussy, tired, and scared. Children who are sick are under added stress, and children with autism may find it difficult to connect with anyone, especially someone they do not know. The treatment of a sick child is obviously an occasion for anxiety for the child and for the parents or caregiver. You can increase your chances of communication success by adopting a number of strategies.

Maintain eye level with the child. Call them by their name. Be positive and simple. Try to get your idea across in one sentence, using simple words.

To better gain cooperation with a request, use the phrase "I want," as in "Alice, *I want* you to show me

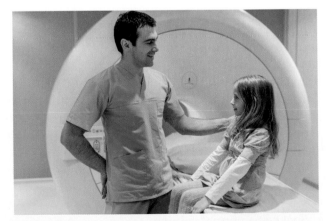

Figure 6.9 A magnetic resonance imaging technician calms an anxious, young patient before the test. (Copyright © istock.com.)

which ear hurts" instead of "show me where your ear hurts." This is not as harsh as a direct order, and it plays into a child's desire to please you as an individual.

You may also gently bargain with a child. For example, you can use the "When-then" strategy: "*When* you have your shot, *then* you can have a cup of orange juice." You can also offer a choice to involve the child in the decision-making. "You can have the insulin shot in your arm or in your leg."

If the child is crying or panicking, calmly ask, "Can I help you?" In almost all cases, the parent or caregiver will accompany the child into the examination room. Ask the parent or caregiver for assistance whenever possible, including gently restraining the child when necessary.

Communicating With Elderly Patients

The communication process in general is complex and can be further complicated by age. One of the biggest challenges health care providers face when dealing with older patients is that they are actually more heterogeneous, or diverse in their character, than younger patients. Their wide range of life experiences and cultural backgrounds often influence their perception of illness, willingness to adhere to medical regimens, and ability to communicate effectively with health care providers and professionals.

Communication can also be hindered by the normal aging process, which may involve sensory loss, decline in memory, slower processing of information, lessening of power and influence over their own lives, retirement from work, and separation from family and friends.

However, in most cases, you will communicate with elderly patients just as you would anyone else. You may be more alert to the possibility of any of the disabilities discussed previously, such as hearing loss. Keep in mind that most elderly people are as able and competent as anyone else. However, there are certain groups of elderly people who have special communication needs.

Communicating With Patients and Co-Workers From Different Generations

For the first time in history, we now have five distinct generations in the workplace as co-workers or patients, with each generation bringing its own set of values, norms, and expectations to the job. The five generations include:
* Baby Boomers
* Generation X
* Millennials or Generation Y

* Generation Z
* Generation Alpha.

In health care, where communication is so important, it is important to understand the dynamics of each generation, so you can adjust verbal, nonverbal, and listening communication skills as necessary. Table 6.1 summarizes each generation and its general characteristics. There is a lot of media discussion that tends to stereotype each generation, defining each age group's values and work styles as the same. However, caution should always be used when stereotyping. Patients should be treated and valued based on their unique attributes and not on the year they were born.

Patients With Dementia and Other Organic Brain Diseases

There are many stages of organic brain diseases affecting memory and function. However, the following strategies are useful for communicating with patients experiencing all but the most profound stages of these diseases:
* Approach patients from the front, within their line of vision, so as not to startle them. Face them as you talk to hold their attention.
* Minimize distracting hand movements, and keep in mind that your body language may convey more meaning than your actual words.
* Smile often; a frown could be misinterpreted.
* Speak in a normal tone of voice and greet the patient as you would any other patient. If anything, speak at a slower pace and in a quieter, more soothing tone.
* Choose a quiet meeting place, one without a lot of stimulation or distractions.
* Respect the patient's personal space. If they pace, walk with them while you talk.
* Refocus a distracted person's attention by pointing back to yourself or to a calm feature, such as plants or a window view.
* Ask only one question at a time and use questions to refocus. For example, "You were telling me about your favorite television show."
* Because many people with dementia have better long-term memories than short-term memories, ask them questions about their past.

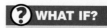 **WHAT IF?**

What if a patient with Alzheimer's disease is arguing with another staff member? How would you intervene to defuse the situation?

TABLE 6.1
General Characteristics of Each Generation

Type	Birth Years	General Characteristics
Baby Boomers	1946–1964	* Value hard work—often working 60 + hours weekly to advance * Less flexible * Loyal to employer
Generation X	1965–1976	* Disillusioned, post-Boomer skeptics * Value work-life balance and seek flexibility
Generation Y or Millennials	1977–1995	* Largest generation in the workplace today * Enthusiastic and collaborative * Embrace technology * Prefer working in groups
Generation Z or iGen	1996–2009	* Optimistic, confident, and happy * Likely to be better off financially than their parents * Technology trend setters * Fastest growing group * Always had access to transformative business models such as Uber, Netflix, and Tinder
Generation Alpha	Born after 2010	* First generation who never knew a time without social media * Most technologically savvy

CASE STUDY 6.2
Advocate for the Deaf

Eva was an experienced dental assistant. She had been working in Dr. Richter's office for about 6 months, having moved to Rochester because of her husband's relocation. She liked the office and the people there, and she was getting to know the patients.

Eva was a little apprehensive today because her 1:00 p.m. appointment, Millicent Marquis, was deaf. Her husband, Tommy, served as her interpreter. Over lunch, Dr. Richter shared some information with her about Millicent.

"She's just coming in for a cleaning, assuming nothing else has come up," Dr. Richter told Eva. "I usually don't bother giving her to one of the hygienists because she is comfortable with me, and we're able to communicate with one another. But she's a big advocate for people with disabilities, and she'll give you a piece of her mind if things go poorly."

Millie was a large woman in her 70s with wild red hair. She walked with two canes and with the assistance of her husband, a wiry man with white hair. "I can't hear without him, and I can't walk without these," she announced, in a voice that was loud and intelligible but somewhat garbled. Dr. Richter greeted her and escorted her to the closest examination room, helping her, with Tommy's assistance, into the dental chair.

Dr. Richter got in front of Millie and made eye contact with her. "We have a new dental assistant, Millie. Her name is Eva Plume," and she pointed to Eva, who moved into Millie's line of sight.

"I guess I'll have to break her in," said Millie. Dr. Richter raised her arm to get Millie's attention. "Go easy on her, Millie. I want to keep her," she joked. Then Dr. Richter said she would be back shortly, and Eva would stay with her.

"I guess you can't hear me," Eva said nervously.

"No, but I can read your lips."

Eva watched in amazement while Tommy gave her a flurry of signs with his hands.

"Oh, she'll survive," said Millie.

"What kind of a dental office is this that I have to bring my own interpreter? He's totally unreliable. You should provide your deaf patients with a professional interpreter."

"That would be nice," said Eva.

"Nice? Did you say nice? It's the law, you know. I have a right to know what's going on."

"Don't take her too seriously," Tommy said to Eva, signing to Millie at the same time. "She definitely knows what's going on, and I'm definitely unreliable."

That made Millie laugh, but then she got serious. "Can you understand me, Eva?"

"Yes. I can."

"Good, because we need a few rules."

"Okay," Eva nodded.

"If you or that Dr. Richter hurt me, I'm going to raise my right hand, and you are going to stop immediately, got it?" Eva nodded.

"If I just want a break from the action, I'll raise my left hand." Eva nodded again.

"Thank you for nodding, Eva. That's something I can understand."

Just then Dr. Richter came back in. She had been wearing a mask, but she took it off.

"Eva knows the rules," Millie told Dr. Richter, and Dr. Richter smiled and winked at Eva.

Throughout the cleaning, Dr. Richter explained everything she was doing, and Tommy translated it to Millie.

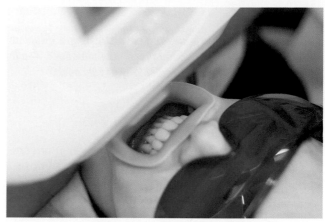

iStock.com/tonefotografia/1376031764

Dr. Richter stopped occasionally to ask Millie if she needed a break.

QUESTIONS FOR THOUGHT AND REFLECTION

1. What would you most worry about it if you were in Eva's position and about to meet a patient like Millie?
2. What actions did Dr. Richter take to make it easier for Millie to communicate with her and Eva?
3. Did Dr. Richter use Tommy appropriately as an interpreter?

A Different Path

Robert was nearing the end of a long day as a medical assistant in Dr. Seldek's office. There was just one appointment left, Ms. Moriarty, and he wanted to get her in and out.

"Moriarty?" Robert asked the elderly woman with a cane.

"Yes, that's me." She replied.

"Are you here by yourself?"

"No, my friend is waiting for me in the car. It's hard for her to walk, and I'm just here to get my, uh, thingamajig checked."

"Sit over there, and the doctor will be with you shortly," Robert said, pointing.

"Where?" she asked as she looked at him through her dark glasses.

"Ma'am, over there," he pointed again.

"Where?" Ms. Moriarty repeated.

Robert was getting impatient. "I need you to sit over there. Can't you see?"

"As a matter of fact, young man, I can't," she says as she smiles and points to her dark glasses.

"Oh boy," Robert said to himself as he moved around the desk to help Ms. Moriarty. He grabbed her arm, which startled her. "Sorry," he muttered. He quickly escorted her to the row of chairs, positioned her in front of the first one, placed one of his feet behind hers, and plopped her down onto the seat. "Oh my," she gasped.

When Robert returned to his station, his colleague Anika approached him. "What are you doing?"

"She's blind," Robert replied.

"I know that. But that's not how you treat a person with a visual impairment."

"Oh yeah? What would you do?"

QUESTIONS FOR THOUGHT AND REFLECTION

1. What would you have done if you were Robert in this situation?
2. What mistakes did Robert make in the way he physically interacted with Ms. Moriarty?

EXPERIENTIAL EXERCISES

Along with a partner, put headphones over your ears or cotton in your ears to simulate a hearing impairment. Talk with your partner for 10 minutes.

1. Have a 10-minute conversation with a partner using only written communication.
2. Take turns guiding each other when one is wearing a mask. Be sure to use touch and provide verbal cues to one another.

⟲ CROSS CURRENTS WITH OTHER SOFT SKILLS

AIMING TO BE ADAPTABLE AND FLEXIBLE: Sometimes you have to think on your feet when communicating with people with disabilities (Chapter 7).

STRIVING FOR TOLERANCE: People with disabilities are entitled to the same high-quality health care as everybody else (Chapter 15).

SHOWING EMPATHY, SENSITIVITY, AND CARING: Caring for people with disabilities gives you an opportunity to practice the values that are at the core of health care (Chapter 13).

PRACTICING PATIENCE: This is when your patience really pays off (Chapter 5).

References

Beckman HB, Frankel RM. The effect of physician behavior on the collection of data. *Ann Intern Med*. 1984;101(5): 692–696.

Managing Conflicts

- Consider Conflict as a Natural Aspect of the Workplace
- Understand the Role of Ego in Conflict
- Understand the Different Types of Difficult People
- Develop a General Strategy for Dealing With All Types of Difficult People
- Learn How to Separate Emotions From Problems

Managing and Resolving Conflict

The art of being wise is the art of knowing what to overlook.

—William James

LEARNING OBJECTIVE 1:
MANAGING AND RESOLVING CONFLICT

- Gain insight into conflicts by being self-aware.
- Name the five conflict management styles.
- Identify other sources of conflict in the workplace.
- Understand how reframing the conversation can eliminate conflict.
- Develop different skills for conflict resolution.

Conflicts

What do you think of when you hear the word "conflict?" Conflict is generally defined as an incompatibility of goals or values between two or more people in a relationship. Conflict arises from differences. It occurs when people disagree over their values, motivations, perceptions, or ideas. It can also occur as a response to frustration or competitive instincts. Conflicts surface because of real or perceived issues, problems, or disputes and rarely go away until they are addressed. If we truly invest ourselves and communicate openly and honestly, we can *resolve* real issues. However, many of us avoid the hard work and choose to communicate politely, superficially, and we only *settle* our conflicts in the moment. By settling, instead of resolving, we are not truly discussing the root of the problem because we are uncomfortable, we feel vulnerable, or we are not skilled at handling our emotions or the emotions of others.

Many workplace conflicts happen because of misunderstandings, miscommunications, or the wrong choice of language or tone. We have the opportunity to resolve our conflicts in a healthy way when we learn how to problem-solve, actively listen, and discuss issues with the intent of finding common ground and a mutual solution.

If you have not received training on how to manage personal or workplace conflict, you are not alone. Most of us receive very little training before we are in the midst of a conflict and forced to confront or, too often, avoid the situation. We will tackle some of the strategies and approaches to conflict management and prevention in this chapter.

Self-Awareness

In every conflict, there is an opportunity to examine our behavior and what we are bringing to the dispute. As discussed in earlier chapters, we need to actively listen, learn, and work together to improve relationships and the culture inside our organizations. We have the responsibility and control to avoid negative and destructive behavior that destroys relationships, teams, and company goodwill.

Once we accept our responsibility in the conflict and let go of the emotional investment of being right, we can truly begin the work of self-discovery and collaboration that is necessary to effectively resolve conflict. Even though conflict can be positive, we are conditioned to think it is going to be a negative experience—something involving winners and losers, so it can be difficult to keep our personal needs at bay. Instead of seeking solutions, we expect to win or lose, and fight and defend.

In managing conflict, our individual personalities will often play a significant role. Sigmund Freud, an Austrian neurologist and the founder of psychoanalysis, famously coined the terms "ego," "superego," and "the id" to describe his personality theories. According to Freud, the id is the most primitive part of our personality and tells us to satisfy our basic needs, such as hunger and sex. The superego, on the other hand, is the moralistic part of our personality and incorporates the values and morals of society learned from our parents and others. The ego works to mediate the id and the superego. The ego prevents us from acting on our basic urges from our id by maintaining our moral and idealistic standards from our superego. For example, your supervisor yells at you about something that was not your fault. Your id may give you the impulse to

yell back and say it was not your fault. However, your superego reminds you that they are your supervisor, and you should not yell back. The ego is the rational part of our mind and balances between the id and superego and stops you from yelling at your supervisor, which may get you fired and unable to pay your rent and bills. Our ego tells us to calmly explain the situation.

Recognizing and Resolving Conflicting Needs

If you are out of touch with your feelings or so stressed out that you can only pay attention to a limited number of emotions, it will be difficult to understand your own needs. In workplace conflicts, differing needs are often at the heart of bitter disputes. When you can recognize the legitimacy of conflicting needs and become willing to examine them openly, it opens pathways to creative problem-solving, team building, and improved relationships. Successful conflict resolution improves when you can:

* **Manage stress while remaining calm and alert.** By staying calm, you can accurately read and interpret verbal and nonverbal communication.
* **Control your emotions and behavior.** When you are in control of your emotions, you can communicate your needs without threatening others.
* **Be aware of and respectful of differences.** By avoiding disrespectful words and actions, you can resolve conflicts much faster.

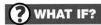 **WHAT IF?**

What if you observed a conflict that was conducted with politeness and civility in your workplace? Would that surprise you? How do you think that is possible?

Conflict Resolution

We all deal with conflict in different ways, and we therefore resort to one of several conflict management styles. There are five common conflict resolution strategies: avoidance, compromise, collaboration, accommodation, and competition (Figure 7.1).

Before we can develop effective strategies, however, we have to learn to recognize old habits—good and bad. By knowing our own default patterns, we can become self-aware and choose more effective conflict management styles. As you read the five types of conflict management styles, which of them is your most common reaction to conflict? Ask yourself if you are trying to resolve or simply settle the conflict.

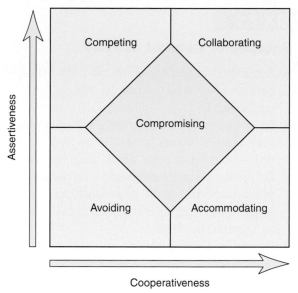

Figure 7.1 Adaptation of the Thomas-Kilmann Conflict Mode Instrument for Conflict Styles (Thomas and Kilmann, 1974).

Avoidance

Avoidance is when we ignore or withdraw from the conflict. When we lack effective conflict management skills, it is normal to try and avoid the conflict or pretend it does not exist at all. We may also choose to avoid conflict when the discomfort of confrontation exceeds the benefits of resolution. However, when conflict is avoided, nothing is resolved. When we avoid the issue, we are not only missing an opportunity to identify and resolve the underlying problem, but it is also likely that the conflict will continue to fester and cause further damage inside the organization.

Avoidance can nevertheless be appropriate when the outcome of the conflict is trivial or when you have no chance of resolution. It can also be effective when the issue would be very costly or when the atmosphere is very emotionally charged, and you need to create some space. In general, avoidance is not an effective long-term strategy to resolve conflicts.

That's what peace is, right? Postponing the conflict until the thing you were fighting over doesn't matter.

—James S.A. Corey

Compromise

Compromise is finding a middle ground or forgoing some of your concerns and needs and committing to others' concerns and needs. It lets everyone give up a little of what they want, and no one gets everything they want. The perception of the best outcome when working by compromise is one that "splits the difference."

Compromise can be an effective approach if the outcome is satisfactory to all parties. As a starting point, compromise can foster creativity and teamwork, which can be positive approaches to a solution. Conversely, compromise will be unsatisfying if one or more of the parties are unhappy with the compromise. In these cases, the parties have settled merely to avoid further conflict. Additionally, overuse of compromise may lead to loss of long-term goals, a lack of trust, creation of a cynical environment, and being viewed as having no firm values. However, refusing to compromise may lead to unnecessary confrontations, frequent power struggles, and ineffective negotiating.

JOURNALING 7.1

Think about a compromise you have made recently and describe it in your journal. How did it come about? Are you satisfied with it? Should you have handled the conflict differently?

Accommodation

Accommodation is a strategy in which one party gives in to the wishes of another. Accommodation takes compromise one step further by addressing the concerns of the other party rather than your own—accommodating another to preserve harmony or avoid further disruption. This approach is effective when the other party is the expert or has a better solution. It can also be effective for preserving future relations with the other party.

Although this approach pays off if the other party possesses the optimal solution, be careful not to be too accommodating, and make sure you are being accommodating for the right reasons. If you always accommodate the needs of others before considering your needs, people may see you as indecisive or easily manipulated. This perception can prevent you from advancing or achieving your goals.

Competition

Competition is a style used by people who go into a conflict planning to win. It is to stress your position without considering opposing points of view. Competition is not generally a productive conflict management approach because its aim is control rather than progress. But it may be commonly used when we need to take quick action, make unpopular decisions, or handle critical issues.

With the competing style, you act in a very assertive way to achieve your goals, without trying to cooperate with or understand the other person. Sometimes competitive people have no idea what they want, just that they want to win. Although being assertive can help you reach your goals, blind assertiveness that lacks cooperation is detrimental. Do not forget that providing health care is a team effort and that your colleagues have valuable wisdom to share.

Collaboration

Collaboration is the optimal approach in most cases. It involves seeking the input of all parties involved in the conflict in order to satisfy both parties, which makes everyone feel validated. This style is frequently appropriate in a team environment.

Collaboration incorporates the positive aspects of compromising, because it encourages developing a broad range of potential solutions through teamwork and creativity. It requires your ability to use active listening, confront difficult situations in a nonthreatening way, and use critical thinking. Although irrational parties may never agree to a reasonable solution, this approach uses problem-solving to implement solutions, even over the objection of irrational parties, in the interests of a higher goal, such as patient safety.

> **JOURNALING 7.2**
>
> Consider a recent conflict either at work or in your personal life. Which conflict resolution style did you use? Was it effective in resolving the conflict and meeting your needs? If not, which conflict style do you wish you used?

Identifying Sources of Conflict at Work

Conflict is centered on disagreements. So, how should we approach conflict when we encounter it? Knowing the source of the workplace conflict is often the first step toward resolving it (Box 7.1). Taking time to understand why a conflict is occurring will allow you to collect the right tools to successfully resolve the conflict.

Take a moment to review what people in the dispute *do* agree on. This helps create a context in which the disagreement seems a little smaller in scope and importance. Resist the urge to criticize, condemn, or complain. Document and describe the current problem and get agreement from both sides. For instance, a dispute might arise in the waiting room as to who arrived first. Assure everyone that they will see the

---

> **BOX 7.1**
>
> ## Sources of Conflict at Work
>
> - Assumptions and expectations both cause conflict when they are not commonly understood.
> - Core values, such as honesty, are not being met. Many conflicts appear to be over surface issues, but these often mask deep issues.
> - Different personal lenses and interpretations of the world based on insensitivity to other's religion, political beliefs, or moral convictions can lead to conflict.
> - Emotions: Once emotions are engaged, logic and common sense can get lost.
> - Gossip and cliques: Whether you are in high school or at work, gossip and "in" crowds are destructive.
> - Miscommunication and vague or thoughtless language can lead to unnecessary conflict. Try to pause and choose the right words the first time. It is extremely difficult to correct a misimpression that you caused with careless language.

doctor shortly. The dispute has not been resolved, but the common ground makes it seem less important.

Try to pretend you are in the other person's position. Encourage conflicting team members to ask themselves, "How does my personal bias affect this relationship?"

Due to interdependency of employee relationships and the real-world effect of decisions in the workplace (e.g., raises, hours, bonuses, promotions), the workplace can be a breeding ground for unhealthy conflict. Left unaddressed, unhealthy conflict can quickly turn into a hostile work environment that results in increased employee dissatisfaction and turnover, absenteeism, poor performance and productivity, and even litigation.

Communication Conflict

The root cause of most conflict is poor communication. Ineffective communication can result in missed deadlines, missed opportunities, and misunderstandings. Miscommunication and misunderstanding can create conflict even where there are no basic incompatibilities. With more employees working remotely and using more electronic means of communication, there is an increase in the number of ways we can miscommunicate. Therefore it is important that we take time to think before we speak, carefully read our emails before we hit send, and always consider the needs and perspectives of others. We also need to know when to have a direct conversation or phone call with a person instead of sending an email that may be misinterpreted, further exacerbating the conflict.

With direct or face-to-face communication, listening and being able to convey body language will help your co-worker or patient feel their concerns are being heard and are more likely to listen to your point of view. This approach creates a deeper, more meaningful relationship and offers the best course toward conflict resolution.

When communicating via email or other written communication, it is important to carefully craft your words and thoughts. Because email can be impersonal, think about ways to humanize your message. The recipient of the email will not have the benefit of seeing your facial expression or hearing the tone of your voice; therefore it is important that you clearly communicate your key message. Lack of skill in communicating what we really mean in a clear and respectful fashion often results in confusion, hurt, and anger, all of which simply feed the conflict process. Avoid any confrontational language when writing emails, such as unnecessarily capitalizing or bolding words. Remember, emails will likely be forwarded to others within the company, so never put anything in writing that you would not say to a group of co-workers or a patient.

Economic and Resource Conflict

Economic conflict involves competing to attain scarce resources. We all need access to certain resources to do our jobs well. This may include office supplies, help from co-workers, reserving a meeting room, and even more compensation. When more than one person or group needs access to a particular resource, conflict can occur. In this type of conflict, each person wants to get the most they can, and the behavior and emotions of each party are focused on obtaining the most resources or the resources they need.

Health care facilities are undergoing unprecedented consolidation through mergers and acquisitions as health care transitions from nonprofit to for-profit entities. Businesses have continually had to use strategies, such as cost-cutting, productivity gains, and efficiencies through automation. All these changes, often unwanted by workers, can lead to conflicts and employee stress and uncertainty.

Relationship Conflict

Difficult co-workers and patients add stress and conflict to any workplace, and health care is no exception. Relationship conflicts occur when two people have incompatible needs, goals, or approaches in their ability to communicate. Relationship conflicts occur because of strong negative emotions, misperceptions, poor communication, or negative behavior.

Relationship problems often fuel disputes that can spiral beyond the initial conflict when they go unresolved. Encouraging a balanced expression of perspectives and emotions for acknowledgment is one effective approach to managing relational conflict.

Relationship conflict can also be the result of strong personality differences. Personality conflict refers to differences in motives, values, or styles in dealing with people. Personality conflict can be more challenging to resolve. For example, if both parties in the relationship have a high need for power and both want to be dominant in the relationship, it is difficult to find common ground that allows both parties to be satisfied, and a power struggle begins.

In a customer-oriented environment such as health care, conflict arises among co-workers when someone fails to act because the co-worker believes a task is not their responsibility—a response seldom acceptable when it comes to patient care (Figure 7.2). Patients and their families are the reason your employer exists, and their care is the focus of your work. Patients and their families are often in personal crisis or acute stress, and their behavior can lead to conflict with the health care providers and professionals they encounter. In health care, customer satisfaction is everyone's job, although people can be difficult at times.

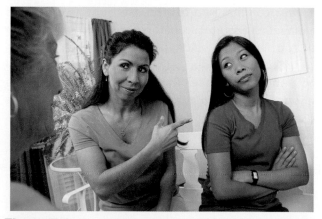

Figure 7.2 Co-workers disagreeing about work duties may lead to conflict. (Copyright © istock.com.)

Nothing gives one person so much advantage over another as to remain always cool and unruffled under all circumstances.

—Thomas Jefferson

Power Conflict

Power struggles occur when each party wants to maintain or maximize its amount of influence in the relationship. It is impossible for one party to be stronger without the other being weaker, at least in terms of direct influence over each other. Thus, a power struggle ensues, which usually ends in a victory and defeat or in a "stand-off" with a continuing state of tension. Power conflicts can occur between individuals or between groups.

Values Conflict

Values conflict is caused by perceived or actual incompatible belief systems. Values are fundamental beliefs that give meaning to people's lives and dictate their behavior, such as honesty, justice, and integrity. Values help us decide what is right versus wrong or what we perceive as unjust.

Employees with differing values work in harmony all the time. However, disputes over values typically surface when people attempt to force their values on others or when their beliefs do not allow for divergent opinions.

Conflict Resolution Skills

The quality of our lives depends not on whether or not we have conflicts, but on how we respond to them.

—Thomas Crum

Once you have identified the source or cause of your conflict, you can choose from a number of management strategies before it escalates. Once you set your emotions aside, the key is to then focus on strategies under your control by reframing (changing your perspective) the conflict and then taking action. Conflict can result in destructive outcomes or creative ones, depending on the approach that is taken. If we can effectively manage the conflict, we can often find new solutions that are satisfactory to both parties.

The first step of conflict resolution is to focus on things that are within your control. These choices will divert your attention from the negatives and give you something positive to focus on.

* **Change your perspective.** In cognitive psychology, this is called "reframing." What if you no longer

cared how a dispute turns out? What if you viewed circumstances from a different perspective? You do not have to be a prisoner of your own preferences or biases.

* **Review your personal goals.** Goals are aspirations that are truly important. How does the outcome of the conflict fit into your larger goals? This perspective might change the importance you attach to a particular conflict, position, or solution.
* **Change your response.** Visualize what happens if you choose a different response. Listen and then restate your colleagues' or patient's concern. Ask yourself if you are responsible in a significant way for what has happened. Are your expectations for a resolution unrealistic, out of line, or just not that important? What can you learn from this calm analysis? What solutions might arise from your thoughtful considerations?
* **Check your impulse control.** Ask yourself why some people you know do not seem to get caught up in certain kinds of conflicts. Ask them for their perspective and advice.
* Finally, **act like a third-party mediator** in your own mind. Step outside of yourself for a moment. Ask questions. Why is this issue so important? If you were a disinterested bystander, what could you see that might help resolve a conflict?

If addressing the issue still feels important once you have tried reframing the conflict, it probably is. In this case, it is time to take action, often collaboratively. All negotiators use well-established skills to help end conflict. By now, these may seem like common sense to you, but it is worth examining them from a health care perspective.

Learning How to Listen

Listen first, talk second. When people are upset, the words they use rarely convey the issues at the heart of the conflict. When we listen for what is felt, as well as what is said, we have an opportunity to connect more deeply to our own needs and emotions and to those of others. Listening in this way also makes it easier for others to hear us. Use a friendly and calm tone of voice. Most team conflicts are rooted in communication breakdowns. Always show respect for the other person's opinions or views.

During a conflict, make sure you understand what the other person is telling you from their point of view. Repeat what the other person tells you and ask if you have understood them correctly. Resist the temptation to interject your point of view until the other person has finished speaking.

Setting a Positive Example

You can exercise leadership simply by holding your behavior to a higher level. This can be challenging at times, and you may ask "Why me, and why doesn't the other person take the high road?" Suppose you observe two nursing assistants standing outside of a patient's room, arguing over whose turn it is to clean the room. "I'll do it since the patient needs our help," you say, going into the room. The conflict is likely to dissipate because of your positive example (Figure 7.3). This may also remind your co-workers that this is not about them but about the patient's care.

Your attitude is essential to the outcome. Stay positive. For example, if you have a difficult team member, try to list five strengths they have and show the team how those traits can benefit the team's goals.

When they go low, we go high.

—Michelle Obama

Exchanging Ideas

Conflicts are not necessarily negative. They can be positive and beneficial when used to effectively solve problems, develop interpersonal relationships, and promote collaboration among co-workers.

You can change a negative conflict into a positive and productive conflict by refocusing the discussion on the issues rather than on the people and their emotions. For example, Andy wants to sterilize the instruments at the beginning of the day, but Susan wants to do it at the end of the day when she has more time.

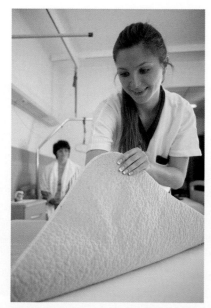

Figure 7.3 A nursing assistant changes bed linen, setting a positive example of patient care. (Copyright © istock.com.)

Before allowing the conflict to escalate, take a moment to assess the situation and make a plan to resolve the conflict. How long does the sterilization take? How many instruments need to be sterilized? Are there other tasks that need to be prioritized? By asking questions about the process and best practices, you have introduced new considerations that may help reduce the tension in the discussion or resolve the conflict all together.

Another method to facilitate ideas between co-workers is changing your perspective. Put yourself in the other's position. Encourage feedback. Use "I" and "we" messages rather than "you" messages. Listen with an open mind, and wait until the other person is finished speaking before speaking yourself. Maintain perspective and a sense of purpose. Look for areas of agreement and ways to negotiate compromise with others.

Evidence-Based Decision Making

By referring to an objective source, personal conflicts can often be abandoned more readily. The best way to do this is using an evidence-based approach, which is a strategic method of applying empirical knowledge or data and research-supported principles to make logical and reasoned decisions. For example, if the conflict has to do with infection control practices, you might suggest that everyone examine the latest universal precautions guidelines issued by the Centers for Disease Control and Prevention or the Occupational Safety and Health Administration, which should resolve the conflict.

Avoid criticizing or passing judgment on ideas and opinions. It is important to remember to allow the person who is incorrect to retreat with dignity. This means not making them feel bad or foolish about being in error. Maintain a rational goal-oriented state of mind. Outline ways to improve accountability for behavior and attitude. Stay fact focused rather than personality focused. Build skills by working through differences and show your willingness to be flexible in achieving your organization's goals.

🔄 JOURNALING 7.3

Can you learn anything from a situation that will help you avoid being drawn into these kinds of conflicts in the future? In most cases, each situation offers insights for the future. Remember a recent conflict and list three things you learned from it—about yourself, the other party, or the situation.

Dominick decided to see a counselor at the hospital's Employee Assistance Program (EAP) before making a final decision about his career. He had been a first responder and paramedic for the Spring Valley Medical Center for almost 15 years. He does not want to resign but feels he has been pushed to his limit.

He admitted it. Lately, he had been difficult to get along with. Over the past year, he had gotten into numerous arguments with his co-workers. The tragedies that he had witnessed as part of his job were starting to affect him, especially those involving children.

About 2 weeks ago, he had been in a really foul mood, and he did not even know why. A call came in as soon as he arrived at work. It was a woman experiencing early labor in a remote area of town. He got into the driver's side of the ambulance and started driving way too fast for the dark conditions and winding roads.

"Slow down! You're going to get us in an accident," yelled Dave, as they slid on some gravel along the edge of a curve.

"Shut up! I'm driving!" Dominick barked back.

On the way back to the hospital, he was even worse. Dave kept telling him to slow down and reminding him that he had passengers this time—a pregnant woman and her husband.

Two days later, Dominick received an email from Dr. Alfred Singh, the head of the Emergency Department, informing him that he was not allowed to drive pending further notice.

Dominick explained all of this to the EAP counselor.

"What did Dr. Singh say when you talked to him about it?"

"I didn't talk to him about it. I'm not talking to him after getting an email like that! What's there to say?!"

"Well, Dr. Singh does have a responsibility to his department and to the safety of his staff and patients. I'm sure he's just following protocol," the counselor commented.

"No, it's not right. I didn't do anything wrong. The mother and baby are fine and I didn't get into an accident. People are getting upset at me for no reason."

"You seem very angry about it."

"Yeah, I am!" he said, raising his voice.

Dominick paused for a moment before saying, "I've been angry a lot lately," almost surprised at his confession.

"Then let's talk about that," she said.

Dominick filled her in on the past year.

"It's understandable that you're going through this. Your job is very stressful, and you witness a lot of traumatic events," she said. "I suggest you try to find techniques to relieve stress and reframe your thoughts to better deal with the conflict and stress you're dealing with," she said.

"I'm open to anything," said Dominick. "I'm not myself and I'm afraid it'll get worse."

She taught him to take some deep breaths. She urged him to hold his reactions to stressors and to think about his response before taking any action. She encouraged him to consider perspectives other than his own. For example, how did the mother or father feel when you were driving so quickly? She also suggested that Dominick apologize to some of his co-workers who were on the receiving end of his rage, and she recommended he meet with Dr. Singh.

Dominick made an appointment to see Dr. Singh in his office.

After apologizing to Dr. Singh about the situation, he explained that he was seeing an EAP counselor to help him deal with stress and conflict.

"I appreciate your coming to speak with me and that you took the initiative to do some personal reflection," said Dr. Singh.

After they finished talking, Dominick decided he was going to apologize to Dave.

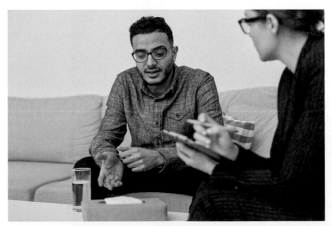
iStock.com/SeventyFour/953262972

QUESTIONS FOR THOUGHT AND REFLECTION

1. What part did emotions play in his conflicts?
2. If you were asked to counsel Dominick, what else would you tell him?

3. In this situation, what would Dominick's response be according to his id, superego, and ego?
4. Have you ever been reprimanded like Dominick, and what was your response? Did it result in a positive or negative outcome?

A Different Path

Southwestern Physical Therapy had just acquired five new continuous passive motion (CPM) machines for total knee replacements. Rick Cervantes, the owner of the practice, was excited about having this equipment to offer to his patients.

"By working with Orthopedics Southwest, we can rent each machine out for $350 a week—that's twice the rate that the local medical supply vendors charge. We can roll it into all the other billing, and nobody will be able to tell."

"I don't know," said Gary Loo, one of the physical therapists." Since Isabelle left, we don't have anyone trained on these things."

"These are patient controlled," scoffed Rick. "Look. They can operate them by themselves."

"It says here you can lock the patient out," said Gary, looking at the manual. "You can set sequence codes that keep the patient from adjusting the settings. What about the Interferential Therapy units? Are you going to use them to subdue the pain?"

"Great idea, Gary. We can add the IT units to the package and charge $450 a week. I can get portable IT units online for $100 apiece."

Gary shook his head.

"Now what?"

"I only brought up the IT units because, if you suppress the pain, the patients won't know that the settings are wrong. That could really damage a knee replacement."

"And what is the probability of that happening, Gary?"

"I really don't know, Rick. But it could happen and we should be concerned about that."

"Low," said Rick. "That's the probability."

Gary just lowered his head.

"Okay, Gary. Do you have any other concerns here? We're just trying to make a little money and run a business, if that's OK with you."

"Well, I understand that. But what if Orthopedics Southwest notices we're gouging the patients on these devices. That's not going to sit too well."

"Are you kidding me, Gary? Do you think they care what we charge? It's the insurance that pays anyways. Besides, we're not going to itemize this stuff."

Within 6 months, a CPM machine from Southwest Physical Therapy tore a patient's knee replacement, and the patient could not feel it because of the Interferential Therapy unit.

Art Kreutzer, the owner of Orthopedics Southwest, asked to meet with Rick. He asked Rick, "Why weren't the sequence keys used to lock out the patient operation?"

Rick explained that the risk was low and that something like this could happen with the new CPM machines.

"But you knew that it was a risk, right?" said Dr. Kreutzer. "Because of your decision, you have made me liable for this patient's injury. I'm sorry to inform you but Orthopedics Southwest can no longer use Southwest Physical Therapy as one of its providers."

QUESTIONS FOR THOUGHT AND REFLECTION

1. What role did Gary have in this situation? Do you think he should have been more assertive?
2. Was Gary satisfied with the decision that was made on the CPM machines?
3. What conflict resolution style did Rick use?

1. Identify people in your life—at school, work, church—who seem able to effectively manage conflicts. Ask them about their strategies.
2. Watch a political debate or a news program featuring people with conflicting views. How much of the exchange is about issues and how much about egos? Were any of these conflicts resolved? Were they able to listen to the other person to gain his or her perspective?

🌀 CROSS CURRENTS WITH OTHER SOFT SKILLS

MANAGING STRESS: Managing conflict shares a lot with managing stress (Chapter 3).

LISTENING ACTIVELY: Conflict cannot be effectively managed without listening (Chapter 6).

CONTRIBUTING AS A MEMBER OF THE TEAM: Whether it is contributing to positive conflict or defusing negative conflict, managing conflict is part of your responsibility to your co-workers (Chapter 15).

SHOWING EMPATHY, SENSITIVITY, AND CARING: These skills will enable you to manage conflict caused by sick, anxious patients and their families (Chapter 6).

Dealing with Challenging People

No one cooperates with people who seem to be against them.

—Rick Kirschner

LEARNING OBJECTIVE 2: DEALING WITH DIFFICULT PEOPLE

- State why extreme behavior can become problematic.
- Name four approaches to dealing with difficult people.
- Recognize the range of difficult behaviors.
- Connect patterns of dysfunctional behavior with their best remedies.
- Identify general tactics for dealing with difficult people.

At work, you will have to interact with a number of different people, and some of them may be dysfunctional or difficult to interact with. In the past, you may have been able to avoid difficult people, but being a health care professional requires collaboration and working with all team members and patients. You often do not get to pick the people you work with, and you do not get to pick your patients. You do not have to like everyone at work. You do, however, have to find a way to work with everyone and be professional.

For the most part, your co-workers will be excellent to work with and your patient interactions will be rewarding. However, in every job you will sometimes encounter people who are challenging to work with. Even those who mean well can take a positive trait too far. For example, good workers may become perfectionists, responsible people may become controlling, and sociable people may want to talk when you are trying to concentrate. Sometimes even nice people will still simply rub us the wrong way.

The trouble with people who have no vices is that they have some pretty annoying virtues.

—Elizabeth Taylor

Approaches to Challenging People

Sooner or later in our personal lives and careers, we will all encounter someone whose behavior itself is genuinely problematic or dysfunctional. What do you do then?

There are several methods for dealing with challenging people. All of them will be effective at one time or another. Your response will depend on the type of behavior you are confronted with.

⬅ JOURNALING 7.4

Record what kind of work environment you have. Is it getting the work done, getting the work done correctly, socializing, or seeking recognition?

Discuss the Problem

It may be best to have a conversation with the person instead of letting the behavior continue. Having a calm discussion about the conflict may deliver a surprising response. Remember to use the communication skills we learned earlier.

Most people do not realize the adverse and negative effects their statements and actions have on others. Try to remain calm, allow them to express their point of view, and be open and honest about how you are being affected by their behavior.

Control Your Own Response

As with any conflict, focus on issues directly under your control. When dealing with challenging people, you can control your own behavior, attitude, and approach. Avoid reflecting the same behavior coming at you, as tempting as that may be. This is the worst thing you can do. By responding in kind, you validate the behavior and encourage the person to continue their inappropriate behavior. Moreover, responding with anger impairs your judgment and is likely to escalate the conflict. It is best to withhold your reaction until you can rationally choose your response.

Learn to respond and not react. When we react, we often panic and proceed, usually poorly. When we respond, we can pause, process, plan, and then proceed. Reacting is quick. Responding is slower. Responding creates more space between an event and what you do (or don't do) with it. In that space, you give immediate emotions some room to breathe, better understand what is happening, make a plan using the most evolved part of your brain, then go forward accordingly. Responding is harder than reacting. It takes more time and effort.

Change Your Attitude

Once you examine your role in a difficult relationship, you may find that your own behavior is contributing to the problem. This calls for a change in your attitude. Other times, you will find that you can improve the situation simply by being more empathetic or understanding.

Empathy is usually the best approach to a challenging patient. Listening actively, validating the patient's concerns, acting calmly, and being empathetic (placing yourself in their shoes) will ease the frustration the patient is displaying.

Change Your Approach

Changing your approach is like pressing the rewind button. First, identify the behavior that is difficult and see it in its more general pattern. Try to understand why that behavior is meeting the person's needs and gain some insight into what those needs are. Then, choose an approach or a strategy that is most likely to be effective, given the dynamics of the behavior you are being confronted with.

Ignore the Behavior

If you have tried all the other approaches and the person is still not being receptive, it might be best to ignore the inappropriate behavior and simply proceed with the work at hand. This is the best approach, for instance, with co-workers who often complain. You are not likely to stop these people from complaining. Ignore the complaining and refocus on your own duties and responsibilities.

Walk Away

In extreme cases, walking away may be your best action. If your co-worker is angry, threatening, insulting, or irrational, remove yourself from the situation. They are out of control, and addressing the problem at that time may not be possible.

In these cases, it may be more appropriate to wait and allow your co-worker to calm down. If the behavior continues, you may want to discuss this with your supervisor or the human resources department at your work.

Problem Behaviors in Co-Workers and Patients

You will encounter many people with different behaviors and personalities at work. Each type of person, whether a co-worker or a patient, presents special issues for you to deal with, and each issue calls for its own approach.

The Bully

In the workplace environment, bullies use force, threats, intimidation, or aggressive actions toward co-workers to get what they want. Bullies may be intelligent and talented, and they may consider themselves much more superior than anyone else they have to deal with. However, most bullies are very insecure. They can be quite charming in the presence of their superiors, but they intimidate their co-workers and subordinates by invading personal space, using aggressive language, and dominating conversations.

Usually, bullying does not have much to do with an actual work issue, although a work-related issue may spark the behavior. Bullying has more to do with a need to dominate or to feel powerful. Bullies work by homing in on your weaknesses or sensitive issues. If you submit to their behavior, the behavior will most likely continue.

Reflect on your personal sensitive areas and try to understand the source of these sensitivities. By recognizing them, you can develop strategies to prevent emotional reactions.

If you are in the presence of a bully when the behavior starts, you must calmly defend yourself. You can listen to gain information, but you must look the bully in the eye and speak in a calm voice without focusing on the bad behavior. Provide facts if the bully does not have them or is making statements not founded on facts, and ask questions to clarify issues. Give the bully feedback on the behavior by saying things such as, "You seem very angry about this. I wish I understood your concerns better." If the behavior is escalating, make the observation, "Your anger seems much worse than the actual problem here. Is something else bothering you?" Often, acknowledging the bully's behavior will shock the bully into controlling the inappropriate behavior.

Being the victim of a bully in a meeting or a public place is a different problem and may require a different approach. The bully's behavior is even more inexcusable because a greater element of humiliation is involved. Ask to speak to the person in private to resolve the issue. If you are being bullied via electronic communication, take the time to calm down before responding. For instance, do not reply to a threatening email right away. Before you reply, gather all of the necessary facts to develop a solution to the problem. Wait until you can craft a diplomatic response. Of course, forward the message to a supervisor if the message is abusive or threatening.

Ultimately, bullies act the way they do to elicit a response or to get what they want. Some bullies are not even aware of their behavior. Thus, it is important to defuse the situation and manage the bully's behavior. For example, if the bully is correct about a situation but is acting in an inappropriate manner, defuse the behavior by saying, "You're right. Here are the steps we're going to take to achieve these results." If the bully is incorrect, you can gain respect by presenting your ideas calmly and firmly without being confrontational.

If the bully's behavior crosses the line from dominating to abusive behavior, you should not tolerate it. In a calm but firm voice, insist that the bully end the abuse.

Although it may be difficult, avoid responding in an angry, argumentative manner. People who approach life from a hostile perspective love to argue;

if you fall into that trap, you lose. If necessary, leave. Approach the person later when the person is in a more rational, receptive frame of mind. Do not be afraid to point out that it is never acceptable to be rude at work. Ask if something else is going on that could account for such rude behavior. If you receive an apology, accept it and work to build a better rapport with this person.

The Provocateur

Provocateurs operate in the background, sniping at others, making them look foolish in public, and lowering others' credibility. They may appear to be innocent contributors, simply bringing up issues or information. For example, they may comment, "It looks like everyone but Mary signed up for the training" or "Gary, do you think all these x-rays are necessary?" Afterward, the provocateur may sit back and watch the action, enjoying any conflict that may arise. Sometimes the provocateur operates by gossiping, spreading rumors, and circulating inaccurate information.

If you are the victim of this behavior, clarify the situation and behavior with the person. If confronted, the person may just deny it and blame you for misinterpreting or overreacting. Calmly and politely ask the person what the purpose was in bringing up this issue.

The Know-It-All

The know-it-all is a person, as the name implies, who claims to know everything. They have a need to feel right and a compulsion to offer their advice on virtually any subject, because they are so knowledgeable and well informed. This person can be more of an annoyance than a danger. Ignoring them, however, even though it may seem the obvious strategy, often provokes an even more assertive effort on the part of the know-it-all to convince you of their vast knowledge. That is because the know-it-all craves attention and appreciation. They usually suffer from low self-esteem and need to be praised.

Now that you know this person's hidden motivation, you are in a position to respond effectively. If the know-it-all is truly knowledgeable, the person can be irritating but also helpful. If you are interested, ask specific questions, not open-ended ones that will prolong the display of knowledge. If you are not interested, do not probe. Change the subject or direct attention elsewhere. If you value the friendship or working relationship with this person, you simply may need to be patient.

On the other hand, if the know-it-all is really a know-nothing, their hunger to be recognized for their supposed knowledge could be dangerous. They could give incorrect information or advice to a patient. In this case, you need to calmly and politely challenge their knowledge. "Where did they get that information?" Or "That's interesting. I'll have to research that." You do not have to be obnoxious about this process, just inquiring and persistent. Once you demonstrate that you do not easily accept the know-it-all's hearsay, they will think twice about giving you information that is based on little more than "well-known facts."

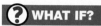 **WHAT IF?**

What if a co-worker you are very good friends with becomes angry because they did not receive the recognition or attention they were seeking? How could you make them feel better without encouraging chronic attention-seeking behavior?

The Liar

People will lie to protect themselves, avoid embarrassment, and take credit for others' ideas and words. Your best defense and response to a person who lies is in the facts. Try to avoid a confrontation, which can lead to arguments, defensiveness, personal attacks, and more lies. Rather, calmly stick to the facts. If you are confronted in public by a liar, ask hard-hitting questions. "Did you record the vital signs, or did you think I was going to do that?" Offer logic or proof. "I don't believe I said anything to give you the impression I was going to."

If a co-worker has proven to be unreliable, document the commitments. Send an email stating your understanding of the commitment and ask if any clarification is needed. In an email, you can state the facts and document your own ideas, contributions, and statements. In a verbal encounter, try to have a witness on hand. People who lie will not last long and neither will their lies, but your careful clarifications and documentation will prove effective as you respond to lies.

The Manipulative or Unreliable Person

Passive aggressive manipulators have an agenda, but they keep it a secret. Instead of being direct, they are often scheming and deceitful. They may try to position you into taking on their work or responsibilities, or they may omit information to get you to do what they want. Do not try to psychoanalyze them or change them, which can only lead to frustration

and even more conflict. However, as with liars, monitor them and be cautious around them. When they tell you something that will have a negative effect on you and your workload, demand proof. Do not make assumptions. Ask questions to reveal motives.

Unreliable people are famous for their excuses. They have excuses for every problem and shortcoming, but they rarely include their behavior among the causes. They find it much more comfortable to use external explanations for everything: the weather, the traffic, the lack of equipment, someone else's tardiness, the lost chart, the unreasonable patient.

Do not back down from people who have excuses for everything. Is their excuse the real cause of the shortcoming? Could something else have been done? What actions did the person take to deal with the situation? If you make it clear that you are not the kind of person who accepts excuses, the other person may think twice before abandoning a problem.

With patients, challenging excuses related to health issues is seldom helpful. Neither you nor the patient can change the parents, their genetics, the cause of the accident, or the source of the disease that is often offered as an excuse for the current state of the patient's health. As a health care professional, you can counsel the patient to take responsibility for future actions. The patient can take medication, get exercise, eat better, or socialize more. Recognize the excuses rather than challenging them and focus on the personal responsibility that can be assumed from this point forward. Box 7.2 offers some insights for combating excuses.

The Complainer

Complainers seldom seem happy. Every problem, issue, or change elicits a complaint. Ignore the complaints. Do not engage. Change the subject to work, and stay focused on the message or the task at hand.

One way to address complainers is to suggest that they put their complaint or concern in writing and give it to their supervisor to address. You can also ask them what solutions they envision or recommend.

The Social Butterfly

Under most circumstances, being friendly and outgoing is usually a plus. However, in a work environment where you are paid to perform a job and people are relying on you, some people may find it difficult to balance their outgoing nature and need to socialize and chat with the need to stay focused and stay on task. This person is commonly referred to as a social butterfly.

BOX 7.2

Combating Excuses at Work

- Do not let co-workers get under your skin or distract you from your own job.
- Do not let a lazy co-worker negatively affect your attitude by making you hostile; hostility is as bad as laziness, and it is much more visible.
- Do not worry that it is not fair; life is not always fair. Focusing on fairness makes you feel bad without changing the situation. Be the best you can be.
- Do not let lazy people set the norm. Do not follow their example.
- Do not do their work for them.
- Do not gossip, complain, or whine about your co-workers.
- Do not tattle or report their laziness to your supervisor or theirs. If their laziness is negatively affecting your ability to get your work done, present it as a business problem to your supervisor and ask for advice.
- On the other hand, do not let your co-worker's laziness hinder your progress. Refuse to take blame when somebody else is slowing down the work.
- Recognize that your "lazy" co-worker may just be disorganized, unaware of deadlines, or preoccupied with a personal problem.
- Communicate and reinforce deadlines.

A co-worker who is a social butterfly is fun to socialize with during breaks and after work. But sometimes the social butterfly can become a pest, interfering with your and their work. For example, when you arrive at work, the social butterfly can stop you from starting your day by chatting about what they did over the weekend.

The solution? If it becomes an issue, politely stop the social butterfly by saying, for example, "I really want to hear what you did over the weekend, but can you tell me at lunchtime? I want to make sure I get this task done." Not only are you not jeopardizing your job by socializing at inappropriate moments but you also may be helping the social butterfly avoid getting into trouble.

The Gossiper

It is usually beneficial to have co-workers get along and engage in casual conversation during break time and when it is not busy at work. There are times that this can result in gossip. Gossip is any casual or unconstrained conversation about someone who is not present and that the details are not confirmed to be true.

Although gossip usually has negative connotations, gossip can be neutral and even good depending on how we use the information. A good gossiper is someone who people trust with information and someone who uses that information in a responsible way. For example, a co-worker tells you that they are about to buy an expensive new car because of a new promotion at work. You inform them that you overheard the office manager discussing that the position may go to someone else. In this case, the information you are sharing is being used in an appropriate way that is helping someone.

A bad gossiper is someone who shares information about others to gain an advantage or just as entertainment. For example, a co-worker is applying for a promotion along with another co-worker. One co-worker starts talking about the other co-worker when they are not present and telling others that they are doing a poor job, make lots of mistakes, and that the office manager wants to fire them. In this case, gossip can ruin productivity, employee trust, and morale, and can create anxiety when determining if the gossip is true or not (Figure 7.4).

When you find yourself in a situation where gossiping is occurring, think twice before engaging in it. Will you be helping or hurting someone by sharing this information? Do not gossip for your personal gain, and consider how true the information is.

The Challenging Patient

A challenging patient, client, or patient's family member warrants a special approach. As someone who is sick or injured, in pain or under stress, it is

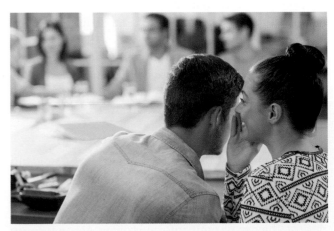

Figure 7.4 Gossiping may ruin productivity, trust, and can morale, and can create anxiety among co-workers. (iStock.com/Wavebreakmedia/813099606.)

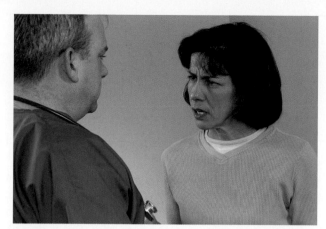

Figure 7.5 A patient expressing anger. (From Proctor DB, Adams AP: *Kinn's the medical assistant: an applied learning approach*, ed 12, St Louis, 2014, Elsevier.)

understandable if the patient is being challenging and difficult. However, every patient should receive the utmost consideration and sensitivity. The same consideration should be given to family members and caregivers who are worried about the patient. Worry and anxiety can make them agitated and more impatient than they are under normal circumstances. It is important to recognize that they are not in their normal state of being, and we are there to help them (Figure 7.5).

In the case of an anxious patient or loved one, follow the same strategies you use in dealing with anyone who is anxious—but with an extra dose of compassion and patience. Start by listening, and ignore the displaced anger. Try to determine what the patient or family member really wants. Sometimes it is not always so clear. For example, a family member may complain about not having enough magazines in the waiting room when, in fact, they are worried about their partner. You might say, "I'll see if I can find anymore magazine for you. But, in the meantime, is there anything else I can get you or your partner?" Often, acknowledging their feelings and offering to help can de-escalate the situation.

Justified or not, upset patients are simply customers with grievances. Box 7.3 suggests ways to deal with challenging patients. If you take the time to see the pattern and understand the motivation, you can devise an effective strategy for dealing with all kinds of difficult people and, as a result, be a better professional.

I do desire we may become better strangers.

—**William Shakespeare**

BOX 7.3

Tips for Dealing With Challenging Patients

- Remain friendly; indicate that you want to help if you can.
- Focus your attention entirely on the patient. Offer to sit together and discuss the issue if necessary.
- Remember that your behavior reflects on your employer.
- Be sympathetic but honest. If you cannot move the patient ahead of others, explain so.
- Promise only what you know you can deliver.
- Be empathetic and on the patient's side to search for a solution.
- Learn the patient's expectations. Ask, "What would you like to see happen?"
- Ask clarifying questions to show interest in understanding the patient's problem or complaint.
- If the patient is being irrational, you may not have uncovered the real problem.
- Thank the patient when the patient shows signs of reasonableness or understanding.
- If you make a mistake, admit it, apologize, and move on.
- Seek information or training that will equip you to handle particular problems better in the future.

 EXPERIENTIAL EXERCISES

1. Apologize to someone who deserves your apology. Reflect on how that makes you feel. How did it make the other person feel?
2. Practice ignoring complaints and poor behavior. What happened?

CROSS CURRENTS WITH OTHER SOFT SKILLS

LISTENING ACTIVELY: With difficult people, one of the best things you can do to manage them is to listen to their content and understand their motivations (Chapter 6).

EXUDING OPTIMISM, ENTHUSIASM, AND POSITIVITY: This is the opposite of being difficult, and it signals that you are not open to the tactics of difficult people (Chapter 5).

CASE STUDY 7.2
Fresh Start

Things were going downhill fast at Banker Street Dental. Last year, there was an audit by the Internal Revenue Service (IRS). As a result of the audit, Dr. Billingsley had to pay a large amount in taxes and penalties. Since then, Dr. Billingsley became a resentful and angry man with a forced smile on his face. He occasionally barked orders at his staff and was not his usual friendly self with his patients. People were noticing, and he started to lose some of his longtime patients, and he experienced rapid turnover among his staff due to his declining customer service and poor management skills.

Rae Martin knew none of this when she accepted the position as the new dental assistant. To her, Dr. Billingsley seemed like a pleasant, if overly formal, person in the interview. On Monday morning, Rae introduced herself to the receptionist, who also handled appointments and insurance. "Hi. I'm Mildred," she said. "We won't be seeing the doctor for another half hour."

The first day was not what she expected. Dr. Billingsley's idea of training Rae was to berate her. "No! Not that one. I thought they would've trained you better at your school," he said, when she handed him the wrong instrument.

Dr. Billingsley continued to reprimand her when the tray was not quite right, when the suction was not at the right angle or place, and when there were not enough cotton pads. "Didn't they teach you this in school?"

That night, Rae reflected on her new job and told herself that she was an excellent dental assistant and she would prove it to him. Further, she needed the job and would find a way to make it work.

The next day started the same way as the first. "Arrange my instruments like I showed you yesterday," he barked at her. "It's not that hard is it?"

"You never showed me how to arrange the instruments, Dr. Billingsley," she said. "But I'll certainly do that from now on."

"Just do as I ask," he barked.

The day continued in the same manner, with Dr. Billingsley criticizing Rae's performance and berating her for minor errors. At the end of the day, Rae knocked on Dr. Billingsley's office door.

"Dr. Billingsley, do you have a minute to talk to me?" she asked.

Dr. Billingsley looked irritated and said, "What is it? I don't have a lot of time."

"I wanted to discuss with you my performance. I'm a very good dental assistant and was top of my class. I understand that every office is different, and I'm ready to be flexible with different procedures here. But it doesn't help me do my job better for you or the patients when you speak to me that way."

"What way is that?" he quickly replied.

"I would absolutely appreciate constructive feedback and work to improve the to best of my ability. But I would appreciate your doing it in a more constructive way," Rae said while keeping a calm tone.

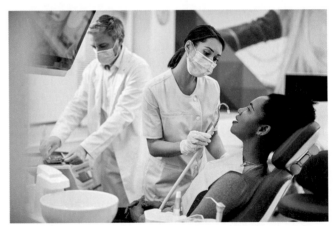

iStock.com/Drazen Zigic/1340829885

QUESTIONS FOR THOUGHT AND REFLECTION

1. Have you ever worked for someone like Dr. Billingsley? What did you do in that situation? Did it improve or worsen?

2. Dr. Billingsley was under an immense amount of stress, and he is Rae's employer. Does that give him a "right" to behave this way? Why or why not?

3. Why was Rae's plan effective?

4. Do you think the results would be better, worse, or the same if Rae yelled back at him and demanded that he stop speaking to her in that way?

Things were going downhill fast at Banker Street Dental. Last year, there was an audit by the Internal Revenue Service (IRS). As a result of the audit, Dr. Billingsley had to pay a large amount in taxes and penalties. Since then, Dr. Billingsley became a resentful and angry man with a forced smile on his face. He occasionally barked orders at his staff and was not his usual friendly self with his patients. People were noticing, and he started to lose some of his longtime patients, and he experienced rapid turnover among his staff due to his declining customer service and poor management skills.

Rae Martin knew none of this when she accepted the position as the new dental assistant. To her, Dr. Billingsley seemed like a pleasant, if overly formal, person in the interview. On Monday morning, Rae introduced herself to the receptionist, who also handled appointments and insurance. "Hi. I'm Mildred," she said. "We won't be seeing the doctor for another half hour."

The first day was not what she expected. Dr. Billingsley's idea of training Rae was to berate her. "No! Not that one. I thought they would've trained you better at your school," he said, when she handed him the wrong instrument.

Dr. Billingsley continued to reprimand her when the tray was not quite right, when the suction was not at the right angle or place, and when there were not enough cotton pads. "Didn't they teach you this in school?"

That night, Rae reflected on her new job and told herself that she was an excellent dental assistant, and she would prove it to him. Further, she needed the job and would find a way to make it work.

The next day started the same way as the first. "Arrange my instruments like I showed you yesterday," he barked at her. "It's not that hard, is it?"

"Dr. Billingsley, you never showed me how to arrange the instruments," she said.

"The matter is resolved," he sneered. "Just get the set-up ready."

"Actually, this matter is not resolved," she said firmly. "The unresolved matter is your behavior, Dr. Billingsley."

"What?"

"Yes. From now on, you do not have my permission to speak to me like that."

"What? Like what?"

"You may not raise your voice to me. You may not berate me. You may not embarrass me in front of the patients or the other staff members."

"Look here, girlie-"

"That's just what I'm talking about. You may not call me 'girlie' or address me in a demeaning tone of voice."

"Young lady, you may not address me with this insolent manner of yours. I think you should leave for today and not come back."

QUESTIONS FOR THOUGHT AND REFLECTION

1. Who do you think is at fault in this situation?
2. Have you ever responded like Rae to a supervisor? What was the outcome? What would you have done differently?
3. What are steps could Rae have taken to improve this situation?

References

Thomas KW, Kilmann RH. *Thomas-Kilmann conflict mode instrument*. Mountain View, CA: Xicom, a subsidiary of CPP, Inc; 1974, 2007.

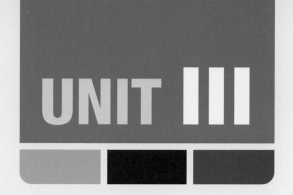

CAREER BUILDING SKILLS

CHAPTER 8

Being a Successful Student

BY THE END OF THIS CHAPTER, YOU WILL BE ABLE TO	<ul><li>Understand the Importance of Developing Good Note-Taking Skills</li><li>Choose a Note-Taking Format and Develop Review Techniques That Work for You</li><li>Use Effective Reading Techniques to Preview and Review Material</li><li>Explain How Tests Are Part of the Daily Life of a Health Care Professional</li><li>Use Tests as Incentives to Learn</li><li>Apply Effective Techniques and Strategies to Improve Your Performance on Classroom Tests and Professional Examinations</li></ul>

Taking Notes

He listens well who takes notes.

—Dante Alighieri

LEARNING OBJECTIVE 1: TAKING NOTES FOR SCHOOL SUCCESS

- Explain why it is important to take good notes in class.
- Describe how to prepare before class to listen actively and take good notes.
- List ways that instructors help you know what to record during their lectures.
- Describe the different types of note-taking methods.
- Explain how students can learn from the notes they take in class.

Skills for Note-Taking

There are many skills and tools to help you become a successful student. One of the most important tools is notes. Note-taking has been shown to improve student learning, where you remember more of what you learn from listening to your instructor and reading a textbook if you take notes. This is because taking notes takes effort rather than passively taking in information, which you will most likely forget the next day. By taking notes, you encode the information into words or pictures, which forms new pathways in your brain and stores it more firmly as long-term memory. Further, notes provide you the opportunity to revisit this information later and reinforce the learning.

Note-taking requires a range of multiple skills, including active listening, critical thinking, and organization skills. Taking effective notes combines the art of listening and the act of selective writing—being able to identify what is important to write down. Many students report having trouble taking effective notes, but it is a skill you can master.

Taking notes in class is just the first step in creating a personalized learning tool. Your notes are not complete when the instructor finishes the lecture. To make them useful, you need to edit and review them on a routine basis. Box 8.1 list the five "R's" of note-taking.

Active Listening in Class

Most of the successful people I've known are the ones who do more listening than talking.

—Bernard M. Baruch

You cannot record what you do not hear, so good listening skills are necessary for taking good notes. As we discussed in previous chapters, being a good listener is an important professional skill, so the classroom is the perfect opportunity to learn information and to acquire a life skill at the same time. Box 8.2 list some good tips on how to develop good listening skills in class.

Learning Styles and Listening

More than half of all people are visual learners. This can make it difficult for many students to pay continual attention during lectures, as most information is auditory. If you are a visual learner, here are some techniques to help you get the most from lectures:

* Complete any reading assignments before class.
* Avoid sitting near visual distractions.
* Keep your eyes on the instructor.
* Pay special attention to visual prompts such as writing on the board, PowerPoint slides, or other visual aids.
* Ask the instructor to write down any words or phrases you do not understand.
* During lectures, refer to your textbook or handouts that relate to the material.

If you are a kinesthetic (hands-on) learner, you can benefit from the physical activity of writing when you take notes. Here are some other ideas to help you improve your listening skills in class:

* Think about how you will use the information you hear during lectures.
* Imagine yourself interacting physically with the topic, such as performing procedures or operating a machine.
* Practice active note-taking by underlining or highlighting important concepts or terms.
* Try using flash cards or sticky notes to create your study materials as you take notes in class.
* Make slight movements that do not disrupt others but keep you somewhat physically active. For example, count off the steps of a procedure with your fingers, stretch your legs, or take occasional deep breaths.

BOX 8.1

The 5 "R's" of Note-Taking

- **Record**—During the lecture, write all meaningful information legibly.
- **Reduce**—After the lecture, write a summary of the ideas and facts using keywords as cue words. Summarizing as you study helps to clarify the meanings and relationships of ideas and strengthen memory retention.
- **Recite**—To study properly, you must recite all the information in your own words without looking at your notes or the text.
- **Reflect**—Think about your own opinions and ideas as you read over your notes. Raise questions, then try to answer them creatively.
- **Review**—Before reading or studying new material, take 10 minutes to quickly review your older notes. Skim over the main ideas and details. Reviewing enhances your retention of old material while adding new material to your memory.

JOURNALING 8.1

What kind of learner are you? How might this affect how you take notes?

BOX 8.2

Developing Good Listening Skills in Class

- Have a positive attitude about learning to listen.
- Leave your mental baggage at the classroom door.
- Sit where you can both see and hear well.
- Concentrate on the content of the lecture.
- Reel in your mind when it wanders and focus on the lecture.
- Keep an open mind about what you hear.

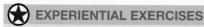

Prepare Before Class

By failing to prepare, you are preparing to fail.

—Benjamin Franklin

Preparing for classes is an important part of taking good notes. If you do not plan ahead and just show up prior to the instructor beginning to speak, you will miss out on a good part of your educational investment.

Be sure to complete any assigned reading and other homework. There is nothing more frustrating than trying to follow a lecture in which the instructor assumes you read ahead and know at least a little about the subject—and you know nothing!

Plan to arrive at class a few minutes early so you can be ready when the lecture starts. Arrive with a positive attitude and be ready to get as much benefit from the instruction as possible.

Note-Taking Systems

There are several ways you can organize lecture content as you record it. When choosing how to take notes, consider your learning style, your instructor's way of lecturing, and the subject. The most important thing is to become proficient at it, so you can focus on the content of the lecture.

Outline Method

The outline method is perhaps one of the most common, but still one of the best note-taking methods. Probably, you have been using it before, maybe without even knowing it had a name. With this method, your notes and thoughts are organized in a structured and highly logical manner, which drastically reduces the editing and reviewing time.

The outline method is one of the most structured note-taking methods and visually looks very organized. Add your main points as bullet points and elaborate on them underneath. For any piece of supporting information, create a nested bullet point below it. Remember to keep your points brief, preferably

around one sentence per point. Your notes should look similar to this:

Title
* Main topic
    * Subtopic
    * Thoughts or supporting facts

Figure 8.1 is an example of notes written using the outline method.

Boxing Method

The boxing method is a highly visual note-taking method. It gives you an at-a-glance overview of your topic. Each section or subtopic of your notes will live in its own labeled box. Using this method, your notes should look similar to this:

Topic
Sub-topic
    Key points
    Key points

Charting Method

The charting method is a great way to organize different items or concepts that all share several properties. For example, if you were studying physical examinations and understanding the different methods of taking temperature, each row would be a different method and the columns would list the normal measurement and when you would use this method. Your notes should look similar to this:

Method	Normal Temperature	Recommendation
Oral		
Axillary		
Tympanic		
Temporal Artery		
Rectal		

Cornell Note-Taking System

The Cornell Note-Taking Method is one of the most popular and renowned techniques, created by Professor Walter Pauk of Cornell University in the 1950s. The Cornell system is a method for laying out, editing, and studying from your notes. A key feature of the system is leaving plenty of blank space on each page, so you can add information when you review and edit your notes. It is designed to make you actively

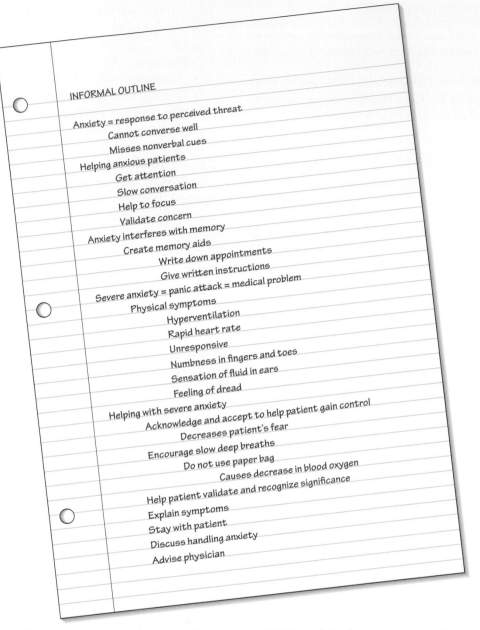

INFORMAL OUTLINE

Anxiety = response to perceived threat
Cannot converse well
Misses nonverbal cues
Helping anxious patients
Get attention
Slow conversation
Help to focus
Validate concern
Anxiety interferes with memory
Create memory aids
Write down appointments
Give written instructions
Severe anxiety = panic attack = medical problem
Physical symptoms
Hyperventilation
Rapid heart rate
Unresponsive
Numbness in fingers and toes
Sensation of fluid in ears
Feeling of dread
Helping with severe anxiety
Acknowledge and accept to help patient gain control
Decreases patient's fear
Encourage slow deep breaths
Do not use paper bag
Causes decrease in blood oxygen
Help patient validate and recognize significance
Explain symptoms
Stay with patient
Discuss handling anxiety
Advise physician

Figure 8.1 Example of notes using an informal outline. This is probably the most commonly used method. (Data from Bonewit-West K, Hunt S, Applegate E: *Today's medical assistant: clinical & administrative procedures*, ed 2, St Louis, 2013, Elsevier.)

think about your notes as you go along, rather than mindlessly jotting things down.

The method has you setting up each page on which you will take notes by drawing a line about 2.5 inches from the left side. Then draw a line about 2 inches from the bottom. Figure 8.2 shows this page layout.

All notes go into the large space in the center of the page. The smaller column on the left side is for key words, headings, questions, and other notes. The bottom space is for writing short summaries and can be done after class to help you review the material.

Deciding What to Record

Instructors can say a lot during a class, and sometimes it is difficult to decide what to write down. You need to write down enough to understand your notes later. At the same time, you cannot and should not try to record every word. Box 8.3 lists note-taking tips that apply to any method.

Use what you have read about the topic to form a mental overview of the material. Listen for the main ideas in class, as instructors often give clues about what is most important. Here are some common instructor behaviors that indicate what you should write down.

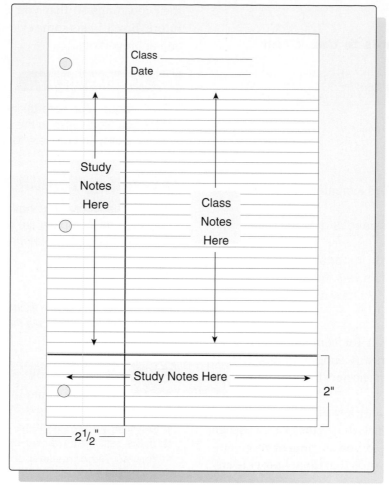

Class _____

Date _____

Study Notes Here

Class Notes Here

Study Notes Here

2"

2½"

Figure 8.2 Example of setting up a page when using the Cornell note-taking system. After class, write additions and revisions on the reverse sides of the pages.

* Saying, "This is important" or "You'll need to know this when you're working."
* Emphasizing or repeating certain words or ideas.
* Expressing extra interest or enthusiasm.
* Illustrating points with stories and examples.
* Asking questions of students during the lecture.

Box 8.4 contains a list of questions to keep in mind as you listen in class and study your notes. They can help you keep yourself on track mentally and help you focus on the main points of the lecture.

Paragraphs and Phrases

Writing in paragraphs can be effective when a lecture is hard to follow. Use phrases. Create a paragraph for each main idea. It is not necessary to write complete sentences. You can use abbreviations and shortened forms of words (e.g., Not nec to write compl sent. Can use abbrev, short forms/words). Mark important points during lectures. Organize and fill in details

---

BOX 8.3

Successful Tips for Note-Taking

- Create your own abbreviations and symbols.
- Leave some blank space between major ideas.
- Write out examples, definitions, formulas, and calculations.
- Write on only one side of the page.
- Write as neatly as possible.
- Use an erasable pen.

BOX 8.4

Guiding Questions When Note-Taking

- Why is this important?
- How does it work?
- What are the main parts?
- Why is it done this way?
- How is it done? How will I do this? When will I do this?

Suggested Symbols to Use When Reading

- → = Leads to or results in.
- ↓ = Decrease.
- ↑ = Increase.
- = = Is equivalent to.
- < = Less than.
- > = More than.
- T = the instructor has indicated you will be tested on this
- ?? = I do not understand and need to ask about this
- * = this information is important
- ** = this information is *very* important
- circled word = this is a new word for me

their meanings so that you can refer to them in the future. Box 8.5 lists some examples of helpful symbols and abbreviations.

JOURNALING 8.2

Think about your note-taking skills. Have the class notes you have taken in the past helped you to learn, master skills, and prepare for tests?

EXPERIENTIAL EXERCISES

Review the notes you have taken in one of your classes. How complete are they? How useful do you think they will be for reviewing and learning?

WHAT IF?

Suppose a classmate was ill and missed class and asked to borrow your notes. Would they find them useful?

EXPERIENTIAL EXERCISES

1. Choose the class note-taking method you believe would be best for you. Try it during the next few class lectures you attend and see how it works.
2. If the first method you chose does not work well for you, either revise it or try another method for a few days.

WHAT IF?

What if you have been taking notes in your classes but have not had time to review them? When you finally get to it, you find that you do not understand much of what you wrote and that your notes seem incomplete. What should you do now?

later. This can be difficult for some students. They must write quickly and neatly enough to read later. It can be good for hands-on learners because it involves activity.

Use phrases and note only key words instead of full sentences, such as not including "the" or "a" when note-taking. This will help you document more efficiently by skipping the words that do not provide any real meaning to you.

Symbols and Abbreviations

Using symbols and abbreviations in place of frequently used words, phrases, or names is an effective shortcut for note-taking in lectures when speed is essential. It is important to be consistent so you remember what they represent and can use them easily. Keep a "key list" of frequently used symbols/abbreviations and

CASE STUDY 8.1
Being a Non-Traditional Student

Jan is excited about starting her practical nursing program. She dropped out of high school to get married and was happy raising her four children. She got her GED a few years ago, but she always regretted not getting more education. Last year, her husband, Joe, was in a serious car accident and spent time in the hospital, followed by weeks in a rehabilitation facility.

During that time, Jan saw the work performed by the nurses who attended to Joe. She could see what a positive difference the good ones made in Joe's attitude and progress.

Jan noticed that the practical nurses seemed to have a lot of contact with him, and a career with direct patient contact and the opportunity to make a difference appealed to her. Going into health care would also give her the training she could use to continue Joe's long-term care at home and provide extra income to replace what Joe could no longer earn.

Her first few days in nursing school are almost a blur. There is so much to absorb: school policies and rules to remember, classes to attend, and people's names to learn.

There was a lot of pressure for her to do well because she had to take out a student loan, and the last thing she wanted was to go into debt and waste any money.

Jan attends all her classes, but it has been many years since she was in school, and she is beginning to panic. She never was a top student and is finding it difficult at times to follow her instructors' lectures. When she gets home and looks over her notes, they do not all make sense. There are gaps, they are unorganized, and she is pretty sure many of the words are misspelled, or at least she cannot find them in her textbooks.

At first, Jan is afraid to say anything. She is older than many of her classmates and believes that she should be able to do this at her age. After all, her children did well in school, and she would be embarrassed to admit she is having trouble. Instead, she works extra hard studying in the evenings and tries to concentrate in class.

In her first semester, Jan does not do well on her quizzes and examinations and begins to question whether she can be successful in this program. She worries a lot about this and even loses a few nights' sleep. Finally, she admits to Joe that she believes she has made a mistake.

"Let's take a good look at this," he tells her. "You've been out of school for more than 30 years. That's a long time."

"You're right about that," Jan admits.

"So, remember when we first got married? Did you know how to cook? How to keep house? Of course, not. You had no experience being in charge of a household. But you learned and ended up being the best cook in the neighborhood!"

"Okay, so what's that got to do with the trouble I'm having in school?" Jan asks.

"I think it means that you have to learn how to learn this new stuff. There are probably some techniques—like when you learned how to manage our household budget—that you just need to know about," Joe says.

"That does make some sense," Jan responds. "Maybe I should talk with my instructors and see if I can get some help learning to learn."

The next day, Jan made appointments to meet with one of her instructors, Bethany. She asked Jan a lot of questions about how she was studying whether she read the assignments in her textbook, and did she take notes in class and were they helping her. Jan was not sure. Bethany asked to see her notes.

After looking them over, Bethany smiled and said, "I think I know where we can start working on your study skills. I have a few helpful tips that I used when I was a nursing student that really helped me." Over time, with work and the help of her instructors, Jan learned to take notes that she could use to help her learn and succeed in her classes.

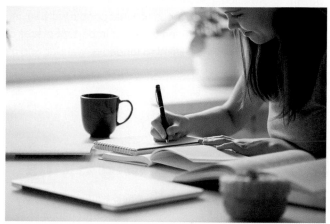
iStock.com/fizkes/1209703879

QUESTIONS FOR THOUGHT AND REFLECTION

1. Do you think Jan's situation is a common one for older returning students?
2. What are some of the reasons why she waited so long to ask for help?
3. Why do you think she was having so much trouble taking notes?
4. How was Joe able to help Jan see her problems more realistically?
5. What suggestions do you think her instructor gave her?

A Different Path

Dan Abrams felt he was lucky. He attended school to become a physical therapist assistant with his girlfriend, Ashley. If it were not for her taking notes in class and helping him review for tests, he probably would not have made it through graduation. Ashley took great notes in class and always gave Dan copies to study. Taking notes just was not his thing. He attended many of the classes, but he was not interested or motivated in learning to take good notes. After all, he would be working with patients, so when would he ever use note-taking again?

After graduation, Dan got a job at a small physical therapy practice and really enjoyed helping patients with their exercises. He communicated well with his supervisor, Teresa, and got along well with the patients.

After he had been on the job for a couple of months, the patient load declined, and Teresa had to let the receptionist and therapy aides go. This meant that many of the staff members, including Dan, would have to be cross-trained to take on additional responsibilities. For example, Dan and the other physical therapy assistants would have to take shifts answering the phones, taking messages, scheduling appointments, and documenting and transcribing patient histories in the medical records.

When the time came for Dan to take on some of these new duties, he decided to give it his best. But after taking down a few phone messages incorrectly and recording patient information inaccurately, he began to panic. He just did not seem to be able to focus on what people were saying and had a hard time capturing the most important pieces of information. Sometimes, his mind tended to wander, and he would lose track of what they were saying before he could get their words or information down on paper.

Teresa was noticing Dan's performance and was growing concerned. She had to tell him that if he did not improve, she would have to let him go. She simply did not have the time to correct Dan's mistakes or take the losses they were causing.

QUESTIONS FOR THOUGHT AND REFLECTION

1. What does Dan's experience demonstrate about the relationship between study skills and job skills?
2. How did Dan benefit from relying on Ashley's notes to study? How did Dan hinder his own progress by relying on Ashley's notes?
3. Do you think Dan will make it as a physical therapist assistant? Why or why not?

Effective Reading Skills

To read without reflecting is like eating without digesting.
—Edmund Burke

LEARNING OBJECTIVE 2: READING TO LEARN

- Explain the importance of effective reading.
- Understand the purpose and benefit of previewing and reviewing.
- Use different resources to research.
- Explain the question-answer method as it is used when reading.

Reading, along with listening and taking notes, is one of the most important ways you will acquire information as a student. Like effective listening, reading to learn requires you to pay attention and actively participate. For example, if you were reading instructions about how to assist in a medical procedure, you should ask yourself, "Do I understand this? What exactly am I supposed to do?" And then you may read it again more carefully to make sure you got it right.

The goal when reading your textbooks and other materials is to understand and comprehend or think about how you will use your new knowledge. Being able to effectively understand what you read has many benefits (Box 8.6).

BOX 8.6

Importance of Effective Reading

- The more ways you take in information, the more likely you are to remember it. Your memory paths are created and maintained by repeated use.
- Reading will give you background information for class lectures.
- Textbooks are a permanent way of saving information. You can review over and over.
- Books usually contain more supporting details, examples, graphics, and organizational aids than lectures.

JOURNALING 8.3

Do you enjoy reading? Why or why not?
Do you read to learn new things?
How would you rate your reading skills?

Preparing to Read

There are several prereading activities or techniques you can do to make reading easier and more beneficial. The first is to clear your mind of clutter. Reading requires concentration. If you have something bothering you that can be handled quickly, take care of it before you start studying. If it will take more than a few minutes, write it down so you will remember to deal with it later.

The next step is to find a place that encourages reading rather than sleeping or daydreaming or may distract you. Many students find that a straight-backed chair at a desk works best versus reading on their bed. Also, make sure there is adequate lighting. An uncomfortable environment can tire you and cut your reading and studying time short.

You need more than just a textbook to read actively. Gather your tools for effective reading: notebook, pen or pencil, highlighter or colored pen, and a dictionary. Getting in the habit of gathering what you need beforehand is a good health care practice. You would not want to interrupt a patient procedure because you forgot to bring something from the supply room.

Previewing

Many methods have been suggested for getting the most from your reading, but they all recommend that you preview the material you are about to read. This means quickly skimming the entire selection, learning any new vocabulary, paying attention to the headings, and using clues in the text to anticipate the content. Pay special attention to the lists at the beginning of chapters: vocabulary, objectives, headings and subheadings, and introduction. Box 8.7 describes the different features of a textbook.

Determine what you want from the assignment. Turn each heading into a question. Write down your questions and look for answers as you read. For example, if the heading is "Patient Confidentiality and HIPAA," ask yourself, "How does this relate to my future profession?"

★ EXPERIENTIAL EXERCISES

Look over your current textbooks. Using the list in Box 8.7, list the features they contain.

When previewing, headings provide a logical structure to guide your reading. Try to relate them to information you already know:

Communicating With Patients
Verbal and Nonverbal Communication
Interference With Communication
Listening Skills
Nonverbal Measures to Facilitate Communication
Interviewing Techniques
   Closed Questions
   Open Questions
   Keeping the Conversation Going
   Drawing Out Patients

Avoiding Responses That Inhibit Communication
Before even reading the chapter, you can learn at least three things from these headings:

1. Interviewing techniques are used when communicating with patients.
2. There are at least two kinds of questions.
3. Some types of responses can interfere with communication.

Knowing this, you create questions in your mind and anticipate what you will be reading. You are now an active reader.

You may be thinking that previewing is a waste of time and that it would be better to just jump into the reading and get it done; however, this is not true, as many studies have shown. Previewing is an excellent use of your time, as it will help you read more efficiently.

★ EXPERIENTIAL EXERCISES

1. From this or any other textbook, write a list of 10 chapter headings or chapter objectives.
2. Convert each heading or objective into a study question.

BOX 8.7

Anatomy of a Textbook

- **Preface:** Introductory section stating the purpose of the book and a list of its features.
- **Table of contents:** Often contains detailed outlines of chapter content.
- **Appendices:** Extra materials at the back of the book. Examples: list of professional organizations, guidelines for infection control, a metric conversion chart.
- **Index:** Alphabetical listing of all the topics in the book and the page numbers on which they appear.
- **Bibliography and/or references:** List of source materials used by the author and/or recommended readings for students who want more information.
- **Glossary:** Alphabetical list of words with their definitions at the back of the book.
- **Vocabulary or key terms:** Lists of words, with or without definitions, usually placed at the beginning of chapters.
- **Learning objectives:** Statements telling students what they should learn or be able to do after studying the material in the chapter.
- **Section headings:** Words or phrases that divide and identify various parts of the text. Serve as a "heads up" about what is to follow.

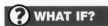

WHAT IF?

What if you find that some of your textbooks contain many words you do not know or are difficult to understand?

Active Reading

When you have finished your previewing and started reading, there are actions you can take to increase your learning. The first, and the one proven to be by far the most effective, is to ask and answer questions, out loud, about the material. To use this method, change each section heading into a question and look for the answer as you read. See Table 8.1 for examples of questions.

Another reading technique is marking your book in some way: underlining, highlighting, writing questions or key words in the margins, or using symbols. Do the highlighting or underlining after you have read a section (Figure 8.3). Otherwise, you are likely to mark too much material, thus defeating the purpose of highlighting.

A tool that combines the features of a highlighter and pen is a colored pen. When it is used to underline, the color draws attention for easy review. Use the same pen to write in your book. This tool saves time because you do not have to switch back and forth between a highlighter and a pen.

Reviewing

The average person forgets half of what was said during a typical class lecture within 24 hours of hearing it. The most important way to use your notes is to review them often—the more often, the better. The key to

long-term memory is repetition. Keep in mind that you are not simply learning to pass the next test, but you are gathering knowledge to succeed on the job.

So, it is important to review your notes within a day of taking them.

You should try to review your notes within 24 hours since this has been shown to move information from short-term to long-term memory. Spend 15 minutes looking over your notes and reciting the main points again. Weekly, spend 5–10 minutes rereading your notes and highlighting portions of your text. This keeps neuron pathways accessing the information for better recall.

Begin your review by reading over your notes and filling in any missing words or writing out the words

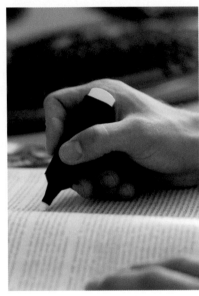

Figure 8.3 Highlighting important passages is a good way to actively study. (Copyright © istock.com.)

TABLE 8.1
Examples Using the Self-Questioning Study Method

Section Headings	Study Questions
Verbal and nonverbal communication	What is the difference between verbal and nonverbal communication? How are the two types of communication used by health care professionals when working with patients?
Interference with communication	Give two examples of factors that can interfere with effective communication.
Listening skills	What are good listening skills? How can good listening skills be developed? Why are good listening skills important when working with patients?
Closed question	What is the definition of a closed question? What is an example of a closed question? When should closed questions be used when interviewing a patient?

you abbreviated. Next, fill in ideas or reorganize your notes as needed. If there are gaps or notes you do not understand, look for answers in your textbook, ask a classmate, or check with your instructor.

Consider rewriting your notes if they are very disorganized or incomplete. This revision will also serve as a good review and reinforcement of the material. Use a highlighter or colored pen or underline to mark key words and phrases. Write questions or notes in the space on the side and bottom of the page. See Figures 8.4 and 8.5 for examples.

Another effective way to review is to write key words or questions in the blank space on the left. Box 8.8 has a list of sample questions. Cover your notes on the right-center of the page and answer the questions or define or explain the key words. This review method forces you to think and helps transfer the content of your notes into your long-term memory. Many experts also

recommend reviewing out loud, especially when you are asking and answering your questions, as the best way to learn and retain new information. Use what

BOX 8.8

Examples of Review Questions

- What is the definition of _____?
- What is the meaning of _____?
- What are the steps in performing _____?
- What is important to remember about _____?
- How does this relate to _____?
- Why must you _____?
- What are the principal parts of _____?
- How does _____ function?
- What is the purpose of _____?

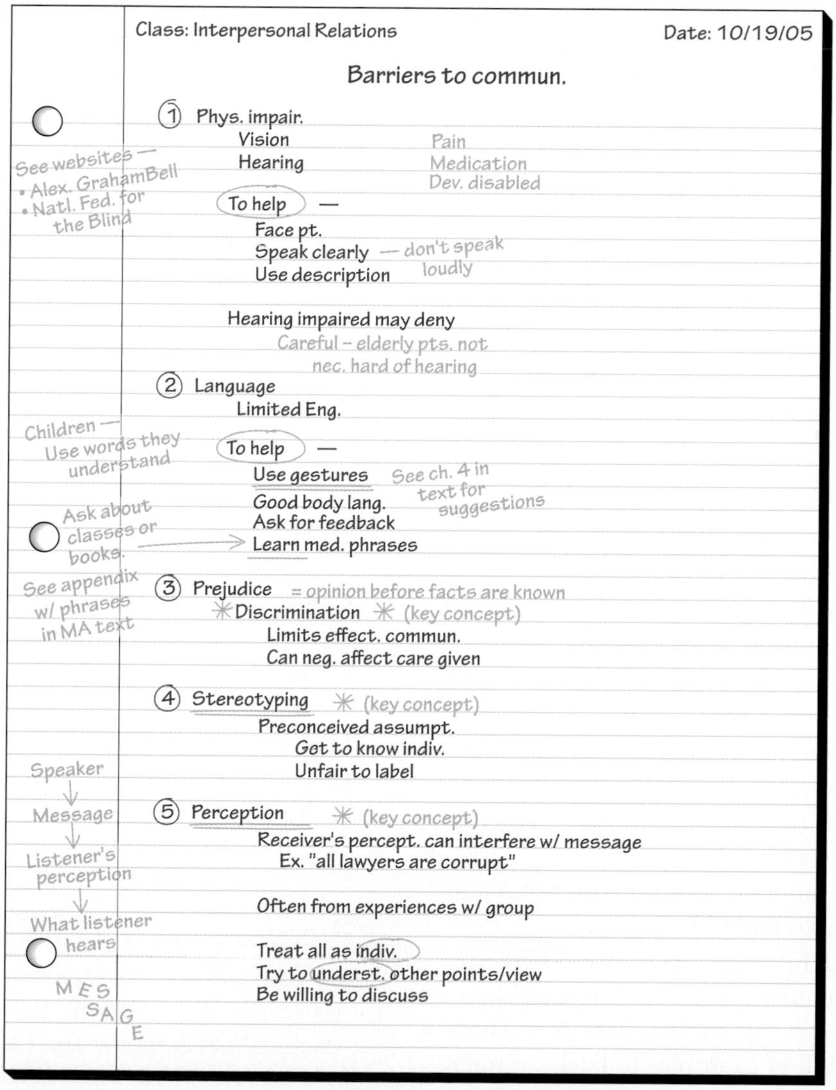

Figure 8.4 Notes are more useful if, when reviewing, you add details, write questions, note sources for more information, and mark key concepts. (From Haroun L: *Career development for health professionals: success in school and on the job,* ed 4, St Louis, 2016, Elsevier.)

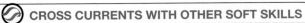

YOUR QUIZ QUESTIONS	LECTURE NOTES
What is the definition of anxiety?	Anxiety = response to perceived threat
How can anxiety affect patient behavior?	Cannot converse well Misses nonverbal cues

What are ways the health care professional can help anxious patients?	Helping anxious patients
	Get attention
	    Slow conversation
	    Help to focus
	    Validate concern

What can the health care professional do to help anxious patients remember important information?	Anxiety interferes with memory
	    Create memory aids
	Write down appointments
	    Give written instructions

What is a panic attack?
What are the physical symptoms associated with severe anxiety?
	Severe anxiety = panic attack =
	        medical problem
	Physical symptoms
	Hyperventilation
	Rapid heart rate
	    Unresponsive
	    Numbness in fingers and toes
	    Sensation of fluid in ears
	    Feeling of dread

What actions can the health care professional take to help patients who are experiencing severe anxiety?	Helping with severe anxiety
	    Stay with patient
	    Acknowledge and accept patient's feelings
	    Help patient validate and recognize significance of anxiety
	    Explain symptoms
	    Discuss ways of handling anxiety
	    Advise physician

Why is breathing into a paper bag no longer recommended for patients who are hyperventilating?	Do not have patients breathe into paper bag Causes decrease in blood oxygen

Figure 8.5 Make up questions based on your notes and write them in the left margin. Cover the main section and review by answering your "quiz" questions. This is reported to be the most effective way to learn from reading. (Data from Bonewit-West K, Hunt S, Applegate E: *Today's medical assistant: clinical & administrative procedures*, ed 2, St Louis, 2013, Elsevier.)

you know about your learning styles when studying your notes. Here are a few ways to do this:

* Visual: Picture the words and concepts in your mind. Label drawings. Draw sketches. Color code your notes by assigning colors to overarching themes or main points in the course material. Use outlines, highlight, or underline to organize your notes and emphasize key ideas.
* Auditory: Review out loud. Record your notes and review by listening to them.
* Kinesthetic: Stand up and move around as you review. Use movements and gestures to emphasize important points. Act out content. Use flash cards for key terms. Think of examples to back up main points and concepts.
* Interactive: Review with a study partner. Discuss concepts you have learned.

* Global: Write out the concepts and create a list of supporting facts. Taking and reviewing notes by hand may improve your recall of important concepts.
* Linear: Look for logical patterns in the material. Use outlines or diagrams to record the patterns in your notes.

CROSS CURRENTS WITH OTHER SOFT SKILLS

SHOWING EMPATHY, SENSITIVITY, AND CARING: You must be able to listen attentively to people in order to demonstrate empathy and caring (Chapter 5).

PROFESSIONAL PHONE TECHNIQUE: Taking accurate notes to record phone calls is an essential workplace skill (Chapter 13).

CASE STUDY 8.2
To Read or Not to Read

Emily Hasbrow did not really know what to do with herself after graduating from high school. After reading an article in the local paper about careers in massage therapy, her mom said, "Emily, you are a perfect fit for this occupation. You've spent the last year moping around the house, not knowing what to do with yourself. You're really good with your hands, and you like people. Maybe you can get a job on one of those cruise ships. That would really be fun."

When her mother agreed to let her continue living at home to save money and to help her with school expenses, Emily finally decided to go ahead and give the massage therapy program a try. She passed the program's entrance examination, bought the necessary books and uniform, and started attending classes the next week.

Emily thought the classes were okay, although not as interesting as she had hoped. And the homework—good grief! Did the instructors really expect the students to do that much reading? After a few days of slugging through her assignments, Emily decided that since she was going to class and taking decent notes, she could not see any reason to waste her time reading the textbook. When her mom asked about homework, Emily explained that there really "wasn't any." All the work was completed in class.

Emily was able to pass the short weekly quizzes in her classes with "C" grades, but she had a surprise when the class had their midterm examination. Where did the instructor get these questions? Emily could not remember having heard anything about some of this information. She had attended every class—had she fallen asleep or something?

When the tests were returned, Emily earned a "D" grade, so she went to see her instructor, Ms. Shepherd, to find out what had happened. Had Ms. Shepherd given them the examination intended for a different class?

The instructor explained, "Emily, looking over your test, it appears that the questions you missed were on the information contained in the readings I assigned. They are in your textbook and in the supplementary reading material. Didn't you ever look at these?"

Emily looked down, not wanting to admit that she had not been doing the reading, as she thought it was a waste of her time. All she could say was, "Well, I guess I messed up. I thought you were covering everything we needed to know in your lectures."

Ms. Shepherd smiled. "There's no way I have the time in class to cover everything you will need to know on the job. That's why I give the reading assignments."

"Okay," said Emily. "I understand. I'm going to have to spend some time catching up, but I will make sure I finish all the reading assignments from now on."

QUESTIONS FOR THOUGHT AND REFLECTION

1. Do you think Emily is really interested in becoming a massage therapist?
2. What mistake did she make when deciding how to spend her study time?
3. What kind of attitude does Emily have about school?
4. Do you think she will stay in school and pursue this career? Why or why not?

A Different Path

Megan is glad to be finished with school—well, almost finished. She is now working at her externship site, a pharmacy located in a large grocery store where she is practicing what she learned in her pharmacy technician program. Megan is glad to be working because, as she told her friend, Amy, "I'm just so tired of reading boring books and doing homework assignments every night."

Amy, who is studying to be a nurse, agreed that studying could become tiring but seemed necessary if they were to learn all they needed to know for their careers.

Megan is not happy to learn that Ted, the pharmacist who is her supervisor, expects her to read the employee procedure manual before she can start working with customers.

"Oh, great," she tells Amy one night on the phone. "Now I have to do *more* reading. I thought I was done with that."

"Well," Amy replied, "there might be important things about the pharmacy that you need to know."

"I just don't think I have it in me to go through that stupid manual," Megan said. "I think I'll just pay attention to what the employees are doing and ask questions when I need to."

Amy did not think this was a good idea, but she had her own studying to do and did not want to argue.

Megan followed her plan. She paid special attention to the actions of the pharmacy technicians and asked them questions about things she was unsure of. She thought she was doing just fine and told Ted that, yes, she had read the manual from "cover to cover" and was ready to work with customers. The first couple of days went smoothly, but on the third day, it seemed that every customer had some kind of question that Megan could not answer. Those that she was unable to bluff her way through, she asked the experienced technicians.

At the end of the day, Ted called her into the office behind the pharmacy. "Megan," he said. "I need the truth. There were questions today you were asking the staff that you would have known if you had read the procedure manual. Did you read the manual?"

Megan answered, "The truth? No, I didn't. I thought it might be a waste of time and that I could learn in other ways."

Ted sighed. "If you had told me this in the first place— the truth, rather than lying about having read it—I would let you have a second chance to read and study the manual and try again. But in this case, I'm afraid I'm going to have to ask the school to end your externship."

QUESTIONS FOR THOUGHT AND REFLECTION

1. What do you think of Megan's decision to learn about the pharmacy procedures by observing and asking questions instead of reading the manual?
2. Should Ted have tested Megan on the material rather than taking her word for it that she had read it?
3. Do you think Ted was fair in terminating Megan's externship?
4. What do you think Megan should do now?

Doing Research to Learn

LEARNING OBJECTIVE 3: RESEARCHING TO LEARN

- Define what information and computer literacy is.
- Become familiar with library resources in your area.
- Explain how to evaluate websites for credibility.
- Use the Internet to research topics of interest.
- List examples of reliable websites that contain health care information.

Research is not limited to finding information for a paper you must write. We do research all the time, such as when we investigate which car to buy or how to find the best auto insurance. Research simply means finding sources of reliable information and obtaining what we need from those sources. The ability to find and evaluate resources for learning is a necessary skill for lifelong learning and effective work in many fields.

With so many resources at our disposal, it is important to understand and develop *information literacy*. Information literacy is the set of skills required to identify, retrieve, organize, and analyze information. It is something all students must learn to effectively complete research. Students with knowledge of information literacy are prepared to find the data or information they need for any decision or task in

life. Information literacy helps students recognize misleading, out-of-date, or false information. It also helps them sort through the data and interpret it intelligently. Information literacy allows students to assess their information needs, searching for possible sources of information, evaluating the credibility and quality of sources, and integrating information across sources and into research and/or assignments.

Information used to be more controlled and now it is more diverse and expansive. Using multiple resources has become a more complex and layered activity. As a result, being able to identify resources and determine their credibility are important life skills to effectively use all these resources.

Libraries

With advancements in technology and the advent of the Internet and a wide range of online resources, libraries were often the main source of information and resources for students. In fact, they still are. You should get to know both your school library and your local public library. If there are other schools of higher education nearby, ask whether they allow the public to use their libraries. Some give checkout privileges for an annual fee. Others might allow interlibrary loan of books to your school's library. Many hospitals and clinics have libraries for employees, as well as for the public.

Today's libraries have many resources in addition to books and journals. Most offer Internet services, DVDs, and other multimedia materials. Every library is different. Walk around and explore. Look for informational brochures and how-to guides and ask the librarian for help. Librarians can assist you in locating relevant sources and answer any questions you may have about the library.

The Internet

You would be hard-pressed these days to find someone who did not know what the Internet is. The Internet is a vast network that connects computers all over the world. Through the Internet, people can share information and communicate from anywhere with an Internet connection. The Internet is a rich source of all types of information. Box 8.9 contains a list of examples of what is available.

The Internet has made it easier than ever for students to access different kinds of resources relevant to their academic work. Students can use the Internet for searching for their study-relevant materials, assignments, quizzes, presentations, and all study-relevant materials available on the Internet. Not only students but teachers also get help from the Internet. They can use the Internet for their research.

If you do not own a computer, check with your school to find out what is available. A complete discussion on how to search the Internet is outside the scope of this book; however, it is easy to use and does not require a lot of computer experience. You can learn more by entering the key words "Internet tutorials" or "online search tutorials." The Internet is a huge

---

BOX 8.9

Examples of What Is Available on the Internet

- Articles from newspapers, magazines, and journals
- Informative papers written by researchers
- Directories
- Dictionaries
- Opportunities to communicate with experts
- Job postings and applications
- Information about diseases and health conditions for both patients and health care professionals
- Career advice

---

source of information and resources, and to access the resource from the Internet, there are several kinds of software called search engines.

As a basic overview, the first is by using a website address. All sites have one, just like houses. If you know the address, you simply type it into the browser. If you do not know which sites have the information you need, you can use a search engine. A search engine is a kind of website through which you can search the content available on the Internet by entering the desired keywords into the search field. The search engine then looks through its index for relevant web pages and displays a list of websites that contain information of various kinds about your topic. Several of the most popular general search engines are Google Chrome, Microsoft Edge, Mozilla, Firefox, Apple Safari, Yahoo!, and Bing.

Some search engines can be limited by focus or subject area, such as:

* Google Scholar: https://scholar.google.com
* Health: www.healthline.com
* Science: www.sciencedirect.com

Evaluating Websites

Once you arrive at a website either by typing in the address in the browser or through a search engine, it is good to evaluate whether the website is legitimate and safe. The Internet is not controlled by any single organization or agency that verifies content or keeps it current. There can be a lot of misinformation or obsolete data. Be sure to check the credibility of the information source, especially for academic research. Here are some questions you should ask about a website:

1. Who is the site owner or sponsor? Universities, government agencies, many professional organizations, research institutes, and established publishers are usually good sources. This is not to say that commercial sites do not contain good information. Just note whether their purpose is to inform or to advertise a product. The endings of the web address indicate sponsorship:
   a. University: .edu
   b. Government: .gov
   c. Professional organization: .org
   d. Commercial enterprise: .com
2. Who is the author? They should have education and/or experience in the subject matter. Can you contact the author?
3. What is the purpose of the website? Many sites are designed to sell products or persuade readers to believe in a cause. The material provided may be biased.

4. How are claims supported? Check for statistics and references to original sources of information.
5. How current is the information? Are dates given? Advances and changes in health care occur continually.
6. What is the purpose of the website and its contents? To present facts? To give an opinion? To sell a product or service?

See Box 8.10 for a list of reliable websites that contain a wealth of information about health topics.

Computer Literacy

Computer literacy is the general knowledge of computers, software, hardware, and how they work and how to use them. This includes typing, powering a computer on and off, learning to use common applications, and knowing how to connect and disconnect your computer. Educating yourself on these basic computer skills can prepare you for hands-on computer demands in the workplace.

Computers are electronic equipment that stores manipulates, and retrieves information. The physical device is called **hardware**. Computer hardware includes the physical parts of a computer, such as the case, central processing unit, monitor, mouse, keyboard, computer data storage, graphics card, sound card, speakers, and motherboard.

The instructions that tell the computer hardware how to work and enable the user to interact with the computer is called **software**. Although application software is thought of as a program, it can be anything that runs on a computer. The software that manages the computer hardware itself is called the *operating system*. Examples of operating systems are Microsoft Windows, macOS, and Linux. The operating system also facilitates the use of other software programs, called applications. Other types of software are word-processing applications, image-editing applications, games, email programs, and much more. The electronic health record (EHR) software is an application designed to input and retrieve information that is used in health care. The application (or a piece of it) is placed or loaded into the working space (memory) of the computer.

The computer uses mass storage devices called hard drives to store large amounts information, such as documents, images, and applications. Random access memory (RAM) is another type of "temporary" storage used to store information the computer is actively working on. External devices can be used to store information outside of the computer and include USB drives (thumb drives), compact discs (CDs), and other drives. When connected to a printer, computers can output paper documents.

Oftentimes, the computers at a facility or organization will have very little information stored on them. Today, the hard drives of each machine can be relatively small, because only parts of the applications and data files are on the individual physical devices. The bulk of the data and the applications to access it are stored on much larger and more powerful computers called *servers*. The server is accessed through an Internet connection. This is configuration is called **cloud computing**.

Computers are used in all aspects of health care. The wide use of EHRs has revolutionized the way health care professionals and administrators access and store patient information. For example, laboratory tests and respiratory ventilators are run by computerized equipment. Magnetic resonance imaging (MRI) and heart monitoring equipment are computer driven. Information about patient services and charges for services are maintained on computer systems in most facilities. Health care professionals must be able to enter and retrieve data from the computer to provide efficient care. Although each computer system has its own specifications for use, some basic rules apply to all units and programs.

★ EXPERIENTIAL EXERCISES

1. Choose a topic in which you have an interest. Locate five sources of what you consider to be reliable information.
2. Briefly describe each source and explain why you believe it to be reliable.

Test-Taking Strategies

LEARNING OBJECTIVE 4:
PART OF SCHOOL, PART OF LIFE

- Explain how the daily tasks and duties of health care professionals are tests of their knowledge.
- List the skills you can learn from preparing for and taking tests in school.
- List the different testing-taking formats and question types.
- List several techniques for preparing to do well on tests.
- Explain how to use study tools to prepare for tests.

Tests: Part of School, Part of Life

Think of a test as a challenge instead of a threat.

—Walter Pauk

Taking tests is not limited to your life as a student. The truth is that life is full of tests. Employment interviews are a form of test with the purpose of assessing your ability to present yourself and your qualifications for the job. To legally work in many occupations, such as practical/vocational nurse or radiological technologist, you must pass a national certification or licensing examination. Other occupations, such as medical assistant, have voluntary examinations to obtain certification or registration that improves your chances of getting a job and may be an employment requirement for some employers.

Once on the job, you are, in a sense, being tested every day. Although you may not always think of your everyday tasks as tests, they are applications of what you have learned, and your ability to perform them correctly will be noted by your patients, co-workers, and supervisor. Table 8.2 shows examples of test-taking in school, during the job search, and on the job.

Learning to perform "when it counts" is a valuable skill. For example, the parent of the infant wants to know that the health care professional giving the injection has "passed the test" and is qualified to safely perform this task (Figure 8.6).

The annual employee performance evaluation is a type of test in which your supervisor writes a report about your work and then meets with you to discuss it. This document is then placed in your personnel file. Figure 8.7 shows a sample employee performance review.

JOURNALING 8.4

What are some other similarities between classroom tests and working on the job? Think about past experiences, outside the classroom, in which you felt you were being "tested."

WHAT IF?

You are on your externship and the physician asks you to do a laboratory test. You learned and practiced this procedure in class, but now, you just cannot remember all the steps. What should you do?

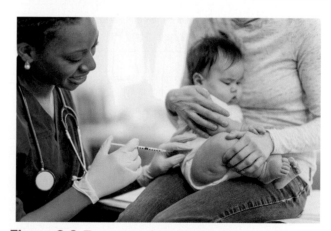

Figure 8.6 The mother of this infant wants to know that the health care professional giving the injection has "passed the test" and is qualified to safely perform this task. (Copyright © istock.com.)

TABLE 8.2
Applications of Test-Taking Skills

School	Job Search	On the Job
Take daily quizzes	Prepare for national and/or professional examinations	Perform daily work accurately and completely
Review and take final examinations	Present self successfully at job interviews	Participate in annual performance evaluation with supervisor
Demonstrate practical skills	Answer interviewer's questions effectively	It's all a test!

Wellness Plus Physicians Group
Employee Performance Review

Name:_____   Position: _____

Hire Date: _____   Date of Last
Performance
Supervisor: _____   Evaluation:_____

Rating Scale: 1 = Excellent   2 = Very Good   3 = Satisfactory   4 = Needs some improvement   5 = Needs much improvement

A. Quality of work performed   Comments:
    Rating   1   2   3   4   5

B. Use of judgment   Comments:
    Rating   1   2   3   4   5

C. Dependability   Comments:
    Rating   1   2   3   4   5

D. Cooperation with others   Comments:
    Rating   1   2   3   4   5

E. Appearance and hygiene   Comments:
    Rating   1   2   3   4   5

F. Attendance and punctuality   Comments:
    Rating   1   2   3   4   5

G. Time management   Comments:
    Rating   1   2   3   4   5

H. Proper use of equipment
   and supplies   Comments:
    Rating   1   2   3   4   5

I. Ability to work independently   Comments:
    Rating   1   2   3   4   5

(1)

Figure 8.7 Sample performance review.

Wellness Plus Physicians Group
Employee Performance Review

Rating Scale: 1 = Excellent   2 = Very Good   3 = Satisfactory   4 = Needs some improvement   5 = Needs much improvement

J. Communication skills

Rating   1   2   3   4   5

Comments:

K. Willingness to take direction
and suggestions

Rating   1   2   3   4   5

Comments:

L. Ability to adapt to change

Rating   1   2   3   4   5

Comments:

Employee's greatest strengths: _____
_____

Progress in meeting goals from last review: _____
_____

New goals for improvement: _____
_____

Plan for achieving goals: _____
_____

Overall evaluation of this employee: _____
_____

Reviewed by: _____

Date: _____

Employee signature _____

Date: _____
      (Signature does not necessarily
       mean agreement)

(2)

Figure 8.7   (Cont.)

Preparing for Tests

The best way to prepare for tests is the same way you prepare yourself for career success: start preparing early and study to learn so you master the content of your courses. Here are a few study techniques that lead to successful test-taking:

* Manage your time so studying is a priority.
* Identify and use study techniques that correspond with your preferred learning styles.
* Use learning techniques that help move information into your long-term memory, such as repetition.
* Take good notes in class and review them often.
* Read your textbooks actively and review them regularly.
* Seek help early if you are having trouble.

Steps for Successful Test-Taking

In addition to practicing good study habits, there are specific steps you can take to prepare for important tests.

1. Find out as much as possible about the test. Gather your notes and handouts and ask the instructor for suggestions on how best to prepare. Suggested questions to ask your instructor include, "What type of questions will be asked (i.e., multiple-choice, true-false, or essay questions)?" "How many points will each question be worth?" "Will there be a time limit?" "Will the test be given at the beginning or end of class?" "Will you review the material first?"

2. Quickly review your notes, textbook, handouts, and any other class materials to check your comprehension. Is there anything you do not understand or cannot remember, even after reviewing? Write a list of questions about the subject to ask in class. (This is why you start your review early, not the night before the examination!)

3. Make a schedule and divide what you must review over the time you have available so you will not run out of time before you have a chance to review everything.

4. Use the study tools you developed when you reviewed throughout the class.

5. Identify and concentrate on the material you find most difficult or have the most trouble remembering.

6. Use the practice questions and quizzes you created from your class notes and from your reading. Try to recall the answers without looking at your notes or textbook. If there will be short answer or essay questions on the test, try writing out your answers. This may be the *single best way* to prepare for classroom tests.

> **JOURNALING 8.5**

Think about your past test-taking experiences. Do you tend to get very nervous? What study techniques have you used to prepare? Do you usually feel prepared?

> ★ **EXPERIENTIAL EXERCISES**

1. Choose at least three study techniques to use when you prepare for your next test.
2. Create a plan for using these ideas, including the actions you will take and a study schedule.
3. After you have taken the test, write a paragraph describing how the strategies worked for you.
4. Are there other strategies you would like to try? If so, describe them.

The Day of the Test

**LEARNING OBJECTIVE 5:
THE DAY OF THE TEST**

■ Explain why you should plan to arrive early on the day of a test.
■ List last-minute pretest actions that can help you perform better on tests.
■ Describe ways to better understand what you are to do on a test.
■ Describe methods for controlling test anxiety.

It is the day of the test, and you feel reasonably prepared. You certainly do not want to perform poorly just because you failed to follow some practical test-taking guidelines. Here are some helpful hints you can apply to any test situation:

* You deserve a good start, so plan to arrive early. Do not stress yourself out by rushing in late, scrambling to find a seat, and missing the introductory instructions.
* Bring your supplies, including books, notes, a calculator (if these are allowed), and pencils or pens. An erasable pen (blue or black ink) works well, because you can make corrections neatly and your instructor will be able to read your answers. Verify with your instructor whether pencils or pens are required for the examination, and plan to bring several.
* Read and/or listen to all instructions. Ask the instructor to explain anything you do not understand. This is not the time to be shy. You have a right to know exactly what is expected.
* Quickly review the entire test before starting. Read all the directions on every page. If you have questions and the test has already begun, go to the instructor and ask them quietly.

* If there are different types of questions, note which ones will take the most time to answer and/or are worth the most points. Then quickly plan how to divide your time among the different parts of the test.
* If the test is longer and/or more difficult than you expected, do *not* panic. Take a deep breath, follow the guidelines, answer the easiest questions first, and focus on doing your best.
* When there are different types of questions, it is usually best to move from the shortest to the longest answers: true-false, multiple choice, matching, fill in, short essay, and then long essay (Figure 8.8). This is like giving yourself a warm-up. Also, the questions that have the answers provided for you to choose from may give you ideas for answering questions in which you must supply the answers from recall.
* Limit the time you spend on questions you find very difficult or do not know the answers to. Mark them and return to them later after you have completed the rest of the examination.
* Proofread your answers before you turn in your test. Did you answer all the questions? Did you mark the correct boxes on the answer sheet? Did you follow all directions correctly? Did you check for spelling errors, words left out, and other careless errors?
* Use all the time allowed if you need it. You do not earn extra points by finishing early, and hurrying may cost you a few correct answers.

Managing Test Anxiety

You have studied throughout the class, you have reviewed for the test, and you feel secure about your knowledge of the material—but you are still panic-stricken by the idea of your final examination. You just know you will freeze up and will not be able to

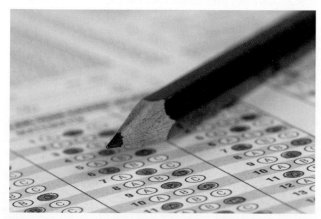

Figure 8.8 A multiple-choice answer sheet.

remember a thing. You may even feel physically ill when you enter the classroom on test days. There just does not seem to be any way around it; you are just "bad at tests." This is a real problem for many students, and solving it is an important step toward achieving your professional goals. Here are some actions you can take to help you manage test anxiety:

* Evaluate your study habits and test review methods. Can you improve them? Are you really using your study time efficiently? For example, some students spend a lot of time reading notes over and over but never actually quizzing themselves without looking at the written information. They think they know it, but without their book or notes, they cannot remember very much.
* Think about your test preparation. It may seem like you are spending a lot of time reviewing because you feel worn out by it. If you engage in a marathon review session the last 2 days before the test, you may feel as if you studied a lot, but you are too tired to remember much of the material.
* Be honest with yourself. Do you have trouble understanding the material covered in your classes but do not ask for help because you are embarrassed? Remember that instructors are there to help you, and asking for help is not nearly as embarrassing as failing a test or finding that you lack information needed to perform your job.
* Do not let your classmates create anxiety. Worrying about competing with them, such as finishing the test first or earning a higher grade, can distract you from focusing on your own performance. Your education is not a race with winners and losers; the goal of a health care program is for everyone to win by graduating as a competent professional. Although the awarding of grades tends to set up a competitive environment, modern health care is delivered by teams of individuals who must work cooperatively, not competitively. Some classmates are even more anxious about tests than you. These people often express their nervousness by talking a lot and predicting total gloom and doom. Be upbeat with them rather than letting their negative talk increase your own anxiety. Avoid participating in catastrophizing conversations around test time.
* Join forces with positive students. Organize a small group to review, share ideas, quiz one another, and cheer one another on. Have each person make up a few test questions and quiz the others. Seek out classmates who are dependable and will contribute to the group. Keep the number small (three to five)

so everyone can contribute. Use visualizations and positive self-talk to promote learning and good test performance.

* Practice good health habits and stress-management techniques. Physical exercise releases endorphins, the body's natural tranquilizers. Do your best to get enough sleep before major tests so you are not exhausted. Take deep breaths to h+elp quiet the mind.

? WHAT IF?

Your medical terminology class is more difficult than you expected. Your classmates constantly complain about how it is "impossible" to memorize so many terms, the instructor expects too much, and so on. Their constant talk is beginning to freak you out. What can you do to reduce your anxiety?

EXPERIENTIAL EXERCISES

Describe five ways you can use tests to your advantage as you prepare for a career in health care.

Desensitization

If you review thoroughly and try the suggestions for relieving anxiety but still find yourself freezing up during examinations, you can try a technique called "desensitization." This is a technique developed for people who have anxieties that interfere with their daily lives. It works by providing exposure to small doses of the source of fear and then gradually increasing the size and number of exposures.

Develop a plan to increase your exposure to tests. Have a friend or family member make up and give you tests, starting with short quizzes. Make them as realistic as possible. For example, set and stay within a time limit. Ask your instructor to give you practice tests. Find out if you can take these in a classroom under conditions as close to those of a real test as possible. Many sponsors of professional examinations have sample tests you can take. These techniques may seem like a lot of work and even a little embarrassing, but if test anxiety is ruining your performance, desensitization is worth trying.

← JOURNALING 8.6

Procrastination is a common problem. Do you tend to put off studying and preparing ahead for tests? If so, can you think of ways to encoura+ge yourself to develop better study habits?

Types of Test Formats

LEARNING OBJECTIVE 6: SPECIFIC TEST-TAKING TECHNIQUES

- Explain the best way to do well on tests.
- Explain why knowing about various test formats can help you perform better on tests.
- List techniques for successfully answering different question formats.

The well-being of patients depends on what and how well health care professionals master the knowledge necessary for their professions. The purpose of studying is to learn for the future, not just to pass tests. And the *best* way to do well on tests is to thoroughly know your material. That said, it is also true that learning about commonly used test formats can help you to be more effective in passing examinations. Students who are unfamiliar with question formats can waste time and miss valuable points on examinations.

If there is no penalty for incorrect answers, go ahead and guess. With true-false questions, you have a 50% chance of answering correctly, whereas with most multiple-choice questions, the chance is only 25%. But the more answer responses you can eliminate, the higher your chance of guessing and choosing the correct answer. However, it is important to remember that the suggestions given in the following sections are only guidelines and *do not substitute for learning the material.*

True-False Questions

Examples

Read each of the following statements. If the statement is true, circle the T. If it is false, circle the F.

T F 1. Classroom tests are always good indicators of how well students understand a subject.

T F 2. Test performance can be improved by cramming as much as possible the day before the test is given.

T F 3. Reviewing material regularly throughout the course is the best way to do well on tests.

Suggested Techniques for Answering

* Be sure that every part of the answer is correct. If any part of it is false, the entire answer is false.
* Watch out for words like "always" and "never." Few things in life are that final, and statements with these words are often false. (There are exceptions, however. For example, there are safety rules in health care that must always be followed and

legal rules, such as those concerning the release of patient records, that can never be violated.)

* Answers with middle-of-the-road words like "usually," "sometimes," and "often" tend to be true (except as previously noted).
* Do not spend a lot of time on true-false questions you are unsure about, especially if they are at the beginning of a test that also contains more time-consuming questions.
* Guess only as a last resort (and only if there is no penalty).

Multiple-Choice Questions

Examples

Circle the letter to the left of the response that best answers each question.

1. Which is the best reason for learning to spell correctly?

A. Patients are impressed by correct spelling.

B. Patient care can be negatively affected if words are misspelled on medical documentation.

C. Students who spell correctly get better grades in school.

D. Good spelling skills increase the chances of receiving a promotion at work.

2. The Cornell note-taking system has proven helpful to students because it:

A. Prevents them from having to review notes after class.

B. Helps them record everything the instructor says.

C. Provides a format that encourages review.

D. Teaches specific active listening techniques.

Suggested Techniques for Answering

* Read the instructions and questions carefully. If the question asks you to identify the "best" answer, it is possible that more than one is correct (Figure 8.8). In the first sample question, all answers are good reasons for spelling correctly. So, you need to think about which is the most important reason, and that is patient safety. Therefore B is the correct answer.
* If the directions state to select the "correct" answer (as opposed to the "best," "most complete," etc.), consider each statement separately, and then ask yourself if it is true or false. (Many professional examinations, such as the Certified Medical Assistant examination, are multiple choice.)
* Read through all the answers before selecting one.
* Immediately eliminate answers that are obviously incorrect.

* If the answer requires a math calculation, do the problem yourself before you look at the answers.
* Match each answer to the question rather than comparing the answers to one another.
* If you are guessing, choose an answer that has information you recognize.
* You can sometimes eliminate choices by using logic. For example, if two answers say basically the same thing, they must both be incorrect. As with true-false answers, if any part of a statement is wrong, the entire answer must be wrong. If the answer is silly or farfetched (instructors sometimes like to have a little fun), eliminate it immediately.
* If you are allowed to write on the test, circle or underline key words in the question to focus your attention when you read the answers.

Matching Questions

Examples

On the line to the left of each number in Column A, write the letter from Column B that explains one of its uses.

	Column A	Column B
____ 1.	Comma	A. Substitutes for letters that are dropped when contractions are formed
____ 2.	Semicolon	B. Indicates a change of thought within a sentence
____ 3.	Colon	C. Connects two sentences into one long sentence when a connective word is used
____ 4.	Apostrophe	D. Follows the greeting in a formal business letter
____ 5.	Dash	E. Connects two sentences into one long sentence without the use of a connective word
____ 6.	Period	F. Is placed at the end of a sentence

Suggested Techniques for Answering

* Read the instructions carefully. Note whether any item can be used more than once.
* Quickly count each column to see if both columns have the same number of items. Sometimes they do not. It is possible that an item may be used more than once or that one item is not used at all.
* Read through both columns before you write in any answers.
* Do the ones you know first.

* Some students find it easier to read the longer answers first (usually placed in the right-hand column) and then look for the shorter match. See which method works best for you.
* Mark or cross out each item as you use it if you are allowed to write on the test paper.

Fill-in-the-Blank Questions

Examples

Fill in each blank with a word or phrase that correctly completes the sentence.

1. The huge group of interconnecting computers located around the world is called the _____.
2. Learners who are both visual and global sometimes find that _____ is a useful note-taking technique to record information in a way that clearly shows relationships.
3. An explanation of why a procedure is performed in a certain way is called the _____.

Suggested Techniques for Answering

* Read the entire statement before attempting to fill in the blank(s).
* Write answers that fit the form and content of the words around them. For example, if the last word before the blank is "the," you know the answer is a noun.
* It sometimes helps to convert the phrase into a question in which the answer is the correct fill in.
* The length of the space may be a clue to the answer, but the length of the spaces may also be uniform or random. Therefore, this is not a reliable way to select an answer.

Short Answer Questions

Examples

Write a short answer to each of the following questions, using the spaces provided. Some questions have several parts. Your answers do not need to be complete sentences.

1. List three reasons why many educators recommend using a three-ring binder to keep your notes and class materials in order.
2. Explain why previewing is a critical part of the reading process.
3. Describe four ways of starting to write a paper when you are having trouble determining exactly what to write and/or how to organize it.

Suggested Techniques for Answering

* Read the instructions to find key words that tell you exactly what is expected in the answer. Are you asked to explain? Give two examples? List five reasons? Define? Give the steps? Be sure to answer all parts of the question.
* If you are asked to write several sentences, answer the question as directly and completely as possible without padding with unnecessary information.
* If you do not know the entire answer, write down as much as you do know. You may receive partial credit.

Essay Questions

Example

Write a well-organized essay at least one page long explaining the meaning of this statement: "Study skills are career skills." Support your answer with examples and references to the National Health Care Skill Standards and the requirements of employers. You will be graded on how well you demonstrate understanding of the concept, as well as on spelling and grammar.

Suggested Techniques for Answering

* As with short answer questions, read the instructions carefully to find out what you are to include in your answer. Provide evidence for your response? Give examples to illustrate? Give the sequence? Explain reasons and purposes? Defend your answer? Compare and contrast?
* Do not write answers that are too short. Even if the question does not specifically ask for examples or evidence, you should fully explain or defend your answer. Providing examples may also help you include important information.
* Do not spend time with a lot of words that do not really mean anything, such as repeating the question or writing a long introduction. Answer questions directly.
* If you have trouble organizing an answer in your head, quickly jot down a few key ideas, an outline, or a mind map.
* Use the rule that journalists use when they write a newspaper article: State the most important information first by answering the question as quickly as possible. Use the rest of the time to develop your answer, write examples, provide evidence, and so on to support your answer. This way, if you run out of time, you know you have included the most important information.
* Include the principal ideas of the course, as appropriate, especially those the instructor emphasized.
* Use the principles of good writing discussed in the chapter on writing strategies: good organization and correct grammar and spelling.

1. Study the strategies given in this section for the various types of test questions.
2. Use the strategies when taking your next quiz or test.
3. Do you believe the strategies were helpful? Explain.
4. Discuss this statement: "Test-taking strategies are not a substitute for learning."

? WHAT IF?

You studied all the material you understood would be on a weekly test. However, some of the questions do not seem to be related to the week's lessons.

After the Test

LEARNING OBJECTIVE 7: AFTER THE TEST

- List the actions that students should take if they perform poorly on a test.
- Describe common test-taking problems and how to resolve them.

Resist the temptation to forget about the test you just took. Just like athletes who analyze each game to learn which plays worked and which did not, you can use the same method to review and analyze your performance to your advantage. As soon as possible after finishing the test, review your notes and books to find the answers to the questions you were unsure about or just did not know.

Continue to review the material from time to time to reinforce and retain important facts and information. If you did poorly, do not lose heart. Instead, try the following:

* Listen to any review the instructor gives of the test.
* If you have to return it to the instructor, take notes on a separate sheet of paper listing what you missed.
* Pay special attention to the questions you missed and write down the correct answers.
* If the instructor explains information, be sure to take notes.
* Ask questions about anything you do not understand.
* If your instructor does not discuss the test with the class and you did poorly, make an appointment to discuss it privately.

At your earliest opportunity, review your notes and the marks you made in your books. Did you miss some of the major points? Study the wrong material? Not really understand it? What can you do to improve your performance the next time? See Table 8.3 for suggestions on how to deal with testing problems commonly encountered by students.

TABLE 8.3
Common Test-Taking Problems

The Problem	What to Do
You did not study at all or waited until the last minute and crammed.	You know what to do!
You studied but could not remember the information when you needed it for the test.	Check your understanding. Information you do not understand well can be very difficult to remember. Did you use prompts to study and review the material without looking at the answers? Or did you simply reread your notes and textbook? Passive review, or simply looking at the material, is not an effective learning technique for most people.
You were extremely anxious during the test and froze.	Review the section in this chapter on anxiety and try using the techniques. If they do not work for you, seek additional help.
You made careless errors.	Allow time to proofread your test before turning it in.
You did not understand what the questions meant.	When you are studying, be sure to look up any words you do not know. During the test, ask the instructor for clarification. If English is your second language, see your instructor for help.
The questions were not what you expected. For example, you memorized a list of facts and definitions, but the test asked you to apply information to new situations.	Review your notes or other information about the test to see if you misunderstood. Be sure to attend all classes so you will hear announcements about test content. If you believe the instructor was unclear about the format and/or content of the test, speak to them privately.

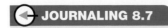

How can you approach tests with a positive attitude? What can you learn from taking tests? How can tests help you become a better health care professional?

Professional Examinations

**LEARNING OBJECTIVE 8:
PROFESSIONAL EXAMINATIONS**

- Explain the purpose of professional examinations in health care.
- Describe who administers professional examinations.
- List the different types of credentials awarded to those who pass professional examinations.
- Explain how students can prepare to be successful on professional examinations.

Many health care professions have examinations they must pass to work in the field. Some are required by the state or federal government or by individual employers. The purpose of professional examinations is to ensure high standards for practitioners by testing for knowledge and skill competency. These examinations may be administered by a governmental agency or a professional organization. Passing them allows the professional to use one of several special designations such as "licensed," "certified," or "registered."

Some professions do not require formal approval for graduates to work in the field. At the same time, voluntary testing is available and recommended for many careers. For example, most states do not have licensing requirements for medical assistants. (Some states do regulate what procedures medical assistants can and cannot perform.) Many medical offices, however, prefer to hire only certified or registered medical assistants, designations earned by passing professional examinations administered by testing organizations, such as the American Association of Medical Assistants and the American Medical Technologists. Additionally, some health insurance companies and government programs, such as Medicare, require only credentialed health care professionals.

Most professional examinations require a fee and usually are taken online. Your school may have included this cost in your tuition or fees. The school may also assist you in applying to take the examination. Some examinations are given year-round and others only on certain dates. Find out whether professional examinations are required for your occupation. Table 8.4 lists examples of different credentials and registrations or certifications for health care professionals. Learn as much as possible about the examination(s) while you are still in school.

TABLE 8.4
Examples of Credentials and Provider Agencies of Health Care Professionals

Professional	Credential	Provider Agency
Electronic Health Records Specialist	CEHRS	National Healthcareer Association (NHA)
Medical Administrative Assistant	CMAA	National Healthcareer Association (NHA)
	CEHRS	National Healthcareer Association (NHA)
Medical Assistants	CMA	American Association of Medical Assistant (AAMA)
	CPT	National Healthcareer Association (NHA)
	RMA	American Medical Technologist (AMT)
	CCMA	National Healthcareer Association (NHA)
	NCMA	National Center for Competency Testing (NCCT)
	NRCMA	National Association for Health Professionals (NAHP)
Medical Biller/Coders	CBCS	National Healthcareer Association (NHA)
	CCS, CPC, CPB	American Health Information Management Association (AHIMA)
	CPC	American Association of Professional Coders (AAPC)
	CPB	American Association of Professional Coders (AAPC)

Tips for Passing Professional Examinations

* Start preparing early. This suggestion is not intended to add further stress to your already busy class and study schedule. It is a reminder that if you prepare over a period of time, you will learn more and experience less stress when the time comes to actually take the test.
* Keep your notes, handouts, and textbooks organized so you can find and use them for review before the examination.
* Pay attention to any information and advice your instructor gives you about the content of professional examinations.
* Some textbooks refer to specific examinations and requirements of professional organizations, and the authors of the textbooks design their content and review questions to help students prepare throughout their courses. Take advantage of these features!
* Find out if there are review books available in your school library or for purchase or online materials to help you focus your studies on mastering the material likely to appear on the examination.
* Practice tests are available for many examinations. Check with your professional organization.
* Find out whether review workshops are available in your area.
* Plan to take the examination as soon as possible after you become eligible. This is usually upon graduation from your program, although some occupations also require work experience. You are less likely to forget information and lose your confidence if you do not wait too long.

⭐ EXPERIENTIAL EXERCISES

1. Learn about the required or voluntary professional examinations for your future occupation. (Sources of information: *Occupational Outlook Handbook* at http://www.bls.gov/ooh/ and your professional organization.)
2. Take practice examinations or study review questions, if they are available.

Academic Dishonesty

LEARNING OBJECTIVE 9: ACADEMIC DISHONESTY

- Explain why cheating is a serious offense for health care students.
- Explain the potential consequences for the patients of students who cheat.

Health care professionals must follow high ethical standards. High-quality patient care and safety depend on their actions, and there is no room for cheating in any form. Furthermore, governmental regulations have increased, and audits of health care facilities are common. The consequences of fraud and taking shortcuts may be severe, including costly fines, termination, and closures of health care facilities.

You may believe cheating on tests in school is not as serious as cheating on the job, but this is not true. Health care graduates who cheat to pass their classes, instead of learning what they need to know on the job, may become dangerous professionals. You are in the process of becoming a professional, and what you do now is setting the groundwork for your future actions. Integrity, honesty, ethics, and trustworthiness are essential characteristics of health care professionals, and cheating undermines your profession.

Even if you do not cheat yourself, helping others to do so promotes incompetence in the health care system. Would you or one of your family members want to be treated by "professionals" who cheated to pass their classes? Do you want to carry the load at work for a co-worker who is used to taking the easy way out? Helping friends cheat allows them to avoid taking responsibility for themselves. This can lead to the habit of dependence and unsatisfactory performance on the job, resulting in negative consequences for everyone.

⬅ JOURNALING 8.8

Have you ever felt tempted to cheat, or have you cheated on a test? How did you feel afterward? Why is cheating in a health care class an especially serious offense? What are some possible future effects on the job for students who passed their classes by cheating instead of studying?

❓ WHAT IF?

A classmate tells you she could not study for an examination because her ex-husband has been harassing her. She asks you to help her out by sharing your test answers during the examination. You sit together in the back row, so it is unlikely the instructor will see you.

CASE STUDY 8.3

Mother Knows Best

Rosa Gonzalez is the first in her family to pursue studies beyond high school. She is enrolled in a dialysis technician program. Although she finds her classes interesting, they are also very challenging. They are much more difficult than those she took in high school. As she told her friend, Amelia, "High school classes were pretty easy. I didn't really have to study that much to get by."

Amelia, who is now working in her family's store, replied, "This is why I didn't go to college. I'm earning enough in the store and don't have the hassle of studying and tests to worry about."

Rosa told her friend that she really thought health care would be really interesting and satisfying. "But," she said sadly, "maybe I've made a mistake."

After receiving a "D" grade on her first major examination, Rosa felt ready to give up. That evening, she said to her mother, "Mama, I'm so discouraged. I'm thinking about dropping out of school." "But Rosa," her mother replied, "I thought this meant so much to you."

"I know," said Rosa. "It did—or I thought it did. But I'm afraid I'm too dumb or something. I'm just not getting it." Her mother thought for a moment. "Rosa, I know that you're definitely not dumb. Maybe you just need to work a little harder or different now that you're in college. Listen, you're paying good tuition money for school. Why don't you talk with one of your instructors and see if they can give you some help?"

Later that night, Rosa thought over what her mother had said. It did make some sense. She did admit that she did not do more than sit in class. She did not take notes or study very much. The next day, she made an appointment with her instructor, Ms. Santori. As they talked, Ms. Santori asked about Rosa's study habits. "Well," Rosa said, "I really don't have a lot of time to study. And in high school, I just paid attention in class and did okay. I didn't have to do that much to get by."

Ms. Santori pointed out, "Getting by won't work anymore, Rosa. You're training for an important career that affects patient health and safety. Everything you're currently learning is preparing you for your profession, and it has to be done correctly and accurately. You've got to be prepared."

Rosa admitted that she had not thought about it that way. She asked Ms. Santori for suggestions about improving her time management and study habits to do better.

"Rosa," said Ms. Santori, "I like your attitude. I'd be glad to help you. We can get started today by looking at your out-of-class schedule and exactly what you do when studying for tests."

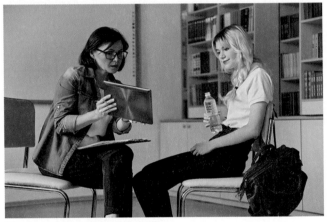

iStock.com/Valeriy-G/1337798085

QUESTIONS FOR THOUGHT AND REFLECTION

1. Why is Rosa having difficulties handling college-level classes?
2. Is Amelia right that Rosa should think about getting a job rather than more education after high school?
3. What suggestions do you think Ms. Santori will give Rosa?
4. Do you think Rosa will complete her program and succeed as a dialysis technician? Why or why not?

A Different Path

Jed Stuart's parents always expected that he would attend college. They hoped he would attend the university where they met and became engaged, thinking he would enjoy living in a fraternity, attending parties and football games, and participating in other college activities. Jed, however, did not really consider himself to be the "college type." He was never very social. He preferred staying home, playing video games, and watching sports and movies on television.

During his senior year of high school, his parents insisted that he start making plans. "Jed," his father told him, "you've got to start thinking about your future."

"Dad," Jed said, "I'm really not interested in going away to school and living in a dorm with a bunch of guys I don't know."

"Well," his dad said, "you know our house rules. After high school, you either need to go to school or get a job and pay some rent if you want to live here. You'll be an adult, and you'll have to act like one."

Jed realized that the only jobs he would qualify for did not pay much. And although he was not crazy about continuing his education, he knew he did not want to be stuck in a dead-end job for the rest of his life. He knew from the career exploration class that seniors were required to take that jobs in health care were promising and in high demand.

Jed talked with the admissions counselor at a local college about the various programs offered. He decided to apply for the medical coding program. He liked the idea of mainly working alone, and the job prospects and salary sounded pretty good. He decided he would enroll in the program after graduation in June.

Once in college, Jed thought his classes were okay. The main thing he did not like was having to work with other students when group projects were assigned. He was also reluctant to ask questions in class when there was something he did not understand. Besides being shy, he believed it was the instructors' responsibility to explain the material well enough so that students could understand the material. This was his reasoning for not spending much time studying his textbooks. If the instructors did not explain it in class, he figured that it must not be that important.

Jed passed the first few short quizzes in his classes, but he failed the midterm examinations in two classes. As he told his parents, "The instructors in these classes really aren't that good. The students haven't worked with this stuff before. How do they expect us to learn it if they can't explain it well?"

QUESTIONS FOR THOUGHT AND REFLECTION

1. What do you think about Jed's reasons for selecting a medical coding program?
2. Do you think he will do well on future tests?
3. Do you think Jed will complete the program?
4. How is his attitude about working with others and speaking up in class affecting his academic success?
5. Is his opinion about the instructors' responsibilities correct? Why or why not?
6. What responsibilities do students have for succeeding in their programs?

Preparing for the Externship

The Importance of the Externship

LEARNING OBJECTIVE 1: THE IMPORTANCE OF THE EXTERNSHIP

- Explain the purpose and benefits of the externship.
- Describe how to prepare for the externship.
- Consider what qualities you can offer to the site where you do your externship.
- Write out goals you want to achieve as you complete your externship.

The difference between ordinary and extraordinary is practice.

—Vladimir Horowitz

Your externship can be one of the most valuable parts of your education. It provides the final link between your education and the skills you learned in the classroom to your future career. The externship helps build an important bridge between school and the real world of work.

The externship is an experiential learning opportunity that is most likely a part of your educational or training program. It allows students to apply academic knowledge in real-world settings. It can have multiple names, such as practicum, internship, or clinical experience, but often encompass the same meaning. Regardless of what it is called, it is when students demonstrate the knowledge and skills they have learned in a supervised, real-world setting. The purpose of the externship is to gain firsthand insight into a career or industry of interest. The externship allows for practical experience and provides an opportunity for students to successfully apply relevant skills and knowledge in a professional setting. It is a great way to gain practical, on-the-job experience before beginning a job in your profession.

Many educational and training programs have some form of an externship, such as nursing, medical assisting, surgical technician, and dental assisting. In most cases, the externship is at the end of the program, and it may be either an optional or a required component of the program.

Experienced professionals and/or externship instructors will guide your work experience in a real occupational setting. Take advantage of this exciting phase of your education to do the following:

* Apply the skills learned in class.
* Gain confidence in performing these skills.
* Learn firsthand about the expectations of employers.
* Practice working with patients.
* Think and problem-solve in real-life situations.
* Gain a clearer idea of what kind of job you would like after graduation.
* Demonstrate your abilities to a potential employer (students are sometimes hired to work at their externship site after graduation).

A successful externship requires your full attention and effort. Some students make the mistake of thinking that this part of their education is just one more assignment, especially if the externship is graded on a pass-fail basis. But nothing could be further from the truth! During your externship, you will deal with real people and real problems. It will be important for you at this time to establish your professional reputation and practice what you have learned.

In addition, the externship allows a student exposure to their future profession. They can understand the pros and cons, which may help them make better informed decisions about their future profession and employer. The externship can also be used as an important component of your resume. Future employers want to see what real-world experience you have after completing your program.

Depending on how you perform on your externship and if there are any available positions, your site may be impressed with your abilities and performance and offer you a position after graduation. Thus, the externship is an excellent opportunity to showcase your skills to a future employer.

Set Goals for Your Externship Experience

What do you hope to learn from your externship? You will increase your chances of benefiting if you write out goals that express specifically what you want to learn, what skills you hope to practice and/or acquire, and what you hope to accomplish by the end of the externship.

It is recommended that you research the facility as much as possible before beginning your externship. This will help you anticipate, prepare good questions for your preceptor, who will be the professional overseeing your on-site experience, and set appropriate goals. Once at the site, share your goals with your preceptor and discuss what the site expects of you.

Ask if you can meet with your preceptor regularly, such as once a week, to discuss your progress and request feedback about your work. At the same time, conduct your own personal progress checks to see if you are meeting your own expectations and goals.

Fully engaging in your externship every day is a necessity and with many personal and professional benefits. It will help you fine-tune your clinical or technical skills you learned in the classroom. It is what you will be employed to do soon, so use this time to become more comfortable and efficient in your techniques and skills.

⭐ **EXPERIENTIAL EXERCISES**

1. Learn as much as you can about your future externship site. Look for a website and/or printed material. Ask your instructor for information.
2. Write three goals for your externship experience.

Before Your Externship

There are many steps before beginning your externship—some must be taken by you while others must be completed by your educational or training institution. In order to be placed at an externship site, your school must partner with a health care organization, such as a medical office, dental office, or hospital, that has sites and staff that are ready to train students. These partnerships often require a formalized agreement called an affiliation agreement. Affiliation agreements are contracts between the school and the organization or business that is providing the externship opportunity and site. They outline the general responsibilities and requirements of each party and often include student requirements. Box 9.1 lists common examples of externship requirements. In some cases, the organization or business may require a resume, cover letter, and interview from the student prior to approving the student's placement. Preparing a resume and a cover letter and preparing for an interview are discussed in later chapters.

Your school or program should have a staff member, called a clinical or externship coordinator or someone in career services, who arranges the externship site and will help you navigate the various steps in preparation for the externship. Prior to being placed at an externship site, there may be opportunities for the student to meet the supervisor who will oversee your externship experience, called a preceptor.

In some cases, you will be required to locate your own externship site. Some good sources for externship sites may be online job postings; contact them to see if they would allow you to perform your externship with them. Or contact or "cold call" a business that is around where you live to see if they would be willing to have you do your externship there. Finding your own site is possible, but it may take time and perseverance. If you have any questions or issues about the externship, you should contact the externship coordinator.

Depending on your program, the duration of the externship may be several weeks or months and will require a specific amount of time for you to commit each week. For example, an externship in a medical assisting program may require you to complete 160 hours. Working with the preceptor and externship coordinator, you will create a schedule and share it. The preceptor may recommend specific days and times for you to be available. For example, the preceptor may require you to avoid Monday mornings because it is the busiest time and there may not be any staff members to work with you. Your externship coordinator may recommend to you to work at least 20 hours a week in order to complete in a specific time frame or to ensure you are present at the site enough each week to experience working in a real-world setting.

Dress Code and Appearance

Depending on your program and externship site, your externship may have a dress code. Some facilities are more formal than others, and what is appropriate in one may be unacceptable in another. Follow the directions you receive during your orientation. As an extern student, it is better to be more rather than less conservative, even if other co-workers seem to be casual about their appearance. For example, an externship student in a medical billing and coding program or medical administrative assistant program may be asked to wear business professional attire, such as dress shirts and pants. Jeans, t-shirts, and other casual clothing are not appropriate for a health care setting unless specifically stated and approved by your preceptor.

For most externships, such as in a medical, surgical, or dental office, students will be required to wear a medical uniform (Figure 9.1). The medical uniform, or scrubs, includes a top and bottom and may include a lab jacket. Some medical offices and health care organizations may require a specific style or color of scrubs. It will be important to ask your externship coordinator or preceptor before the externship. Your school may provide the scrubs, or you may need to purchase them yourself. You should ensure your scrubs are clean and

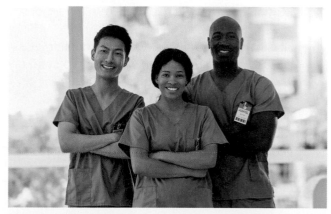

Figure 9.1 Students doing their externships may be required to wear a medical uniform. (iStock.com/PeopleImages/ 1388256621.)

wrinkle free. If you are provided with an ID badge, ensure it is visible and worn at all times. Generally, tennis shoes are appropriate but must be close-toed to prevent exposing skin to spills or needlestick injuries.

Your appearance during the externship must always be professional. Hair must be clean and neatly styled. Long hair must be pulled back so that when the students bend over no hair falls into the face. Students should avoid extreme styles or artificial colors. Any facial hair should be clean and neatly trimmed. Box 9.2 includes other important tips for appearance during the externship.

Students are expected to be free from body odor, tobacco, and scents, such as strong-smelling lotions, perfumes, and aftershaves. Avoid chewing gum or tobacco during the externship.

Students should wear a wristwatch with a clock face that has a sweeping/ticking second hand. Watches that only display digital numbers are not recommended. Smartwatches are allowed only if the watch can be set to show a clock face with a sweeping/ticking second hand that does not time out, does not require the student to touch it to activate it, and does not show incoming notifications while the clock face is active. Make sure you bring all the required supplies during your externship, such as a stethoscope, a small notepad, and a pen to take notes.

During the Externship

During your externship, you work side-by-side with health care professionals in the field you have chosen to study. You will help real patients with their individual needs, just as you would once you are employed. Although you are not an employee and should never be asked to fulfill a paid employee's position or duties, take this opportunity to learn as much as you can and work as closely as possible with your preceptor and the other staff members.

Your classroom experience has provided you with occupational knowledge and skills. Still, there will be a lot more to learn when you start your externship, because each facility has its own policies, rules, and procedures. In addition, you will need to know the proper operation of equipment, the location of supplies, and the correct way to fill out forms.

Start by learning about the job. Ideally, your preceptor should introduce you to the facility and the employees with whom you will work. Your on-site orientation should include the following:

* Tour of the facility
* Location of supplies, files, and anything you will need to do the job
* Safety rules
* How to use equipment
* Job description or list of your duties

As an externship student, you will be expected to perform your best and learn as you gain experience. If you approach your externship with a "can-do" attitude and apply the same skills that helped you succeed in school, you can learn and master your job systematically and effectively. Ask questions and be proactive, professional, flexible, and courteous. This is your prime opportunity to learn about your chosen profession.

Be prepared to meet expectations, such as working the required hours and being punctual. See constructive criticism as a chance to learn and improve. Remember, the people you are working with have experience to share with you.

Other responsibilities you may have during the externship are tracking the hours you completed at the externship site and documenting them, using either

BOX 9.2

Externship Appearance and Dress Code

- Jewelry: Students may wear two stud earrings (one in each ear only, if desired) and wedding ring, if desired. Dangling or loop style earrings pose a potential hazard and may not be worn in the clinical or lab areas. No other jewelry permitted.
- Piercings: Students may not wear any jewelry in any other areas, other than the lower ear lobe. If students have upper ear cartilage piercings, or face/neck piercings, then students may wear clear body piercing retainers in all those pierced areas.
- Headgear: Hats and caps should not be worn. Head scarves may be worn for religious reasons.
- Glasses/contact lenses: Only prescription glasses and/or readers are allowed, no sunglasses or darkly tinted glasses. Only clear or natural colored contact lenses are allowed, no extreme colors.
- Tattoos: Tattoos that are showing on the neck and arms and wrists must be covered at all times by white undergarments and/or white arm sleeves. Tattoos on the hands and fingers may remain uncovered.
- Make-up: Should be limited to neutral shades.
- Nails: Must be clean, short, and free of polish.

a paper form or an electronic submission. Your preceptor may be required to complete a mid- and final evaluation. You may need to remind your preceptor to complete, sign, and approve these forms.

Throughout your externship, it will be important for you to continually be in contact with your externship coordinator and preceptor. Whatever schedule you agree upon with your preceptor, do your best to meet your commitment; show up on time and when you are scheduled. If you are unable to show up, it will be important to inform your preceptor as you would any job. If there are issues or concerns at the externship site, inform your externship coordinator and, in certain situations, your preceptor as well. It is recommended to let your externship coordinator know first of any issues before notifying your preceptor.

Remember, the externship may result in a job offer. If it does not, ask your externship site preceptor for a letter of recommendation and be sure to add the experience to your resume.

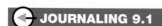 **JOURNALING 9.1**

Think about your personal characteristics. Which ones do you believe will most help you have a successful externship experience? Which ones do you need to work on to increase the benefits you will receive from your experience (e.g., shyness, impatience, or difficulty being on time)?

Preparing for the Externship

LEARNING OBJECTIVE 2:
PREPARING FOR THE EXTERNSHIP

- Explain what is meant by "shift your focus" as you begin your externship.
- Develop the habit of practicing empathy as a health care professional.
- Explain the importance of developing and maintaining a positive attitude.
- Describe ways of making a good first impression as you begin your externship.
- Use your study skills to help you learn during your externship.

By failing to prepare, you are preparing to fail.
—Benjamin Franklin

You should think of your externship as the bridge between what you have learned in the classroom to what you will be doing in your professional career. This may be a difficult transition for some students. In the classroom, it is a more controlled and comfortable environment with instructors who you are familiar with and classmates who you know. During the externship, the real-world, medical setting will most likely look different than the classroom, and there will be many new co-workers to get acquainted with.

In some cases, you will acquire new skills during your externship. Some externship sites may provide time and a staff member to assist you in mastering new skills. However, almost all sites will expect you to be competent in the basic skills of your professions, for example, taking vital signs if you are a medical assistant student, how to count pills if you are a pharmacy technician student, or how to complete an insurance claim if you are a medical biller or coding student.

The first days of your externship can be busy and stressful. Being able to practice your clinical and practical skills is one of the most important objectives of the externship. However, it is important to remember that, during the externship, you are still a student and learning. Do your best, but at the same time be patient with yourself. It takes time to make the adjustment from school to workplace. As an extern student, you may not be 100% confident of your abilities and may feel a little anxious about your performance. Keep in mind that no one expects you to know everything. Be okay with and ready not to know everything and admit when you do not know something and when you need help or have questions.

Several important things to remember:
1. Shift your focus.
2. Develop and maintain a positive attitude.
3. Make a good first impression by arriving on time, acting friendly and cooperative, and showing your enthusiasm for the work.
4. Learn all you can about the externship site and your duties.

Shift Your Focus

As a student, your main concerns are mastering new material, learning new skills, completing assignments, and performing well on tests and evaluations. Your principal responsibility is to yourself, perhaps to a family and a job, and to your personal progress. On your externship, you will need to shift your attention to the goals and needs of others: the externship site, the patients, and your co-workers. You are now accountable to people who are depending on what you do and how well you do it. Keep in mind that patients and others consider you as part of the staff. You now represent the organization, as well as yourself.

Empathy

Understanding the feelings and experiences of others—patients, preceptors, and co-workers—is essential. People who have experienced an illness or injury sometimes feel as if they have lost control of their lives. The empathy expressed by caregivers and other support personnel can be a critical component of their recovery. Empathy is also important in relationships with preceptors and co-workers. Mutual understanding promotes effective working relationships.

Each of us will interpret a given set of circumstances differently. Your externship will give you opportunities to work with people with different cultural and social backgrounds, levels of education, religious beliefs, and life experiences. Difficulties and misunderstandings arise because most of us take our assumptions for granted and do not see them as only one possibility out of many.

Here are some suggestions for developing empathy:

* Listen carefully to what the other person is saying. You must know their view before you can begin to understand, and you cannot know unless you listen.
* Do not judge what you hear. You are gathering information to help you understand the other person, not to decide if they are right or wrong.
* Ask questions or give feedback to ensure that you have received the other person's message as it was intended.
* An important point to keep in mind is that it is not necessary to agree with the beliefs of others. You must simply be aware of them and how they influence their perceptions and actions.

? WHAT IF?

What if a patient who has a common cold complains to you because the physician would not prescribe antibiotics? They do not understand that viruses cannot be killed by antibiotics and insist that the doctor is unwilling to help them.

← JOURNALING 9.2

Describe a situation in which someone made you feel as if they understood and respected you. How was this communicated to you?

Having a Positive Attitude

Approach your externship with enthusiasm and a positive attitude. Look forward to putting your skills into practice, meeting and learning from interesting people, and securing a good recommendation from your preceptor.

We can choose our reactions to people and events. If you find a staff member at your externship site to be especially annoying, it is natural to become angry or frustrated. But how does this benefit you? Negative feelings drain energy and may interfere with your focus on your work. This person is now not only annoying but also has, in a sense, taken over your emotions. Do not give negative people that power.

Choosing to approach life with a positive attitude releases you from the control of circumstances and frees you to focus fully on what has meaning for you. See Box 9.3 for suggestions on how to develop a positive approach to life.

Making a Good First Impression

The saying "You have only one chance to make a first impression" is worth thinking about. People tend to make judgments about others very quickly and often based on very little information. During your externship, others will be forming opinions about the level of your professionalism and competence. There are some key factors under your control that influence first impressions: punctuality, appearance, and courtesy (Figure 9.2).

It is critical that you arrive on time at your externship site, especially on your first day. Plan to arrive at least 15 minutes early on that first day. If you have not been to the externship site already, do a trial run during similar traffic conditions before your start date. Absenteeism and lack of punctuality are two major complaints of employers who accept students as externs.

Most people are strongly influenced by first impressions. Health care professionals, including

BOX 9.3

Focus on the Positive

- Do an inventory of the good things in your life, or start a gratitude journal in which you regularly record everything for which you are grateful.
- Keep things in perspective.
- Fix your sights on your goals.
- Distinguish between what you can and cannot change and concentrate your efforts on what you can change.
- Find sources of help and inspiration.
- Visualize the satisfaction you can receive by overcoming a difficult situation.
- Challenge your negative beliefs.

Accepting Criticism and Feedback

Always keep in mind that the main purpose of your externship is for you to *learn*. You have just completed your classroom training, and no one expects you to perform perfectly all the time. You may make mistakes or not handle situations ideally. In these cases, you may receive criticism from your preceptor or the staff members, or even a patient. Consider this criticism as instruction and an opportunity to learn.

No one likes to be criticized, and it is natural to react emotionally. Dismissing the criticism as unfounded, becoming angry, or taking the criticism to heart and feeling worthless are common reactions. Although these reactions are natural, they are not very helpful. A more constructive response is to pay attention to the message, examine the criticism, and consider it carefully. Then decide, honestly, if any or all of it applies to you. If it does, you can choose to benefit from it and work on self-improvement. If it does not, consider talking over your feelings with the person who gave the criticism to see where the misunderstanding lies.

Becoming a Competent Extern

LEARNING OBJECTIVE 3: BECOMING A COMPETENT EXTERN

- Describe transferable skills you have as a student to the externship.
- List different ways to manage yourself in the workplace.
- Explain the importance of teamwork and working as part of a team.
- List the six steps that are useful for solving problems.
- Explain how personal management habits influence your externship experience.

Employers have contributed to surveys about the competencies they value in their employees. As an extern student, you can work on developing these competencies. Doing so will help you best contribute to the success of your externship, as well as prepare you for a future job.

Transferable Skills as a Student

Being in your externship means still being a student and using many of the different skills you learned as a student. This may include note-taking, keeping a journal, and being an active reader.

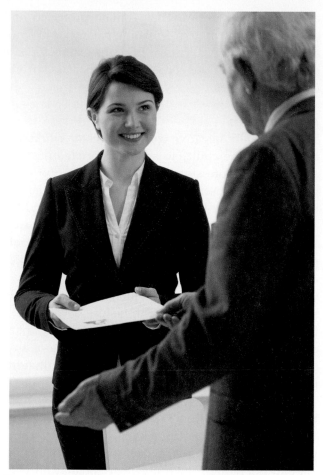

Figure 9.2 A courteous job seeker makes a good impression. (Copyright © istock.com.)

extern students, should follow the following dress and grooming guidelines:

1. Conservative—out of consideration for patients
2. Clean—for the safety and consideration of others
3. Safe—for the benefit of self and others
4. Healthy—to provide a good example of wellness

Courtesy, politeness, and manners are other factors in making a good first impression. Much more than simply using good manners, courtesy refers to being considerate and helpful. It means respecting the feelings of others and showing appreciation for the help you receive. Remember that you are there to learn, so do not get offended when others offer help or show you how to do things. Introduce yourself to anyone you do not know and be courteous to everyone at your site, whether you work with them or not.

◀─ JOURNALING 9.3

Describe a time when someone made a negative impression on you when you first met. Did your impression change after you got to know the person? Why and how? Did it take a long time to change?

Use Your Reading Skills

Printed or digital materials are the source of important job-related information. The following examples highlight a few of the most common ones:

* **Employee manuals.** These contain policies and rules regarding employee conduct, holidays and vacations, and other topics related to the employer-employee relationship. As an extern, some policies may not apply to you, but you should ask your preceptor if you can review the manual.
* **Policy and procedure handbooks.** Facilities create manuals to provide standard instructions for routinely performed tasks. Although it may not be necessary for you to read the entire manual, you should study the sections that apply to your duties. Pay special attention to procedures to follow in emergency situations.
* **Regulatory and approval agency standards.** Health care facilities are regulated by a variety of government and private agencies. Following the standards and rules set by these agencies is critical to the success—even survival—of a facility. See Box 9.4 for a list of important regulatory agencies.
* **Instructions and technical manuals.** Being able to read and follow instructions (often called documentation, especially when applied to computer software) is an important job skill. Misusing equipment or performing a procedure incorrectly can result in serious consequences, including injury to the extern and/or patient.
* **Professional publications.** These include general health care newsletters and journals and those that apply to your specialty. They help you keep up to date in your field, which is essential in health care.
* **Library.** Many large facilities, such as hospitals, have libraries with resources you may find of interest.

It is important to note that you should *not* read patient charts, unless given permission or direction as part of your duties. They contain protected and confidential information. Violating patient confidentiality may result in dismissal from the externship site and even more serious consequences, such as civil and criminal penalties.

Ask Questions

The potentially negative consequences of workplace errors make the ability to ask appropriate questions an essential professional skill. Whenever possible, use resources, observe, and think through situations to find the answer for yourself. If you cannot find the answer, there is no time to do research, or if the situation is urgent, do not hesitate to ask an appropriate person for help. See Box 9.5 for situations in which asking for guidance can be critical.

Knowing *when* to ask questions is important. In situations that are not urgent, choose a convenient time for the other person. It is also important not to ask questions about patients in the presence of anyone else, including other patients. Remember that the patient's right to privacy is protected by law.

Use Your Observation Skills

There may be important things you need to know about your externship site that no one will think to tell you. They are not written down anywhere and may not even be discussed. Everyone simply takes them for granted. Here are some examples of customs and expectations:

* **Level of formality:** Does Dr. Patricia Abrams want the staff to call her "Dr. Abrams" or "Dr. Pat"?
* **Amount of at-work socializing among employees:** Does everyone go out to lunch to celebrate birthdays and holidays, or do individuals who have become friends at work plan these events on their own time?
* **Organizational values:** What are the most valued employee/extern characteristics?

BOX 9.4

Important Health Care Regulatory Agencies

* Occupational Safety and Health Administration (OSHA): Oversees worker safety
* Clinical Laboratory Improvement Amendments (CLIA): Regulates laboratory testing on humans
* The Joint Commission: Evaluates the quality and safety of care for more than 15,000 health care organizations

---

BOX 9.5

When to Ask for Guidance

* Direct patient care in which the physical safety of both you and the patient is at risk
* Use of equipment, chemicals, and other materials that can be hazardous if handled incorrectly
* Administrative responsibilities in which errors can jeopardize the facility's standing with a regulatory agency
* Coding and billing tasks in which errors can cause rejection of payment by insurance companies, Medicare, and other agencies

* **Management styles:** Are student externs closely supervised or given lots of freedom?
* **Methods of communication:** Does your preceptor prefer all requests in writing?
* **Daily customs:** Who goes to lunch first?

You can learn the organizational culture and discover how to fit in as an extern student by observing carefully and asking questions. At the same time, student externs should maintain some professional distance and avoid getting involved in office politics or employee cliques. It is also best to avoid developing close friendships or dating employees until your externship has ended.

Observe in order to learn from the staff. Note how they perform their work. Pay special attention to employees who seem especially competent and effective in their work.

You may notice that some of the procedures and methods used at your externship site are different from those you learned in school. Often, a certain procedure can be performed in a variety of different, but correct, ways. Some experienced professionals develop preferences or acceptable (in terms of safety and effectiveness) shortcuts. Your facility may have specific reasons for using a different method. If you observe an employee using a method with which you are unfamiliar, increase your learning by asking the person to explain why it was done that way. Then use the method that is most comfortable for you *and* meets facility requirements.

Never suggest that an employee is wrong because they are not doing something the way you learned it in school. The only exception is if you believe a law or safety measure is being violated. Under these circumstances, it is usually best to speak first with the employee. Then, if necessary, speak with your preceptor. And never feel pressured, just because you are an extern, to perform a task in a way you know to be unsafe.

Use Your Note-Taking Skills

Your preceptor and co-workers will be important sources of useful information. Just as you took notes in class, you can profit from taking notes on your externship. Some note-taking situations will be formal, such as structured orientation sessions and employee training programs. Informal situations include receiving explanations and demonstrations from your preceptor and other staff. Taking good notes will prevent you from asking the same questions over and over, something that others will find annoying. Other benefits of taking notes at your externship site are listed in Box 9.6.

BOX 9.6

Benefits of Taking Notes in the Workplace

- It helps you to concentrate on what you are hearing.
- It reinforces what you hear, through the act of writing it down.
- It creates a record of information you can study later.
- It enables you to put together a personal reference guide.
- It demonstrates to your employer and co-workers that you care about your work and want to learn.

Recall that a key factor in effective note-taking is active listening: clear your mind of distracting thoughts, focus on what the speaker is saying, and ask questions to clarify anything you do not understand.

★ EXPERIENTIAL EXERCISES

Start preparing a list of questions or information you think you will need as you begin your externship. Take the list with you during your first few days to note the answers you receive by being told, observing, or asking.

Create a Workplace Reference Guide

There is a lot of information to remember during your externship. You may need the contact information of your externship preceptor in case of an emergency or if you are unable to show up on a day you are scheduled. There may be passwords you will need to remember for the facility's electronic health record software. You will be given this information when you first start your externship, and it will be important for you to save this information for later. There is nothing worse than to have to continually ask your preceptor or your co-workers for this information because you forget it.

Creating a reference guide would be an effective tool to save important information you want to refer to later. Your reference guide can be paper or digital. The important thing is to include information that will help you succeed in your externship. The following items you might find useful to include are:
* The name and telephone number of the person to contact if you must be absent or late
* Materials given to you during orientation or training sessions

* Notes taken during training sessions
* Schedules: holidays, vacation, meetings, and weekly schedules if they vary
* Facility staff directories and important phone numbers
* Maps and floor plans if you work in a large facility
* Notes from meetings attended
* Printed instructions and other how-to information
* Instructions about what to do in case of an emergency
* Procedures to follow during inclement weather

Do not record any patient names in your journal or any other identifying information to protect patient confidentiality.

Manage Yourself

Managing your personal habits effectively will help you succeed in your externship. As discussed in previous chapters, self-management skills include:

* Attitude
* Personal organization
* Time management
* Stress reduction techniques

Failure to maintain control in these areas can negatively affect your work in several ways, such as:

* Arriving late can disrupt the schedules of patients and co-workers.
* Running out of energy before the workday is over can delay the completion of important tasks.
* Repeatedly calling in sick because of stress-related illnesses may force others to fill in for you, disrupt schedules, and/or leave tasks undone.
* Failure to prioritize tasks can result in missing deadlines.
* Feeling tired can reduce your ability to concentrate and complete work assignments accurately.

This does not mean, however, that your life should be entirely devoted to work. In fact, just the opposite is true. You need to take time out to attend to your personal life. The key is to achieve a balance between your needs and those of others in your life: your preceptor, co-workers, patients, family members, and friends. If you continually ignore your needs, you can deplete your physical, mental, and emotional resources. The result will be that you have nothing left to give others.

At your externship site, self-management means the ability to work without constant supervision. Working without being reminded and told what to do will help you achieve a reputation as an excellent extern. If you are unclear about what you are supposed to be doing,

ask your preceptor. Never simply sit around, spend lots of time visiting with others, or engage in personal matters such as emailing friends or talking on your phone.

Believe in Your Self-Worth

To be beautiful means to be yourself. You don't need to be accepted by others. You need to accept yourself.
—**Thich Nhat Hanh**

Believing in your self-worth means that you value yourself and your actions. You consider both to be important and deserving of respect. You understand that you and your work truly make a difference. These beliefs provide the foundation for all other career competencies, because they generate the self-confidence necessary to ask questions, learn new skills, and build positive relationships with others.

⭐ **EXPERIENTIAL EXERCISES**

1. List five things you like about yourself.
2. List five accomplishments that give you pride.
3. List five things you believe will make you a good extern.

Demonstrate Integrity

Integrity means being guided by sound moral principles, such as sincerity and honesty. Following are some examples of workplace behavior that demonstrate integrity:

* Admit when you make a mistake. Covering up errors in the health care environment can have serious consequences.
* Conduct yourself ethically. This means conforming to established standards for moral and correct behavior. In addition to ethical standards that apply to society, each health care profession has a code of ethics that serves as a guide for proper conduct. You should become familiar with the code for your profession.
* Develop a strong work ethic. This means taking a positive approach to your duties and giving each task your best effort. As an extern, you have responsibilities, just as the paid employees do.
* Show appreciation to your externship site. You may not be paid as an extern, but the site has agreed to take the time to help you continue your training. See Box 9.7 for examples of ways to demonstrate loyalty.

BOX 9.7

Demonstrate Loyalty to Your Externship Site

- Dedicate your time on the job exclusively to work. Personal tasks and telephone calls should be limited to the lunch hour or break time.
- Do not use the site's computer to send personal emails or to surf the Internet at any time. Remember, anything that occurs online can be traced back to you.
- Never take anything that belongs to the employer. Do not contribute to the rising cost of health care by increasing the site's expenses.
- Do not speak badly or complain about your supervisor or the facility. If you have problems, seek solutions by discussing legitimate concerns directly with your supervisor.

★ EXPERIENTIAL EXERCISES

1. Obtain a copy of the code of ethics for your profession.
2. Read the code and describe if and how it addresses human dignity, loyalty, honesty and sincerity, and responsibility to patients.

Respect Confidentiality

You have an ethical and legal responsibility to respect patient confidentiality, including both oral and written communications. You must be willing to monitor your work habits and conversation to make sure this important patient right is constantly guarded. Serious or habitual disregard of this principle can be a cause for dismissal from your externship site, as well as fines and disciplinary action against the facility.

All health care facilities have developed policies and procedures to ensure that medical privacy is maintained. It is essential that you learn and strictly follow these policies to prevent problems for yourself and for your externship site. See Box 9.8 for suggestions to help you avoid unintentional "leaks" of private information.

In addition to patient confidentiality, you have an obligation to protect the privacy of the facility where you are doing your externship. You also need to respect your own privacy. This means that personal problems do not belong at work and should not be discussed there, not with staff members and *never* with patients.

BOX 9.8

Avoid Unintentional Breaches of Confidentiality

- Never discuss patient issues with anyone other than health care professionals who are directly involved in the care of the patient, and confine discussion to matters pertaining to this care.
- Limit allowable discussion to locations where you will not be overheard.
- When speaking with patients about personal matters, do so in a voice that only they can hear.
- Take care when speaking to and about patients on the telephone so as not to be overheard by others in the area.
- Leave patient-related matters at the externship site. Although it is natural to want to share your work with family and friends, any reference to patients and "interesting cases" is illegal.
- Clear computer screens containing patient records when you leave the computer.
- Do not leave paperwork or files containing patient information on reception counters and other areas where they can be viewed by unauthorized individuals.
- Do not discuss a patient's health information with anyone, even with a patient's spouse or relative, without the written permission of the patient.

Be Responsible

As an extern, you will be performing tasks that contribute to the workplace, and the employer will be depending on you. Acting responsibly means that your actions include the following:

* Be on time. If you have not already visited the site, make a trial run before the first day of your externship so you will know what time to leave home to arrive on time. Then be sure to arrive at the site on time every day, return promptly from lunch and breaks, and get to meetings on time. Absences should occur only for real emergencies. Have backup plans for child care, transportation, and anything else that could interfere with your attendance. If you are going to be absent, call your preceptor as far in advance as possible.
* Complete all tasks. This includes returning equipment and supplies to their proper places for the next person who needs them.

* Strive for accuracy. Examples of the many health care tasks in which accuracy is critical include patient charting, medical coding and billing, filling out compliance reports and laboratory reports, preparing sterile fields, and providing patient education.
* Assist when needed, even when it is not specifically your job. The unexpected must be anticipated in health care. Co-workers are sometimes absent, emergencies occur, and situations can quickly change from routine to urgent.
* Follow through with everything you are directed or have offered to do. If you cannot perform a task or need assistance, let your preceptor know so they can reassign the task or provide you with more help.

? WHAT IF?

What if the medical assistant who works in a busy pediatric office fails to autoclave the instruments as directed? As a result, the physician cannot perform minor elective surgery scheduled for a young patient. What would be the effect on the patient, parents, physician, and medical assistant?

Becoming Part of the Team

Failure to work well with others is a major cause of employee dismissal, because it reduces the health care facility's capability to provide high-quality service. Your externship will provide you with the opportunity to practice good interpersonal and teamwork skills (Figure 9.3).

Providing good health care requires the cooperation of many specialized individuals. In addition, new types of professionals, in response to medical advances and increasingly complex delivery systems, continue to join the team. Whatever your occupational field, you will be working with a variety of people who will bring different personalities, work styles, personal goals, and skill levels to the job. Your challenge will be to work in harmony with them all, because each one is important to successful care delivery.

Working With Your Preceptor

The externship provides you with a valuable opportunity to learn how to become a member of a team of professionals. How well you get along with your preceptor can make the difference between looking forward to each day and benefiting from your externship or dreading the thought of showing up and not getting much out of your time there. Take the time and effort to get to know this important person and do your best to maintain a positive relationship with the preceptor (Figure 9.4).

Just as instructors have their own teaching and classroom management styles, preceptors also are characterized by a variety of management styles. These are shaped by the preceptor's personality, beliefs about management, personal experiences, and the organizational culture in which they work. Table 9.1 contains examples of different management styles.

Your work style may not match the management style of your preceptor. This is not uncommon. Consider these differences as opportunities rather than obstacles. Several constructive ways to work effectively with your preceptor in spite of differences include the following:

1. Keep communication open. One of the worst things you can do is avoid someone with whom you disagree or have difficulty with, especially if it is your preceptor. Cutting off contact is likely to increase distance and decrease understanding.
2. Do not complain to the employees at your externship site. This does not resolve problems and can

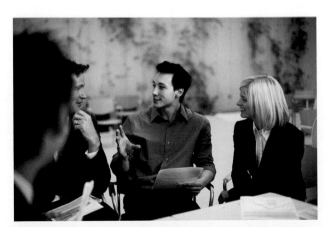

Figure 9.3 Health care professionals collaborate and discuss creative solutions. (Copyright © istock.com.)

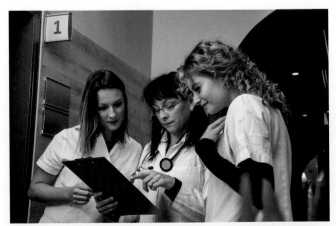

Figure 9.4 An important aspect of the externship is working with the preceptor. (Istock.com/Pokec/1209806626.)

actually create new ones: lowered morale among those who hear your complaints, lost work time, decrease in the quality of service to patients, and worsened relationships with the preceptor who hears about the grumbling through the grapevine.

3. Be empathetic. Your preceptor may have pressures and problems that you are unaware of.

4. Ask questions to learn your preceptor's priorities and find out what is most important. Box 9.9 contains examples of questions to ask your preceptor.

5. Ask for clarification if you are unclear about your duties or exactly what is expected of you.

6. Realize the bottom line is this: you must work with your preceptor, and this means adapting to their style. Do your best to make the situation positive. Focus on learning as much as possible from both the preceptor and the situation.

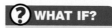
Mr. Cardenas, who does not understand English well, is scheduled for a laboratory test that requires him to follow certain directions the day before the test. The medical assistant gives him a written instruction sheet in English.

Use Problem-Solving Skills

A problem well stated is a problem half solved.

—Charles F. Kettering

Every day, we are confronted with situations that require us to solve problems and make decisions. You should expect to practice these actions during your externship, both at home and in the workplace. Having an organized way to approach problems

---

BOX 9.9

Questions to Ask Your Supervisor

- What are your expectations of me?
- What do you most value in an intern?
- How can I best contribute to the success of the organization and/or facility?
- How often would you like me to report to you?
- What is the best time to report to you, ask questions, and receive progress reports about my work?

TABLE 9.1
Common Management Styles

Management Style	Examples of Supervisor's Actions
Micromanages	Closely monitors your work. Frequently checks on you and wants regular progress reports.
Believes interns and employees work best on their own	Does not appear to pay much attention to your work unless something goes wrong.
Likes a friendly work environment	Conversation is warm and friendly. Interested in your family and other aspects of your personal life. Birthdays and holidays are celebrated in the workplace.
Maintains a businesslike environment	Keeps most conversation work-related. Co-workers who become friends engage in social activities outside the workplace.
Disorganized or too busy to keep order	Loses reports you have turned in. Forgets scheduled meetings. Does not give you promised follow-up in a timely manner. (Caution: Do not assume that because your supervisor is disorganized, they will tolerate *your* disorganization and accept actions such as completing assignments late.)
Values and practices order	Rarely misses deadlines and expects you to meet them, too, correctly and efficiently. Keeps lists, calendars, and orderly files.
Communicates directly	Lets you know how you are doing. Offers suggestions and criticism as needed. You know where you stand.
Communicates indirectly (or not at all)	Does not want to hurt your feelings. Avoids confrontations. May not tell you if you are doing something incorrectly or not to his or her liking. (Caution: May complain about you behind your back, thus depriving you of the opportunity to learn and resolve the problem.)

makes it easier to find effective solutions. One commonly used problem-solving method consists of six steps:

1. Define the problem.
2. Gather information.
3. Brainstorm solutions.
4. Consider possible results and consequences.
5. Choose a solution and act on it.
6. Evaluate the results and revise as needed.

Good problem-solving skills involve both reasoning and creativity. Start by examining what you believe to be the problem. Try to see it from different angles. Mentally walk around the problem, looking at it from all sides.

Try using brainstorming to come up with potential solutions. This means thinking of as many ideas as possible, from the sensible to the extreme. Think creatively. Original methods often provide innovative solutions to problems.

Whereas creativity generates ideas, reasoning helps you to put the ideas together in ways that work. It also helps you to test potential outcomes mentally. Use it to check "What would happen if …" scenarios for the possibilities you have brainstormed.

Before you approach your preceptor with a problem, think it through. Do your best to come up with solutions to suggest. This demonstrates your initiative and willingness to take an active part in solving workplace problems.

⭐ **EXPERIENTIAL EXERCISES**

1. Start now to prepare backup plans for your life during your externship. Consider transportation, childcare, and/or any personal responsibilities that could interfere with your attendance.
2. Develop organizational strategies that will help you balance your professional and personal lives.
3. Consider which of your self-management skills need improvement and develop a plan to improve them.

Overcoming Challenges and Issues

LEARNING OBJECTIVE 4: OVERCOMING CHALLENGES AND ISSUES

- Describe potential difficult situations that may occur during the externship.
- Identify different ways to handle difficult situations during the externship.

Despite your best efforts to learn and benefit from your externship, difficulties may arise. These can range from the annoying to the intolerable. Some problems can be handled with your own resources. Others require the assistance of others to resolve. In either case, approach problems with the intention of finding solutions. Choose actions that are appropriate for the situation and that will build your professional reputation.

Some situations must simply be tolerated. For example, patience may be required when working with people who have annoying habits. Actions, such as refusing to work with them and/or complaining to others behind their backs, may hurt you professionally and ruin your chances for a good recommendation from your preceptor. On the other hand, if you note serious situations, such as unsafe or illegal actions, taking place and not being corrected, you will want to report this to your school and discuss with your coordinator how to handle the situation.

The following are examples of problems that students may encounter during their externship:

1. You are asked to perform duties that fall outside your scope of practice, tasks for which you were not trained, or tasks that are illegal.
   Fortunately, this problem is rare. Unfortunately, when it does happen, it places the student in a difficult situation. The best advice in these cases is—do not do it. Even if you are pressured by your preceptor or are assured that it is okay and "everyone does it," this is too big a risk to take. Inform your preceptor that you were never trained to perform this and report this situation to your school.
2. You find it difficult to get along with your preceptor. Begin by taking an honest look at your own behavior to see whether there is something you are doing—or not doing—that contributes to the problem. Speak privately and frankly with your preceptor about how important your externship success is to you. Tell them that you want to have a good working relationship. Ask if there is anything you need to do to improve your performance.
   When trying to communicate with your preceptor, keep in mind that your purpose is to promote mutual understanding and get the information needed to perform your duties effectively. It is not to prove you are right or to tell your preceptor off—actions that will most likely make the situation worse. Look for ways to relieve your stress without venting your frustration at your preceptor.
3. You observe low employee morale. The employees at your externship site are unhappy and complain a

lot. You would like to get along with everyone and fit in, but the conversation and atmosphere are getting you down.

This can be a tough situation because you are there only temporarily, and it is unwise to become involved in negative conversation and office politics. Do your best to avoid participating in complaint sessions.

4. There is too much to do and you cannot finish all your work.

Start by reviewing your work habits. Are you taking too much time to complete each task? Are there some tasks that you are still learning? Are you practicing good time management skills?

You may be able to draw on the experience of your preceptor and/or the employees to help you increase your efficiency. If more than one person is assigning you tasks, make sure they are each aware of your other responsibilities and talk with your preceptor about prioritizing your work. If you cannot complete everything, which tasks are the most critical? What help is available?

5. Patients do not want to be attended to by a student extern.

Some patients will insist on being seen by someone they know: the physician or the long-time medical assistant they are most comfortable with. Do not take this personally. Patients may be in pain, upset, or experiencing difficult medical conditions.

After Your Externship

LEARNING OBJECTIVE 5:
AFTER YOUR EXTERNSHIP

- Explain how to evaluate your externship experience.
- Describe ways to show appreciation to the externship preceptor.
- Demonstrate how you can document your externship experience in your resume.

Once you complete your externship, congratulations, but you are not completely done. Take advantage of the fact that you successfully completed your externship and graduated from your program by leveraging them to launch your career.

Evaluating and Documenting Your Experience

Use your journal and task log to write a summary of what you learned. Marianne Ehrlich Green, author of *Internship Success*, suggests that students consider the following questions:

1. Did you meet your learning objectives [goals]? Explain how.
2. What was your most important contribution?
3. What new skills did you develop?
4. What were the highlights of your externship?

When asking yourself these questions, consider areas that need improvement and how you plan to improve them.

Showing Your Appreciation

In addition to verbally thanking your preceptor and everyone else who helped you, write a thank-you letter or email to your preceptor after completing your externship. Include a statement about what you learned and how they helped you to achieve your goals.

Be sure to ask your preceptor if you could receive a letter of recommendation or use them as a reference. This is important, especially if this is your only experience in the health care field. Keep this in mind as you do your externship: the skills and professionalism you exhibit here can influence your future employment prospects. Make copies of your letter of recommendation to include with your resume or to put in your professional portfolio.

Preceptors and even some team members who you worked with can serve as references when you are job searching. References are people who can talk about your work experience, work habits, character, and skills.

Career Opportunities

Some students are hired at their externship sites, although students should not expect to be offered a job. Some sites prefer to continue offering opportunities to students from local schools and, therefore, cannot hire every good student who works with them. Regardless, there is no harm in asking. In fact, if you have developed a good working relationship with the staff during the externship, your preceptor may inform you of future job opportunities and you may be a favored candidate.

Include your externship experience on your resume in the Education section. This will enhance your marketability when you are job searching. You can write a brief description of what you learned, the skills you practiced, specific accomplishments you achieved, or anything else that supports your job objective. List the name of the externship site, the beginning and end dates of your time there, and the total number of hours you completed. You should also list the duties in which you were trained and performed. Make sure to use proper medical terms to avoid any misspellings.

CASE STUDY 9.1
Advice From a Professional

Students in the medical assisting class at Goodhealth College are attending their first externship workshop conducted by Ms. Gutierrez, the school's externship coordinator. To help the students prepare for their first days at their externship sites, Ms. Gutierrez has invited Betty Stanford, a nurse with 42 years of experience, for a question-and-answer session.

Q: What advice would you give students who are starting their externship?

A: The basics are still very important for success. Things like professional appearance. In the last 10 years or so, trends like tattoos and facial piercings have become a problem, because some older patients find them objectionable. They don't understand they are just a fashion statement and no longer have the negative connotations they had years ago. Another style that's a problem is low-cut blouses and tops for female employees. These are seen just about everyplace these days, but they just aren't appropriate on the job in health care.

Q: Along with appearance, what other recommendations would you offer?

A: It's important to show an interest and initiative in your duties. Students should want to learn, and they can do this by asking questions—and then following up. By this, I mean writing the information down and making an effort to learn and remember it. We had a student recently who would ask questions and then fail to pay attention. She ended up doing the work her way, which unfortunately wasn't always correct.

Q: There are instances in which students with recent training believe their current education actually makes them more qualified than experienced health care workers. Have you run into this problem?

A: Yes, unfortunately. Although we want students to feel confident about their skills and what they learned, they're still students and still learning. What most students forget is that it takes years to be fully competent in your profession, and they may be working with people who have decades in the profession. They need to do their best to perform efficiently and correctly, while also being willing to learn and be open to feedback. Not being able to take feedback and criticism is not only detrimental to being a student and learning but to the care we give to patients.

Q: What other advice do you consider essential for success in a health care externship?

A: In a few words, be prepared to meet the needs of others, and I don't just mean your patients. I used to work in the ER. When there was a seriously injured accident victim, for example, I was not only helping the patient but also dealing with family members and friends and working with other hospital personnel. There were lots of things to consider, and they all dealt with people. Regardless of the situation, good social skills are really a must.

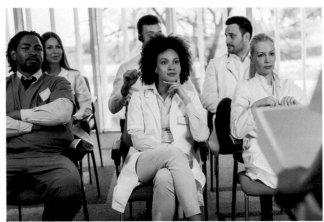

iStock.com/Jovanmandic/1212725864

QUESTIONS FOR THOUGHT AND REFLECTION

1. Why do some people find tattoos or facial piercings objectionable?
2. Why would health care staff find it inappropriate for students to wear revealing, low-cut tops when working at their externship site?
3. How do you plan to learn from the experience of others when doing your externship?
4. If you think you know how to perform a procedure in a better way than what you see employees doing at your site, what should you do?
5. What are the possible consequences if students neglect people skills and focus only on their practical skills while on their externship?

A Different Path

Paul worked in construction for many years before deciding it was time to hang up the hammer. The climbing, bending, and reaching were starting to get to him, and he wanted to be able to enjoy his later years without the injuries he witnessed in older co-workers.

Paul was not ready or financially able to retire, so he spent some time thinking about what he wanted to do next. As a teen, he had considered the medical field, but his family did not have money for college. So, he had followed his hobby of building things and went into construction with his uncle Pete. Now in his 50s, Paul thought it might be interesting to check out a health-related career. He ended up enrolling in a medical assisting course and discovered that he really enjoyed the technical aspects of the program.

Being the oldest student in his class bothered him a bit. His study skills were pretty rusty and concentrating on reading took some effort. But he made it through his program and was happy to be assigned to a large orthopedic clinic near his home for his externship.

As the only clinic in the area specializing in orthopedics, the clinic was a busy one. Paul's preceptor, Ms. Adams, only had time to greet him and give him a very brief description of his duties. Paul spent the first couple of days trying to orient himself. In school, it seemed like everyone was younger than he was. This made him self-conscious and hesitant to ask questions about his duties and how he was to perform them. He believed that at his age, he should be able to figure things out for himself. He tried observing

the employees and thinking about what he had learned in school. The confusing thing was that much of what went on at the clinic was either unfamiliar to him or done in ways he had not been taught. Still too embarrassed to ask for help, he did what he believed were his assigned tasks as best he could, keeping to himself much of the time.

Paul believed that his work had been satisfactory. But a couple of weeks into his externship, his preceptor called him into her office and informed him that some of his work was not up to par—that he was not following the protocols of the clinic. At this point, Paul became upset, raising his voice and telling Ms. Adams, "I can't believe you're telling me this! I've tried hard to figure out what I'm supposed to do here—and how to do it. I really believe I've done my best."

Ms. Adams replied, "That may be—that you've tried. But if you were having trouble, why didn't you ask for help? You never said anything, so we just assumed you were doing okay. Unfortunately, that's not the case."

QUESTIONS FOR THOUGHT AND REFLECTION

1. Whose responsibility was it to explain Paul's duties when he started his externship?
2. Whose responsibility was it that Paul understood his duties after the first week?
3. What could Paul have done to make his experience at the clinic more positive?
4. What do you think he should do now?

CHAPTER 10

Starting the Job Search

BY THE END OF THIS CHAPTER, YOU WILL BE ABLE TO

- Understand Transferrable Skills Needed to Succeed in School and on the Job

- List Three Actions You Can Take to Get the Most Out of Your Health Care Training

- Describe What Employers and Patients Expect From Health Care Professionals

- Know What Skills You Have to Offer an Employer

- Use a Variety of Resources to Locate Health Care Job Leads

- Create a Product—Your Professional Self—That You Can Offer With Confidence to Prospective Employers

- Develop a Professional Appearance That Is Appropriate for the Health Care Field

- Begin Professional Networking Activities

Your Career in Health Care

Your First Step on the Road to Success

Congratulations! By choosing to study for a career in health care, you have taken the first step toward achieving a fulfilling and rewarding future. You have made a significant commitment to yourself and your community.

By enrolling in an educational or training program, you have demonstrated your ability to set your sights on the future, make important decisions, and follow through with action. You have proven that you have a strong personal foundation on which you can build the skills and habits needed to ensure your success in school and in your career.

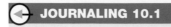

Connecting School and Your Career

- List ways that study skills, such as note-taking, writing, and taking tests, are useful in life and on the job.
- Describe the work habits you want to develop while you are in school.
- Practice asking questions that help you better understand your subjects in school.
- Investigate the resources your school has to offer and use the ones that can help you.
- Dedicate yourself to learning as much as you can from your school experiences.

The process of becoming a health care professional began the day you started classes. In addition to providing you with opportunities to learn important technical skills, your education will help you acquire the attitudes, personal characteristics, and habits of a successful professional. Students who practice good work habits in school generally carry those same habits into the workplace.

A powerful first step you can apply to your life is to act as if you already are what you hope to become (Figure 10.1). Practice behaviors now that you know will be expected on the job. For example, because accuracy and efficiency are important characteristics for the health care professional, complete all class assignments as if the well-being of others depended on your ability to be accurate and efficient.

You can apply the organizational, personal, and study skills discussed in the previous chapters to achieve success in school, during the job search, and on the job. Below are four examples:

1. Time Management

   Your success in school depends heavily on how well you organize your time. Effective use of time is also an important health care job skill. Many health care professionals are responsible not only for their own time but also for planning other people's schedules. Administrative medical assistants, for example,

may be in charge of the health care provider's daily appointment scheduling. Medical coders and billers must submit claims on time to ensure the facility gets prompt reimbursements and avoid denials and any financial losses.

2. Communication

   Expressing yourself clearly and listening attentively are important for participating in class and asking and answering questions, as well as for establishing and maintaining relationships with your instructors and classmates. A critical part of the job search is the interview, in which you combine your ability to think and use verbal skills effectively. Good communication skills are necessary for health care, because most positions involve interaction in some form with others, including patients, co-workers, supervisors, and the general public.

   Physical and occupational therapy assistants are examples of the many health care professionals who provide patient education. The effectiveness of their explanations of exercises and self-care techniques influence their patients' rehabilitation progress.

3. Taking Notes

   You may think note-taking is limited to your courses, but this skill is used extensively outside the classroom. During the job search, it will be important to record information about job openings, interview appointment dates, and times and directions to facilities accurately. During and after interviews, you may want to make notes about the job requirements, additional information you need to send to the prospective employer, and other important facts.

   Note-taking is also an important health care job skill. Many professionals are responsible for interviewing patients and taking patient histories. Another specialized form of note-taking is called charting, which is making notes and documenting the patient's health status on medical records in either written or electronic form. The notes include information about symptoms, treatments, and medications prescribed. These medical records not only affect patient care but also are legal documents. They must be clear, accurate, and complete.

4. Taking Tests

   You may think you are done with taking tests once you leave school, but testing is not limited to the classroom. The truth is that life is full of tests. Job interviews are a form of testing designed to assess your ability to present yourself and your qualifications. To legally work, there are many health care professionals, such as licensed practical nurses,

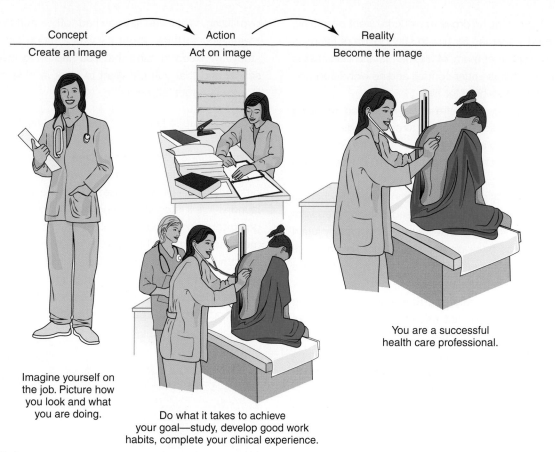

Concept → Action → Reality
Create an image → Act on image → Become the image

Imagine yourself on the job. Picture how you look and what you are doing.

Do what it takes to achieve your goal—study, develop good work habits, complete your clinical experience.

You are a successful health care professional.

Figure 10.1 Become what you visualize. (From Haroun L: *Career development for health professionals: success in school and on the job*, ed 4, St. Louis, 2016, Saunders.)

radiological technologists, and physical therapists, who must pass a professional examination. Other occupations, such as medical assistant, have voluntary examinations to obtain certifications or registrations that make them more marketable to employers. In fact, many employers only hire certified medical assistants.

Once on the job you are, in a sense, being tested every day. Although you may not think of your regular tasks as tests, they are applications of what you have learned, and your ability to perform them correctly will be noted by your patients, co-workers, and supervisor. The annual employee performance evaluation is a type of test or a "grade" in which your supervisor writes a report about your performance and then meets with you to discuss it. Learning to perform "when it counts" is a valuable skill and represents the ultimate ability to take and successfully pass a test. For example, the mother of an infant wants to know that the health care professional giving the injection has "passed the test" and is qualified to safely perform the procedure.

CASE STUDY 10.1
Control of Time, Control of Life

Sam was late again. He had overslept and could not find his car keys. On top of everything else, he discovered that he did not have clean clothes ready for the day. He dreaded the look—and possible lecture—he would get from his boss, physical therapist Angie Johnson.

The tough part was that Sam really liked his job as a physical therapist assistant and did not want to lose it. He had worked hard, and in fact struggled at times, to complete his program at Wellness College, and he did not want to lose everything now because of his tardiness.

Feeling stressed as he drove to work, he went over in his mind how hard it seemed for him to stay on top of things in his life. He noticed that many of his friends and classmates seemed to have things under control, and he wondered why everything seemed so hard for him.

Today felt like the last straw. He was tired of being rushed and worried, so he decided to see if Angie had any advice. After all, she was well aware of his problem. Maybe if he talked with her, she would realize that he was serious about improving.

There were already patients waiting in the office when he arrived, so he knew Angie would already be annoyed with his tardiness. Everyone got to work, however, and by lunch time the office was back on schedule. Sam asked Angie if they could talk in her office. "Sure," she answered. "It's probably a good idea for us to meet."

Once in her office, Angie told Sam that, despite being good with patients, it did not help her or his co-workers when he was not there on time, especially with the early appointments. "Sam," she said, looking directly at him, "you've got to get yourself organized, or you're not going to make it in this office, or in this field, for that matter."

Sam looked down at his hands and said in a soft voice, "I know, Angie, and that's what I wanted to talk to you about. I love this job, but I just can't seem to get my act together. I thought maybe you'd have some suggestions."

"Well," she said, "you seem to have a lot of trouble with time management. Tell me, do you write lists and prioritize your tasks, so that you get the most important things done first?"

"No," said Sam. "I just keep stuff in my head and do what seems right at the time."

Angie asked Sam how he was able to finish his homework and the studying needed to pass his examinations at school.

Sam laughed. "I pulled at lot of late nights—even some all-nighters. There always seemed to be other stuff to get done, so a lot of times I didn't sit down to study until maybe 10 or so at night."

Angie thought for a few moments and said, "We may have identified part of the problem, and it has to do with prioritizing. When you say you had "other stuff to get done," I want you to think about it—was it more important than studying? Keep in mind that you had a big investment in school and that you did want to work in physical therapy. Do you like your job here?"

Sam sat up in his chair. "Absolutely. I really like working here."

"I thought so," said Angie, "and you are good at it. But you've got to get in control of your time, arrive at work promptly, and—," she smiled, "—make time to do your laundry. We'll start by talking about prioritizing. I'm also going to recommend a couple of books on time management that I think will help you."

Sam was so appreciative that he had found someone to help him—his boss, no less. He promised himself that he would do his best to learn about and practice time management and personal organization. He had so much to gain.

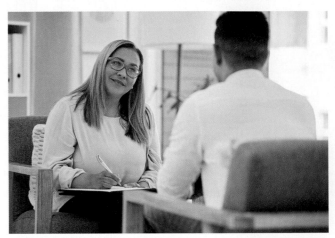

iStock.com/PeopleImages/1369683259

QUESTIONS FOR THOUGHT AND REFLECTION

1. What made Sam finally seek help for his tardiness and disorganization?
2. Why do you think Angie was willing to help him?
3. How would learning to prioritize improve Sam's life?
4. How do you think Sam's habits as a student now will affect him as a professional?

A Different Path

Until today, Christie had been pleased with herself and her life. Just 6 months ago, she completed her nursing training and passed the state licensing examination. Now, at age 22, she is a registered nurse and has a job at a long-term nursing facility.

While in school, she studied hard and took pride in the grades she received in most of her courses. She especially enjoyed anatomy and physiology and classes on nursing procedures. But as she told her friend, Nadine, one day on the phone, "I just don't understand all the emphasis on communication skills. It seems like the instructors are always going on about it. I mean, I'm great at communicating, and people think I'm funny."

"That's true. You always have something interesting to say, including the latest news and gossip," Nadine laughed.

"Right! In fact, I've got something good to tell you about right now. Remember Gerry, the girl I told you about in class—I thought she was carrying on with Jim? Well, I heard she's pregnant."

"Get out!" exclaimed Nadine.

"No kidding! But listen, I've got to go. My next class starts in 15 minutes."

Once on the job at the nursing home, Christie applied what she believed to be her "good communication skills" by befriending other staff members, chatting with the patients, and sharing juicy stories to keep everyone entertained. She noticed that not everyone, especially her co-workers, seemed interested in spending much time visiting with her, but she figured these people were simply too busy working or not the friendly type.

Christie thought things were going just fine until today when Sarah Caldwell, the nursing director, called Christie into her office. "Christie," she said. "I've got to talk with you about how you are communicating with the other staff and patients."

"You must be kidding," exclaimed Christie. "I'm one of the best communicators around here. Some staff don't even talk—"

"Christie!" interrupted Sarah. "I'd like to know how you are defining 'communicate,' because what I'm hearing about you certainly does not fit my definition, especially for a professional."

"I like people. I like to talk. I like to share the news," Christie explained.

"Well, the 'news,' as you call it, that you are sharing often involves personal information about patients, as well as about staff members. Patient confidentiality is critical in health care. It is our legal and professional responsibility. You simply cannot share information with anyone who is not on the patient's care team. And even then, it must be discussed in private, out of earshot of others."

For once, Christie did not know what to say. She was not sure she agreed with Sarah. After all, what kind of an impersonal place would this be if people could not talk to one another and make "small talk"? She told Sarah she would think about what she had said.

"I certainly hope so," said Sarah. "In other ways, you are a good nurse. But, if this doesn't stop, it could be grounds for dismissal. I won't have a choice."

Christie did not say anything. But a thought did pass through her mind: Maybe her instructors were right when they encouraged her to work on her communication skills.

QUESTIONS FOR THOUGHT AND REFLECTION

1. Describe what Christie means by "good communication"?
2. What could be the consequences for the nursing home if Christie continues to share confidential information about others, especially the patients?
3. Other than confidentiality, what issues is Christie having with her communication skills?
4. How would you describe Sarah Caldwell's definition of good communication?
5. Describe a situation in your future profession where good communication and "soft skills" may be more important than clinical or technical skills?

Maximizing Your Education

You are making a significant investment of time, effort, and money in your education. A worthy professional goal is to do everything possible to become the best health care professional you can be. Both you and your school have responsibilities to ensure that this happens.

Your Rights as a Student

That's the very reason they put erasers on the end of pencils ... because people make mistakes. Phoebe Waller-Bridge.

1. Make Mistakes
   You may think this sounds a little strange. After all, are you not supposed to do the best you can,

earning the highest grades possible? Yes, but many students see grades as ends in themselves, rather than as signs of having mastered the skills they will need in the future. Good grades do not always guarantee mastery, nor do you receive grades for all the skills that will determine your future success. Many students want to know "what's on the test" so they can focus their efforts on learning only what they will be tested on. But think about it—can you possibly be tested on everything you will need to know and do to perform your job? If you were, all class time would have to be devoted to testing, leaving little or no time for learning! Studying only what you need to pass tests and earn grades may make you a "good student," but a good student is not necessarily a good health care professional.

Compare your educational experience with learning to ride a bike. First, you use training wheels, go slowly, and tip over occasionally. Eventually, you become a proficient cyclist, able to go faster, and stay upright. Learning is similar to this. School offers you a rehearsal for professional life, providing you with opportunities to learn from mistakes that would be unacceptable if you were to make them on the job. A health care professional may have made mistakes when they practiced working with a classmate in the laboratory, but they learned from them and are now able to use correct techniques to help their patients (Figure 10.2).

The one who knows all the answers has not been asked all the questions.

— Confucius.

2. Ask Questions

You are attending school to benefit from the knowledge and experience of your instructors. So, take advantage of this opportunity by being an active participant in your classes. Do not be an invisible student. If there is something you do not understand, ask questions.

Never be afraid of looking stupid or hesitat to admit you do not understand or are confused. Keeping quiet when you are having difficulty understanding material not only decreases the chances of maximizing your education but also prevents you from learning a critical health care skill—how to ask good questions. Consider, for example, the serious consequences for a medical assistant who is not sure of drug dosages or the steps in a procedure but is

afraid to ask the supervisor for direction. In these situations, risking the safety of patients is indeed foolish and dangerous, whereas asking questions demonstrates professionalism and an understanding of the critical nature of your profession.

Of course, you should not use questions to substitute for reading your textbook or studying the assigned material before each class meeting. This results in the misuse of class time and is unfair to students who are prepared. A related on-the-job example is employees who arrive late and unprepared for meetings, thus wasting their co-workers' time. Develop habits now that show consideration for others.

3. Take Advantage of School Resources

Every school wants every student who enrolls to graduate, and considerable resources are spent on services to support this effort. Find out now what services are available to you, the hours they can be accessed, and whether appointments are necessary. Two of the most important services that all students should become familiar with are the library (or resource center) and career services.

If you are having personal problems or academic difficulties, ask whether your school provides counseling and/or tutoring (Figure 10.3). Some schools refer their students to outside agencies that offer assistance and resources for problems, such as domestic abuse, substance issues, mental health, and childcare.

The school catalog or student handbook is an often-overlooked source of information that can help you succeed in school. Inform yourself about the resources your school offers by spending a few minutes reading these documents and other printed information produced by your school. On the job, you will likely be expected to read organizational handbooks and procedure manuals. Getting in the habit of reading informational literature is a good job skill.

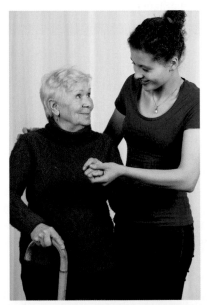

Figure 10.2 The time to learn and even make a few mistakes is while you are in school. You want to be competent on the job when you work with patients who depend on your knowledge. (Copyright © istock.com.)

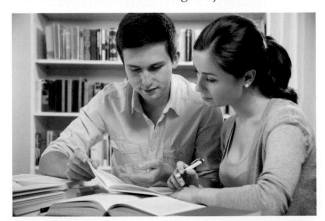

Figure 10.3 Being a student in the health care field is not easy. If you find yourself falling behind in class, it is important to seek assistance from counselors and tutors. (Copyright © istock.com.)

What if a classmate with whom you are friends confides in
you that their partner has been physically abusing them?
What would you do to help them? What resources are
available to help your classmate?

EXPERIENTIAL EXERCISES

1. Take a tour of your school and list the resources available for students.
2. Read a copy of your school catalog and highlight important policies that apply to you.

Your Responsibilities as a Student

1. Attend All Scheduled Learning Activities

   Health care educational programs feature a variety of learning opportunities, including lectures, laboratory sessions, guest speakers, field trips, and hands-on experiences in medical facilities. These activities are designed to help you understand and gain knowledge and skills necessary for your future work.

   Learning to perform essential tasks, such as giving injections, requires you to spend time and put forth effort under the guidance of your instructors. Now is the time for learning, not when you are faced with your first patients.

   Employers routinely request information about a student's attendance record. Good attendance is considered a valuable job skill, because health care services are driven by time requirements. The success of a clinic or hospital and the well-being of patients depend on treatments, procedures, and surgeries being completed in a timely way.

2. Apply Your Best Efforts to Learning

   As a student, it is your responsibility to complete all reading, writing, and laboratory assignments and to participate actively in class. To be successful in your future work, you must now focus on your studies, work hard, and be persistent. Your willingness to prioritize what you need to do over what you want to do will be a major determinant of how well you do in school. Being a college student is not always easy. Keeping your long-term career goals in mind will help you find the self-discipline to stick with it.

3. Ask for Help When You Need It

   Take responsibility for requesting assistance. Ignoring problems will not solve them; they often only get worse. Do not wait until you are hopelessly lost in a class and cannot possibly be ready for the upcoming final examination before asking for help. Remember that asking for help when you need it is a sign of strength, not weakness, and it is one of the actions that distinguishes a graduate from a dropout. The flip side of asking for help is being willing to give it. Offer your assistance to others in the school community. Volunteer to hand out papers for the instructor. Give a student who lives in your area a ride to school. Tutor a classmate who is struggling with a subject you find easy. You have chosen a profession that is based on giving service, and this is a habit you can start practicing now in all areas of your life.

JOURNALING 10.2

List any obstacles that might interfere with your school attendance (e.g., problems with childcare, transportation, work). What can you do now to overcome these obstacles?

? WHAT IF?

You find yourself struggling in one of your classes. You attend class and do the homework as best you can, but you just do not understand the material. Who would you turn to for help?

CASE STUDY 10.2
Fed Up

Keisha has just about had it. She is tired of her friend and classmate, Julie, asking for help. It started with their anatomy homework. At first, Keisha did not mind. She enjoyed learning about the body and was doing well in the class, and helping Julie was also helping her reinforce information. She also liked Julie and wanted to help her succeed.

After finishing their anatomy class, with Julie just scraping by, another request came for help with drug calculations, and it was for more than just tutoring this time.

"Keisha," Julie begged, "if you could just let me see your homework. Jimmy was sick last night, and I just didn't have a chance to do the assignment."

Keisha felt sorry for Julie. She was a single mom, and there always seemed to be problems with her kids. Sometimes, the babysitter did not show up, someone was sick, or they bothered her when she was trying to study. So, the first few times, she gave her a copy of the anatomy homework. After all, it mostly required memorizing a list of medical terms and body parts. What harm could it do if Julie learned them in a way other than doing the reading and the fill-in exercises that comprised most of the homework?

It was when they got to the hands-on courses that Keisha started to wonder if she was doing Julie any favors. Or doing anyone any favors? If Julie did not master the material and understand exactly why and how they were doing certain procedures, would she be safe in the workplace? Would Keisha want to be in the hands of a medical assistant who gives an injection without knowing something about the underlying muscles? Or why this drug is being given? Or how to calculate how much medication to administer?

These questions bothered Keisha, and she decided to discuss the situation with her friend, Stephanie, a nurse at St. Francis Family Clinic.

"I see what you mean, and I can see why you're concerned, Keisha," said Stephanie. "And frankly, you are right. Someone who performs clinical procedures, especially invasive ones like injections, and doesn't really understand what they're doing could be dangerous. I really wouldn't want someone like that on my team or around any of my patients."

"I know," said Keisha, "this is really a tough one. Julie seems to want this so much, but she just isn't doing the work."

"It's hard when it's a friend, I know," said Stephanie. "But you've got to take a broader view. What does it mean to the community if our health care professionals just get by in

school without really knowing what they are doing? It could be dangerous."

Keisha sighed. "You're right. I know what I need to do, but it's good to hear it from someone else."

The next day, Keisha told Julie she could no longer share her homework assignments. Julie was upset and accused Keisha of not being her friend. Keisha tried to explain why she decided that Julie must do her own work, but Julie was not interested in hearing what Keisha had to say. They both completed their medical assisting program, but they are no longer in contact.

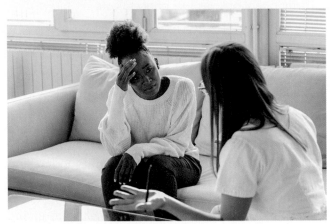
iStock.com/stefanamer/1182390029

QUESTIONS FOR THOUGHT AND REFLECTION

1. Did Stephanie give Keisha good advice?
2. Do you think Keisha was right in refusing to continue helping Julie?
3. Was it worth losing Julie's friendship for Keisha to be honest with her?
4. Could Keisha have done anything else to salvage the friendship and do the right thing?

A Different Path

Julie does not give up. She finds another student to befriend and starts in with her requests for "help" with class, "help" with the homework, and "help" with the tests. She ended up finishing her program after just barely passing her finals, and she did okay on her externship by being extra friendly with the site preceptor.

She was able to find a job at a local clinic, and things went well for the first few days; however, Julie soon realized that there is much she does not know. In school, she depended on others rather than learning things on her own. She tries the same strategy at work, frequently interrupting

her co-workers with questions, such as how to perform a simple procedure or how to determine proper drug dosages.

Soon enough, Julie's frequent requests for help with drug dosages draws the attention of her employer, Dr. Kent. He is concerned that she does not seem to have mastered many of the important skill needed for the clinic. In fact, it was her classmate, Keisha, who did the drug calculations that got Julie through that class. Dr. Kent calls Julie into his office.

"Julie, I've noticed that you always seem to be unsure of the drug dosages you are preparing for patients. Tell me about this."

Julie responds, "Well, Dr. Kent, I'm only a recent graduate, and I really need more time to master all the duties of this job."

Dr. Kent says, "I agree that it does take time to get experience and confidence in these skills. But some of these skill you should have learned in your medical assisting program. When I hired you, I knew you were just starting out. But I expected you to have basic mastery of certain skills, especially for an entry-level medical assistant."

"Well, I think your expectations may have been a bit unreasonable," Julie mumbled.

"I will say that drug dosages can be confusing, and I understand that you might be nervous about making mistakes with pharmaceuticals. But this isn't the only thing. I've received a lot of complaints from my staff about your constant questions when they are working. It seems to have gotten out of control and is affecting some of their work."

"You know what, Dr. Kent?" Julie says. "If this is the kind of unfriendly atmosphere you've got in this office and no one wants to help anyone, I don't think it's a place I want to work." And she stomped out the door. Dr. Kent sighed and called in his office manager. "Louise," he said, "I think we're going to need to look for another medical assistant."

QUESTIONS FOR THOUGHT AND REFLECTION

1. How did the "favors" from Keisha and others contribute to Julie's on-the-job struggles?
2. Was Dr. Kent right in being concerned about Julie's lack of knowledge? Why or why not?
3. Was Julie's response to Dr. Kent appropriate? What could she have done to improve the situation?
4. What must Julie do if she wants to have a career in health care?

Planning for Your Future Career

LEARNING OBJECTIVE 2: PLANNING FOR YOUR FUTURE CAREER

- Start researching your occupational field and jobs for which you might qualify.
- Explore the needs of potential employers.
- Consider the needs of patients and how you might fulfill these needs.
- Make a list of what you are looking for in your first job and in your career.
- List the advantages of a career in health care.

Your future job search can be compared with marketing, or a multistep process that begins with an idea for a product and ends with the sale of that product. When you apply for a job, you are presenting yourself as a product, with the combination of your skills, characteristics, and talents.

You can start developing your own personal marketing plan now as you begin your health care training. The first step is market research or studying the needs of customers. Your "customers" will include your future employers, co-workers, and patients. Now is the time to find out about their needs and expectations for you. You are investing time, effort, and money in the development of yourself as a "product" just as a business would, so it makes sense

to make sure you are creating a product that is both wanted and needed.

What Do Employers Want?

In recent years, employers in all industries have expressed concerns that entry-level workers are not adequately prepared for the modern workplace. Employers are looking for job candidates who not only are qualified technically and with the proper skills but also bring essential professional or "soft" skills, such as the ability to effectively communicate, work cooperatively with others, manage time, critically think, and solve problems (Figure 10.4). (Many of these skills and concepts were discussed in the previous chapters.) These "soft skills" are especially critical

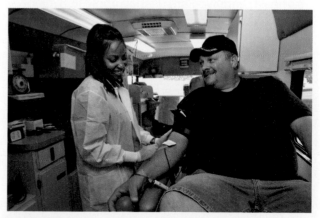

Figure 10.4 A phlebotomist communicates with a donor while collecting blood. (Copyright © istock.com.)

in the health care industry because it is service-based and depends heavily on the quality of its personnel.

National Health Care Standards

The National Consortium for Health Science Education (NCHSE) is a nonprofit education organization that represents state education agency leaders responsible for middle school, secondary, and post-secondary career technical education (CTE) health science programs. NCHSE promotes best practices and career success for future health care professionals. As the national authority for health science education, the NCHSE publishes a series of health science standards, called the National Health Science Standards. These standards are periodically updated.

The standards' objective is to offer an answer to the question, "What does a worker need to know and be able to contribute to the delivery of safe and effective health care?" The standards represent core expectations transferrable to many health professions and outline a list of entry-level worker competencies. Box 10.1 contains examples that apply to all health care occupations. You can see that they are not limited to technical skills, such as taking blood pressure, but include the ability to communicate and work on teams. Some employers report that these types of skills are as important as technical skills in the provision of good health care.

BOX 10.1

Examples of the National Healthcare Foundation Standards and Accountability Criteria (NCHSE, 2022)

Health care professionals will:

- Apply speaking and active listening skills
- Summarize basic professional standards of health care workers as they apply to hygiene, dress, language, confidentiality, and behavior
- Exemplify professional characteristics
- Employ safe work practices and follow health and safety policies and procedures
- Apply ethical standards in health care
- Demonstrate respectful and empathetic interactions with diverse age, cultural, economic, ethnic, and religious groups
- Recognize methods for building positive team relationships
- Apply behaviors that promote health and wellness
- Utilize and understand information technology applications in health care

---

⭐ EXPERIENTIAL EXERCISES

1. The next time you visit your own physician, dentist, or other health care provider, ask what they believe is necessary to succeed as a health care professional.
2. If this person is also an employer, ask about what characteristics they look for when hiring.

❓ WHAT IF?

What if you do not know much about the employers in your area and what they are looking for in potential employees? How could you find out more about them?

Professional Organizations and Associations

Many of the professional organizations that represent specific health care occupations have statements outlining the professional standards and conduct needed to work successfully in their fields. For example, the American Health Information Management Association (AHIMA) is a professional organization that represents health care professionals in health information, such as medical coders and billers. AHIMA publishes standards for Ethical Coding, which includes demonstrating ethical behavior, integrity, and professionalism. Below is AHIMA's standard for: *Demonstrate behavior that reflects integrity, shows a commitment to ethical and legal coding practices, and fosters trust in professional activities.*

Coding professionals shall:

10.1. Act in an honest manner and bring honor to self, peers, and the profession.

10.2. Represent truthfully and accurately their credentials, professional education, and experience.

10.3. Demonstrate ethical principles and professional values in their actions to patients, employers, other members of the health care team, consumers, and other stakeholders served by the health care data they collect and report.

⭐ EXPERIENTIAL EXERCISES

Find the website of the professional organization for your chosen occupation. What personal characteristics are needed to succeed? What qualities do you think you need to work on to be successful in this occupation?

What Do Patients Want?

Patients do not care how much you know until they know how much you care. Patients want to receive competent care delivered with consideration and respect. When seeking health care, people are often at their most vulnerable and are experiencing considerable stress, anxiety, and may be in pain. They may worry about what might be discovered during a diagnostic test or that they will experience pain during a necessary treatment. Patients may also experience a feeling of powerlessness, as their illness or injury and even some aspects of their treatment are beyond their control.

Making decisions about their care can help restore a sense of control. They have the right, both ethically and legally, to be fully informed about their condition, treatment options, and possible outcomes. Health care professionals must give clear explanations in everyday language and offer patients the opportunity to ask questions. At the same time, patients want and have the legal right to confidentiality.

Over the years, the US health care system has undergone changes that have brought special challenges for both patients and health care professionals. In the past, many people had the same physician throughout their lives. They belonged to the same community, and a sense of trust developed over the years.

Patients today may not only see a different physician each time they visit their health care facility, but they may now see different health care providers, such as nurse practitioners and physician assistants. In many cases, this has improved the access and quality of care. However, in some cases, this lack of continuity of care may result in patients feeling more anxious and alienated from their own care while having to face a serious illness or life-threatening condition.

As a health care professional, you can demonstrate a caring attitude that helps create a bond of trust with patients by being attentive, listening carefully, and practicing empathy. Studies have found that even if a health care professional excels in one area, poor communication skills, the lack of empathy, and the appearance of not caring can cause patients to view that person and experience negatively.

Many patients are from different ethnic backgrounds, some of whom have beliefs about health care practices that differ from traditional medicine. Patients also come from a variety of socioeconomic backgrounds. They may have lifestyles or personal beliefs with which you disagree, but they all want and deserve the highest level of patient care and your best efforts. An important aspect in patient care is defining the rights and responsibilities for both the patient and health care provider. For patients, the American Hospital Association (AHA) created the original Patients' Bill of Rights in 1973, which provides guidelines for ensuring the protection and safety of patients. Although the Patients' Bill of Rights was originally intended for the hospital setting, most medical practices, hospitals, insurance companies, and even governments have adopted some form of the Patient's Bill of Rights.

The purpose of the Patient's Bill of Rights is to help patients feel more confident in the health care system in the United States, to strengthen the relationship between patients and their health care provider by defining their rights and responsibilities and those of their health care provider, and to emphasize the role patients play in their health. With that, the Patient's Bill of Rights outlines the guarantees for all patients seeking medical care in a health care organization and basic rights and responsibilities for effective patient care. Box 10.2 lists the Patient's Bill of Rights.

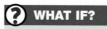 **WHAT IF?**

What if you just arrived at an urgent care facility with a suspected broken arm?

BOX 10.2

Patient's Bill of Rights

1. You have the right to be treated fairly and respectfully.
2. You have the right to get information you can understand about your diagnosis, treatment, and prognosis from your health care provider.
3. You have the right to discuss and ask for information about specific procedures and treatments, their risks, and the time you will spend recovering. You also have the right to discuss other care options.
4. You have the right to know the identities of all your health care providers, including students, residents, and other trainees.
5. You have the right to know how much care may cost at the time of treatment and long term.
6. You have the right to make decisions about your care before and during treatment and the right to refuse care. The hospital must inform you of the medical consequences of refusing treatment. You also have the right to other treatments provided by the hospital and the right to transfer to another hospital.

7. You have the right to have an advance directive, such as a living will or a power of attorney for health care. A hospital has the right to ask for your advance directive, put it in your file, and honor its intent.

8. You have the right to privacy in medical examinations, case discussions, consultations, and treatments.

9. You have the right to expect that your communication and records are treated as confidential by the hospital, except as the law permits and requires in cases of suspected abuse or public health hazards. If the hospital releases your information to another medical facility, you have the right to expect the hospital to ask the medical facility to keep your records confidential.

10. You have the right to review your medical records and to have them explained or interpreted, except when restricted by law.

11. You have the right to expect that a hospital will respond reasonably to your requests for care and services or transfer you to another facility that has accepted a transfer request. You should also expect information and explanation about the risks, benefits, and alternatives to a transfer.

12. You have the right to ask and be informed of any business relationships between the hospital and educational institutions, other health care providers, or payers that may influence your care and treatment.

13. You have the right to consent to or decline to participate in research studies and to have the studies fully explained before you give your consent. If you decide not to participate in research, you are still entitled to the most effective care that the hospital can provide. You have the right to expect reasonable continuity of care and to be informed of other care options when hospital care is no longer appropriate.

14. You have the right to be informed of hospital policies and practices related to patient care, treatment, and responsibilities.

15. You also have the right to know who you can contact to resolve disputes, grievances, and conflicts. And you have the right to know what the hospital will charge for services and their payment methods.

⭐ EXPERIENTIAL EXERCISES

1. Make a list of your personal qualities that you believe will help you succeed in your health care career.
2. Now make a list of attitudes and habits you would like to change to increase your chance of success.
3. Take some time to observe people you believe are successful in their careers. Do they have qualities in common?

What Do You Want?

If you don't know what you want, you will probably never get it.

—Oliver Wendell Holmes, Jr.

In addition to exploring the needs of your future employers and patients, an important part of planning is to identify what you want. You must consider your needs and desires as you create your professional self. The clearer you are about your career goals and expectations, the greater the chance you have of achieving them.

Hopefully, you spent some time thinking and "soul searching" about why you wanted a career in health care. A career in health care is often considered a top career choice and for good reason. Health care careers are often in high demand and offer stability in comparison to other professions in other industries. However, training to be a health care professional can be a long road and may often require you to continue that training to maintain your license, certification, or registration. It may also be emotionally and physically taxing since you are dealing with patients who are ill.

Beginning now to think about your goals and priorities will also keep you alert to employment possibilities. Observe, ask questions, and read about your occupational area. Many fields in health care today have newly created positions and expanded responsibilities for traditional jobs. A wide variety of choices may be available for new graduates.

Although it is important to try to meet your personal needs when seeking employment, you must also have realistic expectations. You will need to compare your work preferences with the needs of employers to see how well they match.

Students sometimes have unrealistic goals for the positions they hope to find immediately after graduation. In most cases, recent graduates are qualified for entry-level positions. You can avoid frustration and disappointment if you understand the workplace and adjust your expectations. Box 10.3 contains a list of goals you should look for in your first job.

> **JOURNALING 10.3**

Why did you choose a career in health care? What do you hope to accomplish? What do you hope to contribute?

The Nature of Work in Health Care

People are generally happiest and most productive when their work provides them with more than material rewards. Health care is a complex, ever-changing field that offers both opportunities and challenges. Here are some of the major sources of satisfaction you can expect:

1. Meaningful Work

Good health is a basic need for both human survival and happiness. Working to promote health gives you the chance to make meaningful contributions to the well-being of others. Whether you provide direct patient care or perform supporting duties, your work directly affects patients, and the quality of your work can truly make a difference in their lives.

2. Opportunity to Serve

People seek the services of health care professionals when they need help. They come with the hope that you can assist them in solving their problems, and they entrust themselves in your care. A career in health care provides you an opportunity to nurture your desire to help others. Regardless of what you do, health care professionals play a crucial part in helping people in significant ways.

BOX 10.3

Goals for Your First Health Care Job

- Apply what you learned in school
- Gain self-confidence
- Work with a variety of people
- Acquire additional knowledge
- Increase your skill base
- Explore specialties within your field of interest
- Network with other professionals
- Demonstrate your abilities

3. Career Stability

The need for health care will always exist, even if job titles change over time. The reorganization taking place in today's health care delivery system is causing continual shifts in the need for specific occupational positions. A decrease in the number of jobs for one position is often balanced by an increase in another. If you are willing to be flexible, you can add the experience and/or training to qualify for new positions.

4. Interesting Work Environment

Health care is changing rapidly, both scientifically, technologically, and organizationally. Advances in our understanding of how the body works, along with discoveries about the causes and treatments of disease, are reported almost daily. Computers and technology have increased our ability to collect and organize information, as well as diagnose and treat disease. Your work will provide a steady stream of new information to learn and apply.

5. Opportunities for Advancement

You are likely to have opportunities for advancement if you are willing to continue learning and adding to your skills. Many employers offer on-the-job training, and many occupational specialties, such as nursing, have career ladders. These are a hierarchy of jobs that require different levels of knowledge, skills, and training. More advanced positions almost always require further education and additional certifications or licenses.

Setting Career Goals

Entry-level jobs, performed well, can be the first step leading to positions that meet all your hopes for a fulfilling career. Adjusting your short-term expectations does not mean giving up your long-term goals. In fact, purposeful planning now can help you arrive where you want to be in the future. Find out now the skills you need to achieve your future goals and look for opportunities to learn as many of them as possible during your studies, externship, and first job.

For new health care professionals who are well prepared and who contribute enthusiastically to the success of their employers, entry-level jobs can serve as launch pads for career success. Serving the needs of others can provide you with opportunities to meet your own needs.

CASE STUDY 10.3
Planning Ahead

Rosa Gonzalez is the first child in her family to go to college. Her parents have worked hard to support their family and encouraged their children to take advantage of all educational opportunities. However, money is scarce, and Rosa has a part-time job to help pay for school expenses. It is not easy working and going to school, but she believes that through a good education she will be able get ahead in life. She wants not only to train for a career in health care but also to serve as an example for her younger brothers and sisters.

Rosa is studying to become a medical assistant. She wants to do well so her parents will be proud of her. Her career goal is to work as a back-office assistant with a plastic surgeon, helping the physician with outpatient procedures. Her interest in plastic surgery began when she saw the miraculous work performed on a young cousin who was disfigured after being burned in a fire.

Early in her program, Rosa did some research and found that there were only a few plastic surgeons in her town, and they all preferred to hire assistants with previous work experience. Rosa decides not to let this information discourage her, and she created a plan of short- and long-term goals to help her achieve her career goal.

While in school, Rosa asks her instructors to recommend books and articles about plastic surgery. Her instructors also allow her to spend extra practice time in the laboratory, so she can reach a high level of competence with sterile technique, surgical instruments, wound care, and other related skills. At the same time, Rosa works hard in her classes, asking for help when necessary and completing all homework assignments.

Upon graduating, Rosa decides to look for a job with a general practitioner or pediatrician who does minor surgery in the office. Her entry-level job goals are to gain experience with sterile technique, standard precautions, surgical assisting, and patient care. She knows that this experience will help her reach her goal of someday working with a plastic surgeon.

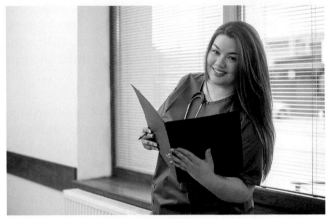

iStock.com/Zdenka_Simekova/823626828

QUESTIONS FOR THOUGHT AND REFLECTION

1. What challenges did Rosa face before even starting school?
2. What would have happened if Rosa had not researched her career goal before she completed her medical assisting program?
3. How do Rosa's short-term goals serve as stepping-stones for reaching her long-term goal?

A Different Path

Greg worked in roofing and construction from the time he graduated from high school. He got a job with a company owned by a friend's father and worked his way up from doing clean up to full-time work as a roofer. He liked the physical nature of the work, being outside most of the day, and having a beer with his fellow workers at the end of the day.

One fall day, as his work team was trying to finish a job before the rainy weather worsened, Greg slipped from a steep incline and fell onto a cement patio. He broke his leg and fractured two vertebrae in his back. He recovered the use of his legs, although he was in pain a good deal of the time. His roofing and construction days were over.

Being unable to work posed a huge problem for Greg. He and his wife, Kathy, had two children to support, and Kathy's job was only part-time and did not provide any benefits. On the advice of a friend who worked at a local clinic, Greg looked into a career in health care. Although the idea of working inside all day was not appealing to him, it seemed as though there were many job openings in health care, and the work was steady.

He and Kathy talked it over, and she encouraged him. "You know," she said, "my friend Louise has been working for Dr. Lewis for years as a medical assistant and really likes the work." Greg had some doubts. "Don't you think there might be lifting and helping patients? My back might not take that kind of work."

"Well," said Kathy, "I did talk with Louise about that, and she said that there are administrative medical assistants. There are also people in the office who do billing and other kinds of paperwork."

"I've never done that kind of work. I don't know if I'd be any good at it," Greg said.

Kathy reassured him. "Honey, I know you can do whatever you set your mind to."

Greg had his doubts, but he enrolled in a medical office administration program at the local college. Kathy's friend Louise gave him some help with his studies, and he managed to complete the program with passing grades. The family's finances were approaching the point of desperation, and he knew he was obligated to finish his program and look for employment.

Greg worked hard at finding a job. He pursued every lead and presented himself well at interviews. It was not surprising that he had a job just a few weeks after graduation. His duties included greeting patients upon arrival and doing front-office work at a medical office. His outgoing personality made him popular with patients, but he found the appointment scheduling, data entry on the computer, and other paperwork tedious and not to his liking. Sitting all day in a small area made him feel closed in and uncomfortable. He stayed with the job and did his best because he did not want to let his family down, but he was never happy with his work and knew that someday he would have to find another profession.

QUESTIONS FOR THOUGHT AND REFLECTION

1. What were Greg's reasons for studying medical assisting?
2. What effect did Kathy and Louise have on Greg's decision?
3. What could he have done to learn more about the profession?
4. Is there anything Greg can do now to improve his situation?

 CROSS CURRENTS WITH OTHER SOFT SKILLS

SETTING GOALS AND PLANNING ACTION: Goals help you achieve academic and career success (Chapter 15).
BUILDING RELATIONSHIPS: Good communication skills will help you work better with your instructors and classmates (Chapters 4 and 6).
MANAGING YOUR TIME AND ORGANIZING YOUR LIFE: Balancing school, work, and other life responsibilities are essential skills for students (Chapter 2).

Beginning the Job Search

LEARNING OBJECTIVE 3:
BEGINNING THE JOB SEARCH

- Understand how much time you will need to invest in your job search.
- List the activities involved in a successful job search.
- Describe job search time management techniques.
- List the supplies you may need for your job search.
- Explain what job search records should contain.

- Describe the purpose and contents of a job lead log.
- Explain how the telephone and emails can be used as job search tools.

The Search Is On

You miss 100% of the shots you don't take.
—Wayne Gretzky

Congratulations! All the studying, assignments, labs, and clinical experience are about to pay off. You are now ready to focus on the job search and reaching your goal of working in your profession. Completing your education and graduating represent important personal achievements. Your attitude played a large part in your success. In the same way, attitude will play an important role in helping you get the right job.

Attitude

Remember that your own resolution to succeed is more important than any one thing.
—Abraham Lincoln

Attitude is the single most important factor in your personal and professional life, including your job search. Keep in mind that you have control over your attitude. You can approach any situation either positively or negatively. Some people are nervous and fearful about looking for a job. They worry about lacking the qualifications needed by employers and see each interview as a chance to be rejected. These are all reasonable and understandable feelings to have. A more positive approach is to look at the process from the employers' point of view. Think about that fact that health care facilities cannot function without good employees. Employers must fill positions with well-trained individuals who can help them serve their patients. You are a recently trained person ready to fill one of these positions.

Knowing what skills and competencies you have is the first step in presenting yourself successfully as the person who fits an employer's needs. Students sometimes do not realize just how much they have learned and underestimate their abilities. Being aware of your accomplishments will build your self-confidence and help you present yourself positively at interviews.

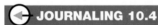 **JOURNALING 10.4**

What do you hope to learn and gain from your first job?

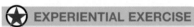 **EXPERIENTIAL EXERCISE**

Write a description of yourself in which you explain what you have to offer prospective employers. Include your skills and personal characteristics that will make you a valued employee.

Focus Your Search

To find out what one is fitted to do, and to secure an opportunity to do, is the key to happiness.

—**John Dewey**

Knowing where to market yourself is the next step in carrying out a successful job search. This means identifying the type of job and facility in which you would like to work. Gaining familiarity with the job market in your area and profession is a process that requires time and diligence and may require multiple steps. Employers may advertise job openings in many ways. Although the Internet is one of the best sources to view job openings and career sites, there are many other sources, which will be discussed in this chapter.

Keep in mind that it is sometimes necessary to set short-term goals to achieve long-term career success. When seeking an entry-level position, you will do better if you are open to a variety of possibilities. School career services personnel report seeing students lose

good opportunities by setting requirements or expectations that are too restrictive. For example, some students do not want to have long commutes. But passing up a good position at an excellent facility by refusing to consider jobs just outside your immediate area may not be a good career move. Driving an extra 10 minutes may, in the long run, be worth the extra investment. You may have higher salary expectations than what you are initially offered. It may be a good idea to initially accept the lower salary and negotiate for more money later or find a new job once you gain more experience. Keep in mind that you have to "walk before you can run."

 EXPERIENTIAL EXERCISE

Create a list of your work preferences that includes the following: type of facility and population served, specialty, work schedule, type of supervision, work pace, amount of interaction with others, range of duties.

? WHAT IF?

You need to start looking for a job, but you have never worked in health care and do not know what to look for in an employer.

Committing to the Job Search

You can't try to do things; you simply must do them.

—Ray Bradbury

Obtaining a new job can be as much work as actually working at a job. It can take a lot of time and effort. You will be most successful if you dedicate a portion of each day to your search and be on call to follow up quickly on leads. Employment professionals recommend that job seekers spend between 20 and 40 hours a week on job search efforts. See Box 10.4 for a list of activities related to your job search. Failure to spend enough time on these activities is one of the major reasons why people fail to get hired.

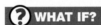 **JOURNALING 10.5**

How strong is my commitment to finding a job? How much time and effort am I willing to spend?

Time Management Tips for Your Job Search

Prioritize. The job search should be your primary focus, apart from caring for your family. Looking for a job is your job. Determine which job search activities are most productive and spend most of your time on them.

Keep a calendar. Missing or being late for an interview is a sure way to lose a job even before you are hired. Take care to note all appointments and follow-up activities accurately and to check your calendar daily.

Plan a weekly schedule. Decide what needs to be done each week and create a to-do list to serve as a guide to keep you on track.

Plan ahead and be prepared. Suppose that one morning you are notified that a hospital where you want to work is scheduling interviews for later the same day. You do not want to miss out because you have not completed your resume or do not have a clean shirt to wear. Make sure your car is in good running order or that you have other reliable transportation.

Plan for the unplanned. The unexpected tends to strike at the worst possible moment. Keep an extra printer cartridge on hand. Have extra copies of your resume printed. Leave early for interviews in case you get lost. Better yet, take a dry run a day or two in advance to learn the route. Check out alternate routes in case of traffic.

Setting Up the Job Search

Set up a space for your job search activities. Gather up your resources and supplies in one location. Check the list in Box 10.5 to see if you have what you need.

Documenting Your Job Search

Keep records of copies of applications you have submitted, a list of professional contacts, employee contact information, and names of the facilities and individuals where you interviewed, and any notes or feedback you have received from potential employers and human resource departments. Use a three-ring binder or a folder on your computer to keep everything organized or create computerized folders and files.

Job Lead Log

A job lead log consists of a document, either paper or computerized, on which you record all job leads and contacts. See Box 10.6 for suggested information to include.

If you have more than one version of your resume (e.g., different objectives to match specific jobs), indicate on your lead log which version you sent, or you can place a copy of the resume on the next page in your binder or in a separate computer file. This way, you will know how to respond if you get a call for an interview. It will also ensure that you take the correct resume to the interview. (More information about interviews and what to take with you will be discussed later in this chapter and in Chapter 12.)

Students who prefer to use a computer for tracking can set up an Excel spreadsheet or other form, such as a table in Word, to record their job search activities. Regardless of the method you choose, design something that is easy for you to use and be sure to keep it up-to-date.

Dialing for Jobs

When you are searching for a new job, it helps to stand out from the competition. One way to do that is by performing "cold calls" to contacts at various organizations who may be in charge of hiring for a particular position that you are interested in. Cold calling is contacting a business that you have no previous interaction with. For example, you call a medical office close to where you live to see if they have any open positions even though they have not posted any job ads. Cold calls give you the opportunity to show your initiative and strong interest in the role. Despite the term, cold calling is most often using the telephone, but it may also include emailing businesses.

The telephone can be a job seeker's best friend. It can also be a barrier if not used properly. Employers form an impression of you based on your telephone manners, so be sure they hear you at your best. The following suggestions for making calls will apply to your telephone habits on the job as well as during the search to get a job:

1. Be prepared with a pen and paper for taking notes.
2. Prepare what you plan to say ahead of time and be as brief as possible without rushing and speaking too quickly.
3. Be courteous, never pushy. If the receptionist cannot connect you to the person you wish to speak with, leave a clear message and ask for a good time to call back.
4. Speak clearly and distinctly. Do not mumble or use slang or nonstandard speech that the listener may not understand.
5. When making appointments or gathering important information, listen carefully and repeat to make sure that you have the correct date and time, address, suite or office number, and so on.
6. Always thank the other party and end the call graciously.

It is important that your school, potential employers, and other contacts be able to reach you in a timely way. Be sure the telephone number you distribute is accurate and includes your area code. If you have voicemail, call your number to make sure

it is working properly and the mailbox is not full. The outgoing message should be simple and professional. Avoid the use of music, jokes, and clever remarks. This also applies to your email address. If it is too cute or strange, it may send the wrong message to any potential employer who sees it. Instruct everyone who might answer the telephone about proper telephone manners and how to write down a message. Every contact represents you, and employers do not have time to deal with rude adults or untrained children.

❓ WHAT IF?

Ms. Adams in career services at your school told you that students have had success in contacting employers, either calling or visiting their offices. But the idea of cold calling makes you extremely nervous. What might you do to become more confident? Are there other ways for you to directly contact employers without cold calling?

Setting Up a Support System

Your job search will be easier and more pleasant if you have people available who care about your success and are willing to help you. They can provide technical support or offer friendly encouragement. Could you use some help with any of the following tasks?

* Proofreading your resume and other written materials
* Role playing to practice interviewing
* Discussing post-interview evaluations
* Keeping things in perspective and not getting discouraged

You may want to work with just one other person who is qualified to help you in many areas, or you might enlist the help of several "specialists." Be sure the people you choose are qualified to spot spelling and grammatical errors and are comfortable giving you constructive feedback. They should know when you need a push and when you need a hug. Consider drawing from friends, family members, classmates, school personnel, and health care professionals. If you have a mentor, this person might be an excellent choice. Be considerate of everyone's time, be prepared when you have meetings with them, and show appreciation for their help.

The career services department at your school provides specific help and support to students as they conduct their job search. Find out what services are provided. In addition, some schools and communities have job clubs or support groups for people seeking employment. Consider using these resources to supplement your support system. They can offer additional viewpoints, encouragement, and helpful suggestions.

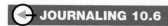

JOURNALING 10.6

Am I nervous about pursuing the job search? What areas do I need to work on to overcome my fears?

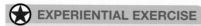

EXPERIENTIAL EXERCISE

Create a list of people who can make up your support system to help with the following tasks: proofread your resume, practice interviewing, review your performance with employer interviews, provide encouragement.

Understanding the Job Market

Employment conditions may vary from one geographical location to the next, and economic conditions change over time. Consider the following factors when planning your job search strategies:

* Local employment customs
* Current economic conditions
* Current employment rate
* Trends in health care delivery
* Medical advances
* Changing government regulations

Local and employer customs vary in what is considered acceptable dress for the workplace. With some employers, health care providers dress casually, with males sporting long hair and even wearing an earring. With other employers, anyone who showed up for work looking like this would be sent home to change. In general, as you have most likely learned in your program, the health care setting often requires a strict dress code of professionalism that must be followed.

Local and national economic conditions affect the job seeker. When the economy is strong and unemployment is low, job seekers have the advantage. When the economy slows down, however, the job market becomes more competitive, and it may become more difficult to find a job.

Health care occupations are also affected by state and federal laws. The demand for certain occupations is influenced by the reimbursement, or payment for services, policies of both government and private insurance carriers. Know what is happening in your area, as well as national trends. Ask your career services department at school for information. Look in the business section of your local newspaper for articles about the economy and local employment trends. Health care trends and major facilities are often featured. Reading articles about major health care employers enables you

to present yourself at interviews as a candidate who has taken the time to learn about the employer.

Many newspapers publish weekly or monthly sections dedicated to employment. They contain articles about resume writing, lists of local agencies that assist job seekers, and announcements of job fairs. News magazines such as *Newsweek, Time, US News and World Report*, and *BusinessWeek* contain many articles about health care topics, and the Internet provides access to a wide variety of topics from literally millions of sources. For example, the Bureau of Labor Statistics maintains a website with reports on employment trends and the national labor market.

EXPERIENTIAL EXERCISE

Use your research skills to write a report that includes the following:
1. Unemployment rate in your area
2. Major health care employers
3. Current hiring trends in health care
4. Current conditions that affect your occupation
5. Influence of all this information on your job search strategies

Locating Job Leads

LEARNING OBJECTIVE 4:
USING CAREER RESOURCES AND SERVICES

- Explain how your job search time should be allocated.
- List and describe the sources of job leads.
- Explain how to best use career services at your school.
- Explain who to include in your network.
- Describe how to best take advantage of career fairs.
- Explain how professional organizations can help with the job search.
- Explain why contacting employers directly can be a good strategy.

Increase your chances of finding the job you really want by using a variety of lead sources. Do not limit yourself to the one or two methods you find easiest or most comfortable to use. Employment experts recommend that no more than 25% of your time be spent on any one job search method (Figure 10.5).

When the economy is slow and there are few job openings, networking and developing personal contacts can be the most effective methods for finding a job. It is possible you will not find the "perfect

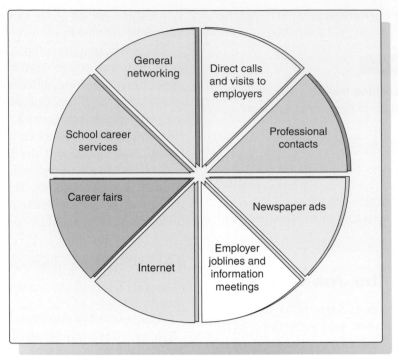

Figure 10.5 Use a variety of job lead sources to increase your chances of finding the right job for you.

job" under these economic conditions. Looking for an opportunity to gain experience in your profession may be the best strategy. When the economy is booming or there is a shortage of qualified workers in your field, you are likely to have a larger selection of opportunities. Under these conditions, you may find that responding to job postings and directly contacting potential employers are effective methods. You will certainly experience all types of job markets during your career. The economy and employment levels run in cycles, and you must be prepared to deal with changing conditions.

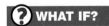 **WHAT IF?**

You live in a small town where there are few medical facilities. How can you increase your chances of finding a job?

Job-Searching Strategies

Employment Ads

Although newspaper classified ads are much less used than in the past, they are still included in today's newspapers. You can see what types of jobs are available in your area by looking at the classified section in the local paper. Writing a cover letter and mailing or faxing a resume in response to job ads may be worth

the time and expense it takes. Every action you take increases your chance of finding the right job.

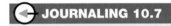 **JOURNALING 10.7**

Am I taking advantage of all sources of job leads? Are there any I need to explore further?

Direct Employer Contacts

Calling, visiting, or writing to specific employers to inquire about job openings can be successful strategies. These actions demonstrate motivation and self-confidence, the very qualities that can help win you a job. They are also a way to discover the estimated four-fifths of jobs that are never advertised-the "hidden job market."

If you are sending a cover letter and resume, find the name of the person who makes the hiring decisions for the department. If you are calling a small medical office, this may simply mean getting the name of the physician or clinic manager. In the case of a large facility, you may have to do more inquiring by phone to find the right person, which may include the hiring director or someone in human resources.

Craft a letter that briefly explains why you would be a good employee for this employer or clinic. The letter should communicate enthusiasm, interest, and a desire to help the employer. Of course, this means that you know something about the employer: specialty or services offered, typical patients, and so on. Include your resume with the letter. Follow up in a few days with a phone call.

Calling employers by phone to inquire about job openings ("cold calling") can be especially helpful if you are relocating. Explain that you will be moving and are unfamiliar with the area. If the facility contacted has no openings, ask whether they can refer you to anyone else in the area.

Visiting facilities that have jobs for which you might be qualified can also be productive. It gives you a chance to introduce yourself to at least one staff member and personally distribute your resume. Ask who does the hiring, leave your resume, and express your appreciation. Even though you should be dressed as if you were attending an interview, do not ask for one at this time if you do not have an appointment.

Large medical facilities, such as hospitals, often coordinate hiring through their human resources office. All resumes and applications must be submitted to this office. It can be worthwhile to also contact or visit the department where you wish to work. Ask for the supervisor and, if available, let them know that you have applied for work through human resources and are very interested in working in that department. Explain why you want to work there and ask that your application be given consideration. If the supervisor is not available, ask to make an appointment. Do not be discouraged, however, if you are unable to make direct contact. Health care professionals today are extremely busy and may not have the time. If they do not, send a letter or email that expresses your interest.

JOURNALING 10.8

1. Do I always conduct myself professionally, including in the classroom?
2. Will people who know me feel confident recommending me for jobs?
3. Are there habits or behaviors I need to improve so people will recommend me?

Career and Job Fairs

Some schools, community agencies, and large health care facilities organize activities to connect job recruiters and job seekers. In a single day, you can meet dozens of potential employers. You can gather information, ask questions, and submit your resume. Check your local newspaper for events in your area. Call large health care organizations in your area or check their websites for information about career fairs or open houses. You can also find upcoming career fairs across the nation on websites such as national-careerfair.com.

Here are suggestions for taking full advantage of job fairs:
* Dress as you would for an interview.
* Prepare a list of questions, such as those in the following list, in advance.
* Take copies of your resume.
* Smile, make eye contact, and introduce yourself to recruiters. Thank them for any information they give you. Leave graciously by telling them it was nice meeting them.
* Take something in which you can collect brochures, job announcements, and business cards. A small notebook is helpful for taking notes.
* As soon as possible after the fair, organize what you collected and use your job lead log pages to record the people you met and what you learned.
* If possible, connect on LinkedIn with the people you met at the job fair. Be sure to include a note with your LinkedIn request.
* Prepare a list of follow-up activities, such as people to call and resumes to send.

Some helpful questions to ask employer representatives at these career and job fairs are:
1. What types of jobs does your facility offer?
2. How can I get more information?
3. What are the most important qualifications you look for when hiring employees?
4. Where can I find a job description for this role?
5. What is the application procedure?
6. Who do I contact to set up an informational session or interview?

Professional Organizations

Some professional organizations include job search tips and job postings on their websites. These organizations are also a good place to network. See Box 10.7 for examples of professional organizations. Many professional journals and publications often contain employment ads targeted to their members.

Government-Sponsored Resource Centers

Governments have established "one-stop" resources for job seekers. They may be called One-Stop Resource Centers, County Career Centers, or possibly another name in your area. Staff members are well informed about employment conditions, as well as specific

BOX 10.7

**Professional Organizations and
Student Associations**

- American Dental Assistants Association
  www.adaausa.org
- American Massage Therapy Association
  www.amtamassage.org
- American Association of Medical Assistants
  www.aama-ntl.org
- Medical Association of Billers
  www.physicianswebsites.com
- American Academy of Procedural Coders
  www.aapc.com
- American Health Information Management
  Association
  www.ahima.org
- National Pharmacy Technician Association
  www.pharmacytechnician.org

employers, in their local areas. Ask your school about these resources or go to the following links to view government jobs:

* www.careeronestop.org
* https://www.usajobs.gov/
* https://www.governmentjobs.com/
* https://www.usa.gov/government-jobs

There are many benefits from a government job, including job stability and security. Government jobs give you a steady income and job security, especially during challenging economic times. Unlike private sector companies that can go out of business anytime, federal institutions remain stable or take new forms over time. In fact, corporate employees are three times more likely to get terminated by employers than federal workers. The government offers jobs in a wide range of fields, such as science, business, health care, or politics.

The government also offers flexible work schedules, telework options, and remote working options for those who work long-hour shifts and have an extended commute. The federal government offers generous benefits, such as health insurance, life insurance, vacation time, sick leave and holiday policies, and retirement plans.

Using Your Network

Career Services

The staff at your school wants you to succeed. The goal of health care educators is to train future workers, and a sign of their professional success is when a graduate

becomes satisfactorily employed. Schools have special personnel who are trained to help students find jobs. These people work to develop relationships with local employers. Employers may contact your school about job openings before they are advertised. How can you be among the graduates who are recommended by your school?

* Get to know the career services staff. Introduce yourself early in your program. Do not wait until you are beginning the job search. Seek their advice about how you can best prepare ahead for successful employment.
* Treat school staff with the same courtesy and respect you would an employer. They cannot risk the school's reputation with employers by recommending students who are rude or uncooperative.
* Maintain an excellent attendance record. Schools report that this is the question asked by nearly every employer about students.
* Participate in career development classes or workshops. Attend every session and complete all assignments. Conduct yourself in practice interviews as if they were the real thing.
* Follow up on all leads you are given, even if you do not think the job is for you. Attend all interviews scheduled for you. Failure to show up embarrasses your school and may result in the employer refusing to consider candidates from your school in the future. And even if the job is not the one for you, the employer may know about one that is.
* Keep your school informed about how to contact you.
* Let the school know when you are hired. Many agencies that regulate and accredit schools require annual reports to monitor graduation and job placement rates. These act as school report cards and are important for schools to stay in good standing. If the staff has taken the time to help you, return the favor by giving them the information they need to complete their reports.

Your Externship Site

Students who perform well during their externship are sometimes offered jobs at the site. Some employers may even create new positions for graduates who impress them with their attitude and skills. Although it is not appropriate to ask your clinical site for employment before completing your training there, you should work as if this were your goal. Even if the site is unable to offer you a position, your supervisor or externship preceptor can serve as a valuable reference and may recommend you to other employers.

Networking

Many people learn about job openings and become employed through personal and professional contacts. Do not be shy about asking for their advice about where you might apply or about the job search in general. People who are successful in their careers are generally happy to help people new in the field and profession. Do show consideration for their time and send a thank-you note when they put forth effort on your behalf. It is critical that you follow up on any leads given to you by professional contacts. Failure to do so is not only rude, but it also may result in the withdrawal of their support.

In addition to professional contacts, general networking can be an effective way to get the word out about your search efforts. Let the people in your life know you are seeking employment. By telling 10 people who each know 10 other people, you create a network of 110 people who know you are looking for a job. Of these 110 contacts, it is likely that a few of them work in health care. When speaking with others about your career goals, present yourself positively and express enthusiasm about your field. People want to feel confident about passing your name along.

Using the Internet

The Internet greatly expands your job search possibilities by being available worldwide and 24 hours a day. It offers a wide range of how-to information, facts about specific occupations and employers, and job postings. So much information is available, in fact, that it is easy to get lost in cyberspace.

Studies have shown that only a small percentage of applicants are actually hired as the result of posting a resume on one of the large employment websites, as

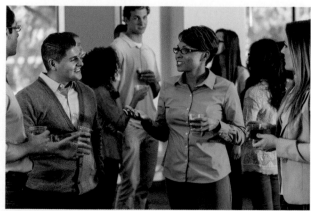

Informal networking can lead to potential employment contacts. (Copyright © istock.com.)

there is simply too much competition. The Internet, however, can be a valuable job search tool. You can read about health care trends, the general economy, and advances in medicine. You can scan job postings to see what characteristics employers mention most, get information about major facilities, and see samples of good resumes.

To access general information, enter key phrases such as "health care trends," "future of health care," "health care providers," and "health care employment" into a search engine. Government agencies such as the Department of Labor (www.dol.gov) and the Bureau of Labor Statistics (www.bls.gov) have information about the national job market, laws that affect employees, and resources for job seekers.

Getting Started

An excellent place to start learning about using the Internet for the job search is The Riley Guide. Available both in print and online, it has provided free, updated career and employment information since 1994 (www.rileyguide.com). Developed by a librarian, the website serves as a gateway to hundreds of other websites on all phases of the job search. Other good sources that have been in business for a long time are Quintessential Careers (www.quintcareers.com) and Career Builder (http://careerbuilder.com).

Health Care Facility Websites

If you are interested in working for a specific employer, you should go directly to the company's website, and there should be a link to their job openings. Many large health care facilities have websites that include photos, maps, information about the services they offer patients, and statements of their goals and overall mission. If you do not know the address, use a search engine and enter the name of the company or facility. Many organizations now list their current job openings, along with online applications. In fact, some facilities accept only electronic applications. Additionally, larger organizations often include a job search page with search filters, enabling job seekers to view vacancies by position type, title, and location.

Employment Websites

Job openings are listed on hundreds of websites. Although some are easier to use than others, most sites organize jobs by occupational fields, such as health care, and geographical location. Box 10.8 lists both general and health care–specific employment websites.

You can view the job listings on these sites without registering. If you wish to post your resume, however, you must register by supplying information such as your name, address, and telephone number. You then select a username and password to access your account each time you visit the website.

In addition to these general health care sites, there are many specialty websites that feature jobs in one career area, such as dental assisting. Links to these websites are available at www.quintcareers.com/healthcare_jobs.html.

Keep in mind that new websites are continually being developed and old ones are merging, being deleted, or being moved to a different web address. Some of the addresses given in this book and in others may have changed by the time you try them, and it is certain that new websites will have been created.

 EXPERIENTIAL EXERCISE

Using websites that list job openings, find and list 10 jobs for which you are qualified.

Networking Online

The Internet provides opportunities for sharing information and ideas with others through mailing lists and newsgroups. Mailing lists (also known as Listservs and email discussion groups) operate through email. Each list is devoted to a specific topic: occupations, hobbies, health conditions, and so on. Once you have subscribed, you receive email messages to which you can respond. Your email is then sent to all other subscribers. Mailing lists offer a way to learn what other job seekers are doing and what is happening in your field around the country. Comprehensive directories of the thousands of mailing lists are available from CataList (www.lsoft.com/lists/listref.html). Another

source of mailing list groups is available from Yahoo! at http://groups.yahoo.com.

Newsgroups offer another way to network online. A newsgroup is basically an online discussion group for a specific topic. Anyone can join and participate by reading and posting messages. Messages that address the same topic are called a "thread," and each time a different topic is introduced, a new thread is started. See "groups.google.com" for a list of groups.

If you decide to use either mailing lists or newsgroups, it is important to learn the proper "netiquette" for participating. Experts suggest that you read a group's messages for at least 2 weeks before submitting anything so that you will know the type and quality of material that is expected. It is also recommended that you check the "Frequently Asked Questions" or FAQs section, if available, to avoid asking something that has already been covered. If you are able to view previous messages, you may also want to use the search field to find previous messages that pertain to your topic of interest. When you do send messages, keep them short and to the point.

Web forums are another form of online discussion group offered through a variety of websites. You need only an email address and web browser to participate. You can ask questions, such as, "How's the job market in San Antonio?" and someone from that area may answer. Lists of discussion groups are available on the Internet. Using a browser, enter the keyword "forum" and a topic of interest to get a list of ongoing forums.

One important rule is to never send advertising or use these groups to ask for a job. You may, however, find someone in the group who you can contact personally via email for possible assistance, just as you would other professional contacts.

See Box 10.9 for Internet success tips.

EXPERIENTIAL EXERCISES

1. Read the article "How to Use the Internet in Your Job Search" at http://rileyguide.com/jobsrch.html.
2. Write a list of the information or suggestions you found most useful.

EXPERIENTIAL EXERCISES

Create an Internet tracking form that includes the following: name and address of the website, your username and password, the date you posted a comment or your resume, and a section for additional information and comments.

Tips for Using the Internet

- **Learn more.** If you are not already proficient at using the Internet, take a class, find online help, or get a copy of one of the many books on how to use it.
- **Be patient.** The Internet is not without its issues. You may get bumped offline just as you find what you are looking for or discover a promising website. If you are completing online forms, be sure to save your work periodically.
- **Monitor where you are.** It is easy to get lost in a maze of links that takes you far from the original site. When you access a major site, write down its name and address so you can find it again. You can also open links in a new tab on your Internet browser, so that you can keep the original site open in its own tab.
- **Mark favorite sites.**
- **Watch the time.** Using the Internet can be addictive. If you find sites that look interesting but are unrelated to the task at hand, note their addresses and return to them later.
- **Beware of scams.** Take care when posting your resume or sending private information. If a website makes claims about jobs that seem too good to be true, it may simply be a means of getting personal information about you. Stick with major employment websites and the websites of employers whose existence you can verify in other ways.
- **Avoid being dependent on it.** The Internet is only one tool for your job search. Use it wisely as a supplement to other methods.
- **Be careful what you post.** Most employers today use social media to screen candidates. If you have accounts on Facebook, Instagram, or other personal social media sites, be *very* careful what you post. Posts complaining about your current or previous employer or photos of yourself drinking alcohol may damage your chances for employment. On professional or public-facing social media sites like LinkedIn or Twitter (now X), avoid posting controversial topics, political views, or other personal information you would not want an employer to see. Some employers admit not hiring candidates based on what they find out about them online. You can, however, use social media to your advantage. For example, if you volunteered for a community fundraiser or serve meals at a community event, you may wish to include photos of yourself participating in these activities.

Job Titles

Regardless of the source—Internet, professional journal, or newspaper—look under every category that might contain jobs for which you are prepared. For example, graduates of health information programs may be qualified for the following positions: coding specialist, health information technician, medical records coordinator or supervisor, and patient records technician. New job titles are constantly being created to describe the many activities performed in the modern health care facility. Job titles can be frustrating and limiting when you are looking for a new job. You want options. You want to be able to evaluate opportunities that are close to what you are looking for.

Even among the same job titles, you will find differing job responsibilities. Starting broadly at the beginning will help. You do not want to miss any opportunities because you were not looking for them. You are increasing the range on your radar. Do not make assumptions that may limit your opportunities. Instead, do your investigative research to determine which will be the best fit.

CASE STUDY 10.4
Career Services Tips

Melva Duran, the director of career services at a large career college, answers students' questions at a workshop she is presenting for soon-to-be graduates.

Student: With so many job seekers out there, how can graduates increase their chances of being noticed by employers?

Mrs. Duran: I think many graduates make the mistake of simply submitting a resume or application. When using the Internet, they may believe that once they've pushed the send button, it is up to the employer. But I have found that this just isn't enough. Graduates need to follow up. Unless requested otherwise in the job posting, this might be a phone call. It can be brief—something like, "I noticed your job posting on the Internet and I've sent an application online. I wanted to let you know I'm very interested in the job and am wondering when you'll be making a hiring decision."

I even had a major health care employer tell me that after he receives resumes, he waits a day or two to see if he receives any follow-up. Then he only reviews the resumes of applicants who have followed up!

Student: You mention the Internet. Are you finding that many graduates are getting jobs by posting their resumes?

Mrs. Duran: Actually, the large job sites often attract too many resumes—there is just so much competition. So, I recommend to students that they browse the job postings to identify where the jobs are and find potential employers. Then they should go in person with their resumes.

Student: So, you believe applicants should go personally to places of employment?

Mrs. Duran: Oh, yes, I think that's even better than a phone call—and certainly better than simply sending a resume electronically. They should do both—send a resume and then follow up. If they notice a large, local employer that seems to have jobs available, they should go to the facility. When talking to a contact person, they should state their interest in employment, ask about current hiring and future jobs that might be available, and ask if there is anything else they should do to apply for jobs.

Student: How about cold calling? Do you recommend it?

Mrs. Duran: Absolutely! In fact, I've had good success with this method when graduates have trouble getting hired. I advise them to dress professionally and go to buildings that have potential employers. This is a better and faster approach than calling on the phone. Employers may be looking to hire, and this saves them time and money spent on posting the job. Even if they don't have an opening, they often take the resume and call later.

This should be a soft sell—that is, don't be pushy and don't ask for an interview on the spot. On the other hand, do be prepared for an interview because that can happen!

Student: Are you suggesting that job seekers should not make telephone calls to seek openings?

Mrs. Duran: No, not at all. With the telephone, you can obviously contact more potential employers.

Student: What is the best way to conduct a phone search?

Mrs. Duran: It's critical when calling to conduct yourself professionally. Second, it's important to speak with someone who has hiring authority. In a physician's office, this is not likely to be the receptionist in a doctor's office, so you need to ask for the office manager.

Student: Many of us are nervous when making these calls. What is the best way to go about it—what should graduates say?

Mrs. Duran: First state your name and say that you are a graduate of the _____ program at _____ school. Then say something like, "I would like to get my resume to you for any jobs you might have now or in the future."

If they are willing to receive your resume, it is best if you drop it off in person. This gives you a chance to see the facility, even if briefly and only the front office, and it gives someone there the chance to see you. So be sure to dress professionally! Before hanging up, ask for the address and any special directions.

QUESTIONS FOR THOUGHT AND REFLECTION

1. What advice do you find most helpful from Mrs. Duran?
2. What is her advice about using the Internet?
3. Why does she recommend making direct contact with employers?
4. How can you best prepare to make a good impression on the phone? In person?
5. What does she mean by a "soft sell"?

A Different Path

Jacob was frustrated and angry when he entered the office of Mr. Gonzalez, Director of Career Services at Met Health Career College. Jacob graduated 2 months before he stopped by to see Mr. Gonzalez and still had not received a job offer. In fact, he had not even had an interview.

"Hi, Jacob," Mr. Gonzalez greeted him. "I haven't seen you in a while. What's going on?"

"Not much, to be honest," Jacob told him. "I'm not happy. I finished my externship two months ago, and you guys haven't found me a job yet."

Mr. Gonzalez looked at Jacob for a moment and then said, "Well, I think there's been a misunderstanding. Our job is to help our students in their job search. We don't get them jobs."

"Look," said Jacob, "When I enrolled at this school, I was told that the majority of students who graduated from my program get placed. I paid a lot of money to go here, and the least you can do is find me a job."

"Let me ask you, Jacob, did you attend any of my job search workshops?"

"No. By the time I graduated, I needed a break from school," Jacob said. "I really didn't feel like coming back for more classes."

"I'm sorry you feel that way," responded Mr. Gonzalez. "The workshops are designed to help students carry out an effective job search. Let me ask you a few questions."

"Here we go," grumbled Jacob, as he flopped down into a chair.

"What have you done so far to look for a job?" Mr. Gonzalez asked.

"A lot! I went to those online job sites and looked for jobs for pharmacy techs," said Jacob. "But most of them were too far away, or didn't look very interesting, or didn't pay enough. I can't take just anything, you know. I've got student loans to pay."

"How about networking? Or visiting pharmacies where you might like to work or closer to where you live?" asked Mr. Gonzalez.

"I thought I was networking by being a student here," explained Jacob. "My instructors know me; you know me. I didn't have time while I was a student to go out and meet a bunch of people. I thought that was your job. Go meet employers and find us jobs."

"Jacob, I'm afraid that you're going to have to take more responsibility and initiative for conducting your own job search," said Mr. Gonzalez. "We can give you leads and connect you to employers who are interested in our graduates. But you haven't been in touch with us at all, not to attend the workshops or ask for help. That's our job, but you have to be willing to do your part."

"Well, I needed time to relax and just hang out after I graduated. And I can see it wouldn't have done any good anyway if you're not going to get me placed in a job I like and that pays well."

Mr. Gonzalez sighs and says, "Well, Jacob, I can see that your finding a job is going to be a struggle since you think a job is going to fall in your lap and you don't have to do anything to get it."

QUESTIONS FOR THOUGHT AND REFLECTION

1. What mistakes is Jacob making in his job search?
2. What part do you think his attitude is playing in his failure to find a job?
3. What do you think about how Mr. Gonzalez handled being confronted by Jacob? Is there anything else he could have done to help Jacob?
4. Based on this interaction, what challenges might Jacob have as a pharmacy technician when he does get a job?

References

Anderson R., Barbara A., Feldman S.: *What patients want: a content analysis of key qualities that influence patient satisfaction,* 2009. http://www.drscore.com/press/papers/whatpatientswant.pdf.

Dickel MR. *Guide to internet job searching 2004-2005.* Columbus, OH: McGraw-Hill; 2004.

Ellis D, Lankowitz S, Stupka E, Toft D, eds. *Career planning.* New York, NY: Houghton Mifflin; 1997.

Graber S. *The everything online job search book.* Holbrook, MA: Adams Media; 2000.

Hansen K.: *Behavioral interviewing strategies for job-seekers.* http://www.quintcareers.com/behavioral_interviewing.html Accessed July 28, 2015.

Lock RD. *Job search: career planning guide, book II.* Pacific Grove, CA: Brooks/Cole; 1996.

Lorenz K.: *Warning: social networking can be hazardous to your job search.* CareerBuilder.com Editor. http://www.careerbuilder.ca/blog/2006/07/12/cb-warning-social-networking-can-be-hazardous-to-your-job-search/. Accessed February 25, 2009.

National Consortium on Health Science and Technology Education: *National Healthcare Foundation Standards and Accountability Criteria.* https://healthscienceconsortium.org/wp-content/uploads/2022/09/NATIONAL_HEALTH_SCIENCE_STANDARDS_with_Blueprint_20220831FINAL-CL-Updated_92422.pdf. Accessed October 29, 2022

Apply for Jobs

- How to Be a Successful Job-Seeker
- Prepare an Effective Resume
- Create a Dynamic Cover Letter
- Learn How to Apply for Jobs Online
- Navigate Talent Management Software
- Complete Employment Tests

Preparing to Apply

In the previous chapter, we discussed beginning your job search. However, multiple steps are involved in the job-seeking process. In addition to researching job sites and available jobs, a critical step is creating your resume and job application and any supporting documents, such as cover letter, references, and even a portfolio. A professional image—in person and on paper—is essential to successful job searching, applying, and interviewing.

Making the First Impression

You never get a second chance to make a first impression.
—Will Rogers

As a job seeker, before an employer even meets you, your first impression is your resume. Your resume is the most effective tool to market yourself to a prospective employer. A resume is a document that provides a prospective employer with a detailed statement and information about your prior work experience, education, skills, training, and accomplishments. The resume is often accompanied by a cover letter, which is a business letter to describe and detail why and how you are qualified for the position you are applying for. The main purpose of a resume is to convince an employer to give you an interview.

There are different types of resumes and ways to submit your resume to apply for a job, such as in person, via email, or online, with the latter becoming more of the standard practice. Regardless of how you apply, you will need to be prepared to navigate the multiple steps to completing a job application in order to ultimately be offered the job.

Starting to plan your resume now will help you:

1. Recognize what you already have to offer an employer.
2. Build self-confidence.
3. Motivate you to learn both the technical and non-technical skills that contribute to employment success.

4. Identify anything you might want to improve about yourself.
5. Know ahead of time what kinds of experiences will enhance your employability.
6. Get a head start gathering information and collecting examples to demonstrate your value and skills.

⬅ JOURNALING 11.1

Before you start reading through this chapter, locate your most recent resume. Highlight and make comments on it as you read this chapter to see where you can improve your resume.

Components of a Resume

LEARNING OBJECTIVE 1: COMPONENTS OF A RESUME

- Define the purpose of the professional resume.
- List the benefits of planning your resume while you are in school.
- List the 10 resume building blocks.
- Describe the contents of each of the building blocks.
- Plan and prepare your professional resume.

You are now ready to gather the information to construct a complete resume. There is no one way to write a resume. The best resume is the one that showcases your unique skills and abilities. Even students who complete the same program at the same time bring a variety of backgrounds and talents that can be presented in different ways. For example, a young person who graduated from high school shortly before beginning a dental assisting program will more likely benefit from emphasizing different experiences than a classmate who worked in sales for 20 years before entering the same program.

You may be tempted to use a standard resume format. Filling in the blanks on a "one-type-fits-all" resume may seem like a fast and easy way to create a resume; however, the time spent customizing your resume can pay off in several ways. For example, you will:

1. Better recognize and review your own qualifications
2. Respond to employers' specific needs
3. Be prepared to support your claims with examples
4. Demonstrate your organizational skills
5. Show your initiative and creativity

There are also local customs and employer preferences regarding resumes. Seek the advice of your

BOX 11.1

Building Blocks for a Resume

1. Professional Profile
2. Education
3. Professional Skills and Knowledge
4. Work History
5. Licenses and Certifications
6. Honors and Awards
7. Special Skills
8. Volunteer Activities
9. Professional and Civic Organizations
10. Languages Spoken

instructors, school career service personnel, and professional contacts. They are likely in contact with local employers and can offer sound advice. Your school may require or recommend that you use a format it has developed.

Box 11.1 lists the most important components or building blocks of a resume. Each component is further explained along with suggestions on how to make them work for you while you are still in school.

Building Block One: Personal Profile

The personal profile, also called the professional summary, is a brief description of what you can offer the employer, highlighting your relevant skills and experience. For example:

* AAMA-certified administrative and clinical medical assistant with 3 years' experience. Reliable, detail-oriented, and passionate about patient care.

As you go through your training, learn as much as possible about the various jobs for which you might qualify. You may be unaware of jobs that closely match your interests. As you discover jobs that might fit your skills and interests, tailor your profile statement to each job. If possible, try to incorporate key terms that are used in descriptions of those jobs or job postings for positions you are interested in.

❓ WHAT IF?

You enjoy your classes but are having a hard time being specific about the kind of job or facility you want. Where could you get more information to help you decide?

⭐ EXPERIENTIAL EXERCISE

Write at least two sentences that describe your objective for your first job in health care.

Building Block Two: Education

The education section lists all your education and training, with emphasis on health care training.

Start your list with the school you attended most recently. Include grade point average (GPA) and class standing (not all schools rank their students by grades) if they are above average; otherwise, leave these out. You may also want to include any honors or certifications you received. Here is an example:

Mental Health Technician Certificate, 2023
Wellness College, Salem, OR

* Graduated with Top Honors
* Grade point average 3.7 on a 4.0 scale
* Received Perfect Attendance Award
* Completed CPR training
* Organized musical program presented by students at Christmas to local extended-care residents

Workshops completed 2022 to 2023
Sunnyville Psychiatric Institute, Salem, OR

* Review of Research on Depression (25 hours)
* Suicide Prevention Measures (20 hours)
* Managing Assaultive Patients (25 hours)

 EXPERIENTIAL EXERCISE

List the schools you have attended, starting with the most recent. Include the name of the program(s) completed; degree(s), diploma(s), and/certificate(s) earned; grade point average; awards and honors; additional training; and any special projects.

Building Block Three: Professional Skills and Knowledge

Professional skills and knowledge refer to the skills and knowledge that contribute specifically to successful job performance.

The way you organize this section depends on your educational program and the number and variety of skills acquired. You can list them individually if there are not too many (such as "Take vital signs") or as clusters of related skills (such as "Perform clinical duties").

Listing individual skills or clusters of skills is a good idea if your previous work experience is limited and you want to emphasize the recent acquisition of health care skills as your primary qualification. It is also helpful if you have trained for one of the newer positions in health care that is not familiar to all employers. For example, "Patient Care Technician" is a relatively new multiskilled worker who can be employed in a variety of health care settings. As you tailor your resume to particular job openings, you should include only information that is relevant to the job you are applying for.

Even if you decide not to include a skills list on your resume (it is optional), maintaining a list for yourself will remind you of what you know and have to offer an employer. You can refer to this list when you go for an interview or attend a job fair. Employers report that many recent graduates do not realize how much they know and, therefore, often fail to sell themselves at job interviews. Reviewing your skills list as part of your interview preparation should help you present yourself effectively and confidently to potential employers.

If you have trouble coming up with a skills list for yourself, find out if your school provides lists of program and course objectives and/or the competencies you will master in the program. Some instructors give their students checklists to monitor the completion of assignments and demonstration of competencies. Other sources of information include handouts from your instructor, such as syllabi and course outlines, the objectives listed in your textbooks, and laboratory skill sheets. You will be amazed by how much you are learning and will have a great skills list to work from. See Box 11.2 for examples of skills.

 EXPERIENTIAL EXERCISE

Create an inventory of the skills you are learning in your program. Update the inventory as you complete your classes.

BOX 11.2

Examples of Professional Skills and Knowledge

- Setting up dental trays for common procedures
- Accurately completing medical insurance claim forms
- Creating presentations using PowerPoint
- Teaching patients to use different ambulatory devices

Building Block Four: Work History

The work history is a list of your previous jobs, including the name and location of the employer, your job title, primary duties and accomplishments, and the dates of employment.

You can benefit from this section of your resume, even if you have no previous experience in health care. There are three ways to do this. The first is to review the duties and responsibilities you had in each of your past jobs, and then determine which ones can be applied to health care work. Highlight these as you list your previous employment experiences.

Skills that are common to many jobs are called transferable skills. See Box 11.3 for examples of transferable skills. Identifying transferable skills is especially important when you are entering a new field in which you have little or no experience. There is a type of resume that emphasizes skills and abilities rather than specific job titles held. It is called a "functional resume," and the format is described later in this chapter. Start compiling a list of your own transferable skills.

The second way to maximize the value of the Work History section of your resume is to state what you accomplished in each job. In a phrase or two, describe how you contributed to the success of your employer. When possible, state these achievements in measurable terms. If you cannot express them with numbers, use active verbs that demonstrate what you did. Here are some examples:

* Reduced costs by 20%
* Designed a more efficient way to track supplies
* Worked on a committee to write an effective employee procedure manual that is still in use
* Trained five employees on the electronic health records system

A third way to add value to this section is to include your externship experience. Although you must clearly indicate that this was a part of your training and not paid employment, it still serves as evidence of your ability to apply what you learned in school to practical situations.

For many new graduates, this is their only real-world experience in health care; however, some students fail to realize the effect their performance can have on their career. Remember that clinical supervisors represent future employers. (In some cases, they are future employers because some students are hired by their externship sites.) Their opinion of you can be a help or a hinderance in your job search, so commit to doing your best during your clinical experience.

Do not be concerned if your work experience is limited or you cannot think of any achievements. You may have finished high school recently or perhaps you spent several years working as a stay-at-home parent. Parents and others who care for family members gain experiences that are valuable to employers (Figure 11.1). Examples include caring for others, time management, and handling family finances. Further, employers understand that everyone starts with a first job, and you are receiving training that will qualify you for work.

? WHAT IF?

The jobs you have held were all entry-level. You cannot think of any real achievements in any of them.

★ EXPERIENTIAL EXERCISE

List the jobs you have had in the past. Include the name and location of the employer; dates of employment; and your job title, duties, and achievements.

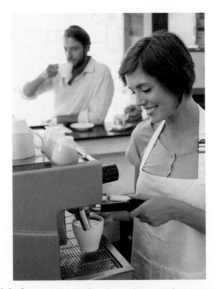

Figure 11.1 Working in food service requires organization, time management, and people skills, all of which are desirable skills that employers seek in new health care professionals. Think about the skills you developed in previous job roles and how they transfer to your new profession. (Copyright © istock.com.)

BOX 11.3

Examples of Transferable Skills

- Work well with people from a variety of backgrounds.
- Provide good customer service.
- Resolve customer complaints satisfactorily.
- Perform accurate word processing.
- Demonstrate empathy.
- Apply ethical standards.
- Apply active listening skills.

Building Block Five: Licenses and Certifications

Some professions require you to be licensed or have specific types of approval before you are allowed to work. Nursing is one example; others include physical and occupational therapy and dental hygiene. Some professions have voluntary certifications and registrations, such as those earned by medical assistants. The kind of approvals needed vary by state and profession. Most licenses and certifications require certain types of training and/or passing a standardized examination. It is important that you clearly understand any professional requirements necessary or highly recommended for your profession.

Learn about the requirements for the occupation you have chosen. Ask your instructors about review classes, books, and computerized material. Check with your professional organization.

Become familiar with the topics on the examinations and plan your studies accordingly. Many testing organizations provide practice exams and study guides for examinations. Knowing the format of the questions (multiple choice, true-false, etc.) is also helpful.

 EXPERIENTIAL EXERCISES

1. Describe the licensing and certification requirements for your occupation, including those that are voluntary.
2. What type of test(s) must you take?
3. What study and review materials are available?

Building Block Six: Honors and Awards

The section on honors and awards is optional. Your school may offer recognition for student achievements and special contributions. Community and professional organizations to which you belong may also give awards. Acknowledgments received for volunteer work should also be included in this section. Examples include:

* Parent Volunteer of the Year for James Madison Middle School, 2020
* Recognition for successful senior center fundraiser
* Perfect Attendance Award, Wellness College, 2023

Investigate what you might be eligible for and use these rewards as incentives for excellent performance. Keep in mind, however, that although awards are nice to report, they are not essential for getting a good job.

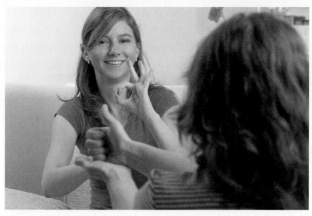

Figure 11.2 Many skills, such as sign language, enhance the value of the health care professional. What skills do you already have that you can use in your future work? (Copyright © istock.com.)

 EXPERIENTIAL EXERCISE

Investigate and list awards for which you might qualify or have already earned.

Building Block Seven: Special Skills

Special skills are those that do not fit into other sections but do add to your value as a prospective employee. Examples include proficiency in desktop publishing or the ability to use American Sign Language (Figure 11.2).

Research the needs of employers in your geographical area. Do you already have special skills that meet these needs? Would it increase your chances for employment if you acquired skills outside the scope of your program, for example, to become more proficient in a particular software application? If time permits, you should try to attend workshops in addition to your regular program courses, do extra reading, or take an online course.

 EXPERIENTIAL EXERCISE

Record special skills you have that might be applicable to a job in health care.

Building Block Eight: Volunteer Activities

Include volunteer activities on your resume if they relate to your targeted occupation or demonstrate desired qualities, such as being responsible and having concern for others. If you are already involved in volunteer activities, think about what you are learning or practicing that can help you on the job. If you are not, consider becoming involved if you have a sincere interest and adequate time. Adult students face many responsibilities outside of class, and the additional activities mentioned in this chapter should be taken as suggestions, not must-dos. Mastering program content should be your main priority.

 EXPERIENTIAL EXERCISE

List any volunteer activities you might use on your resume.

Building Block Nine: Professional and Civic Organizations

Professional organizations provide excellent opportunities to network, learn more about your field, and practice leadership skills. Participation in civic organizations, groups that work for the good of the community, promotes personal growth and demonstrates your willingness to help others. Consider joining and participating actively in a professional or civic organization while you are in school. See if your school or community has a local chapter.

 EXPERIENTIAL EXERCISE

List professional and civic organizations you might include on your resume. Include offices held, committees served on, etc.

Building Block Ten: Languages Spoken

In our multicultural society, the ability to communicate in a language other than English is commonly included on the resume. Find out whether many patients speak a language other than English in the area where you plan to work. Consider acquiring at least some conversational ability or a few phrases to use to reassure patients. Patients benefit greatly, during the stress of illness or injury, when health care professionals know at least a few phrases of their native language. Also, consider learning about the customs, especially the ones related to health practices, of ethnic groups in your community.

 EXPERIENTIAL EXERCISE

List languages you speak other than English, including your ability level in speaking, reading, and writing.

 JOURNALING 11.2

As I put together my resume content, do I feel more confident about what I have to offer an employer?

 WHAT IF?

You want to put together a good resume, but you are not very skilled with word-processing software. What should you do?

Preparing Your Resume

LEARNING OBJECTIVE 2:
PREPARING YOUR RESUME

- List the 10 steps for assembling your resume.
- Describe the three types of resumes.
- Explain when to use each type of resume.
- Understand the importance of grammar and spelling in the resume.
- Determine the best layout for your resume.
- Learn how to use "power" words in your resume.

You are not your resume; you are your work.

—Seth Godin

The steps described in this section will help you create a document that best highlights your qualifications, which can be used in your resume. Following a step-by-step process will help you assemble a resume to fit the job you are applying for. Box 11.4 summarizes the steps that are explained in the following sections.

BOX 11.4

Nine-Step Checklist for Assembling Your Resume

1. Prepare the heading.
2. Add the profile.
3. Select the best type of resume for you.
4. Choose which Resume Building Blocks to include.
5. Plan the order of your Building Blocks.
6. Decide whether you want to add a personal statement.
7. But leave out personal information.
8. Plan the layout.
9. Create an attractive and professional-looking document.

Step One: Prepare the Heading

Clearly label the top of the page with your name, address, telephone number(s), and email address. You may also wish to include the address for your LinkedIn account or personal website. Center your name on the page. Capitalizing, bolding, and/or using a slightly larger font size than the rest of the document helps your name stand out. Be sure that all contact information and numbers are correct.

JAIME RAMIREZ
3650 Loma Alta Lane
San Diego, CA 92137
(619) 123-4567
jramirez@outlook.com

The following format is an option if your resume is long and you are trying to save space:

JAIME RAMIREZ
3650 Loma Alta Lane San Diego, CA 92137—
(619)123-4567—jramirez@aol.com

After submitting your resume, you may receive a response from the hiring manager by email. Make sure your email address is professional, easy to remember, and somewhat easily identifiable to you, such as your full name or some of your name. Make your email address easy for potential employers to find you and remember you.

Avoid email addresses that are flirtatious, silly, funny, or lewd. In some cases, you may need to create a new email account if you have one that is too personal. Once you do, make it a practice to check it daily in case a potential employer is trying to reach you. For some positions, time is of the essence in replying to an interview or job offer.

Resume Credentials

Depending on your health care profession, it is recommended to add your credentials after your name at the top of a resume. Resume credentials often refer to the skills, experiences, and strengths to an open job or position and, as a result, may bring attention to your resume. Below is an example of a resume credential for a certified pharmacy technician:

Heather Donal, CPhT
151 Rainier Way, Unit #5
Maple Valley, WA 98038

When you apply for a job, it is important to identify the credentials that are most relevant to the position. This allows the employer to see how you can be a strong fit for their company while keeping your resume short and focused. For example, you are applying for a medical coding position and have certifications as a

Certified Professional Coder (CPC), Certified Medical Administrative Assistant (CMAA), and Certified Electronic Health Record Specialist (CEHRS). You should include the certification that most applies to the job after your name and include the other certifications in the Licenses and Certification section.

Step Two: Add the Profile or Summary

The profile or summary should be near the beginning of the resume so prospective employers can quickly see whether there is a potential fit between your background and their needs. (Personal profile was also discussed in Building Block One.) This part of the resume may change slightly if you are trying to adapt your profile to the stated needs of each employer. You may wish to change certain terms to match the wording of the job posting.

Consider writing a targeted profile for each job. For each application, your profile should mirror the employer's language and draw attention to how your skills and experience fit that particular job. The following example shows how to write a targeted profile or summary statement:

Job Posting: "X-ray tech with strong patient relations skills for orthopedic practice. Great opportunity to join an established team environment."

Key Words in the Posting: X-ray tech, patient relations skills, orthopedic, team

Targeted Profile Statement: Skilled x-ray tech with experience in an orthopedic office. Highly adept at patient relations and eager to contribute to a team.

Step Three: Select the Best Type of Resume for You

The three basic resume formats are chronological, functional, and combination. They provide different ways to present your work history, skills and training, and professional qualifications. Your particular background determines which type you should choose.

Chronological Resume

The most common type is the chronological resume that emphasizes work history. It shows the progression of jobs you have held and how you have gained increasing knowledge, experience, and/or responsibility. This type of resume is recommended if you have:
* Held previous jobs in health care
* Had jobs in other areas in which you had increases in responsibility or a strong record of achievements

* Acquired many skills that apply to health care (transferable skills)
* No major gaps in your employment history

In the chronological resume, each of your past jobs is listed in reverse chronological order, with the most recent job first, followed by the duties performed and your achievements. The Work History or Experience section is well developed and likely to be longer than most other parts of your resume.

Figure 11.3 shows an example of a chronological resume.

Functional Resume

The functional resume emphasizes skills and traits that relate to the targeted job, but which were not necessarily acquired through health care employment. They can be pulled from work, volunteer, and

---

RUDY MARQUEZ
1909 Franklin Blvd.
Philadelphia, PA 19105
(610) 765-4321   MAmarquez@aol.com

OBJECTIVE   Position as a clinical medical assistant in an urgent care setting

QUALIFICATIONS
* 13 years experience as a certified medical assistant
* Current certifications in CPR and Basic Life Support
* Proven ability to communicate with patients and staff
* Proactive employee who anticipates office and physicians' needs
* Fluent in Spanish and Italian

WORK HISTORY   Medical Assistant   2005-present
Founders Medical Clinic   Philadelphia, PA
* Perform clinical and laboratory duties
* Assist physicians with exams, procedures, and surgeries
* Reorganized patient education program, including selection of updated brochures, videos
* Provide patient education and present healthy living workshops
* Train and supervise new medical assistants

Medical Assistant   1999-2005
North Side Clinic   Pittsburgh, PA
* Performed clinical and laboratory duties
* Developed system for monitoring and ordering clinic supplies that resulted in annual savings of over $25,000
* Received commendation for providing outstanding patient service

Medical Assistant   1997-1999
Dr. Alan Fleming   Erie, PA
* Assisted Dr. Fleming with procedures and minor office surgeries
* Prepared treatment and examining rooms
* Took vital signs and administered injections
* Performed routine laboratory tests
* Handled computerized recordkeeping tasks
* Assisted in researching and purchasing new office computer system

EDUCATION   Associate of Science in Medical Assisting   1997
Emerson College of Health Careers, Erie, PA

Recently Completed Workshops and Continuing Education Courses
* Health Care Beliefs of Minority Populations
* Medical Spanish
* New Requirements for Maintaining Patient Confidentiality

ORGANIZATIONS   American Association of Medical Assistants (AAMA)
Pennsylvania Association of Medical Assistants
Philadelphia Lions Club

Figure 11.3 Example of a Chronological Resume. This type of resume, which lists a detailed work history, is recommended for applicants who already have experience working in health care.

personal experiences. For example, if you cared for a sick relative for an extended period of time or perhaps were a child care provider, this is an experience you might include. Once you have identified and listed qualifications that fit your target jobs, organize them into three or four clusters with descriptive headings. Figure 11.4 shows three clusters developed by a graduate who wants to find a job in health information technology. The applicant has drawn from their experiences as a parent, active member of the community, and bookkeeper.

Functional resumes are recommended if you:
* Are entering the job market for the first time
* Have held jobs unrelated to health care
* Have major gaps in your work history
* Have personal experiences you can apply to health care work

The Work History section of a functional resume consists of a simple list of job titles with each employer's name, city and state, and the dates of employment. In this format, your Skills section will be longer than your Work History section.

COMPUTER SKILLS

- Created electronic spreadsheet to track fund raising for Lewison Elementary School PTA

- Taught self to effectively use leading brand software programs in the following areas: word processing, database, spreadsheets, and accounting

- Set up and managed electronic accounting system for family construction business

- Teach computer classes at Girl Scout summer day camp

ORGANIZATIONAL SKILLS

- Created system to monitor all church collections and fund-raising projects

- Initiated and developed computer career awareness program for Girl Scouts

- Secretary for college HIT student organization

- Completed HIT associate degree program with record of perfect attendance while working part-time and managing family life

CLERICAL/ADMINISTRATIVE SKILLS

- 7 years bookkeeping experience

- Keyboarding speed of 78 wpm

- Excellent written communication

WORK HISTORY

Bookkeeper 2008-Present
Buildwell Construction Company, Yuma, AZ

Bookkeeper 2003-2008
Perfect-Fit Cabinetry, Yuma, AZ

Secretary 1999-2003
Caldwell Insurance Company, Yuma, AZ

Figure 11.4 Work History section of a functional resume for a recent graduate seeking a health information technology (HIT) position. The graduate does not have experience in this field, so the applicant has clustered other skills that support work in HIT, such as bookkeeping and tracking details.

A functional resume may take more time to develop than a chronological one, as you will need to spend time developing descriptions and examples of relevant skills gained from different experiences or jobs. However, the extra effort can pay off; it allows you to highlight the qualifications and transferable skills that are most applicable to the job you are applying for rather than focusing on the details of jobs you may have held in an unrelated field. If your relevant skills were gained primarily from your education, training, volunteer, or other activities rather than from formal employment, a functional resume may be your best choice.

Figure 11.5 shows an example of a functional resume.

HEATHER DIETZ
10532 Cactus Road
Yuma, AZ 85360
(520) 321-7654   thedietz@linkup.com

OBJECTIVE   Entry-level position in health information management in which I can apply up-to-date knowledge and skills. I especially enjoy applying my organizational skills and working on challenging tasks that must be complete and accurate.

EDUCATION   Associate of Science in Health Information Technology   2009
Desert Medical College   Yuma, AZ

COMPUTER SKILLS
- Created electronic spreadsheet to track fund raising for Sage Elementary School PTA
- Taught self to efficiently use leading brand software programs in the following areas: word processing, database, spreadsheets, and accounting
- Set up and managed electronic accounting system for family-owned construction business
- Teach computer classes at Girl Scout summer day camp

ORGANIZATIONAL SKILLS
- Created system to monitor all church collections and fund-raising projects
- Initiated and developed computer career awareness program for Girl Scouts
- Secretary for college HIT student organization
- Completed HIT associate degree program with perfect class attendance while working part-time and managing family life

CLERICAL/ADMINISTRATIVE SKILLS
- 7 years bookkeeping experience
- Keyboarding speed of 78 wpm
- Excellent written communication skills

WORK HISTORY
Unpaid Internship at St. John's Medical Center, Yuma, AZ   2009
Medical Records Department

Bookkeeper   2003-2007
Buildwell Construction Company, Yuma, AZ

Bookkeeper   1998-2003
Perfect-Fit Cabinetry, Yuma, AZ

Secretary   1995-1998
Caldwell Insurance Company, Yuma, AZ

ORGANIZATIONS
Desert Medical College Health Information Technology Student Organization, Secretary
Sage Elementary School PTA, Treasurer
Faith Community Church, Member of Social Service Committee

Figure 11.5 Example of a Functional Resume. This type of resume, which lists skills that support a health care job, is recommended for applicants who have not worked in health care.

Combination Resume

The combination resume, as its name implies, uses features of both chronological and functional resumes. The details of the job(s) held in health care or closely related fields are listed, along with clusters of qualifications or a list of supporting skills. This resume is appropriate if you:

* Have held jobs in health care, and
* Have related qualifications you gained through other, non–health care jobs and experiences, or
* Have held a number of jobs in health care for which you performed the same or very similar duties.

Here is an example of how a recent occupational therapy assistant graduate who worked for 2 years as a nursing assistant and for 3 years as a preschool aide might create a combination resume. The applicant:

* Includes a list of the duties performed in the nursing assistant job
* Creates clusters to highlight teaching and interpersonal skills, both important in occupational therapy
* Lists skills from teaching and other experiences under each cluster heading

Figure 11.6 illustrates how the applicant organized the material to best show their qualifications.

NURSING ASSISTANT   2005-2010
GoodCare Nursing Home, Denver, CO

* Encourage patients to achieve their maximum level of wellness, activity, and independence
* Demonstrate interest in the lives and well-being of patients
* Assist patients with prescribed exercises
* Organize and participate in activities with patients
* Help patients carry out basic hygiene and dressing

TEACHING SKILLS

* Teach swim classes to all ages at YMCA
* Conduct CPR instruction for the American Heart Association
* Organize holiday programs and outings for nursing home residents (volunteer)
* Planned and supervised craft and play activities for preschool children
* Tutored ESL students at Salud College while in OTA program

INTERPERSONAL SKILLS

* Provided daily care for parent with Alzheimer's disease for 18 months
* Answered telephone, directed calls, and took messages for busy sporting goods manufacturer
* Received Connor Memorial Award for graduating class for making positive contributions and assisting classmates at Salud College

WORK HISTORY   **Preschool Aide** 2002-2005
                          Bright Light Preschool, Denver, CO

                          Swim Instructor 2002-Present
                          YMCA, Denver, CO

                          Receptionist 1999-2002
                          Sportrite Manufacturing Co., Denver, CO

Figure 11.6 Work History section of a combination resume for a recent graduate seeking an occupational therapy assistant position. The applicant details the one health care–related job they had held while organizing other skills that support the new career into clusters.

Figure 11.7 shows an example of a chronological resume.

Choosing the Best Resume Format for You

Review your skills and experiences and use the guidelines in this section to choose the best type of resume for you. If you decide to use a chronological format, copy what you prepared for your Work History in Building Block Three.

If a functional resume would serve you better, use the following guidelines to create the clusters:

1. Consider the current needs of employers. Check the websites of local companies and online job boards, such as Glassdoor, Indeed, or LinkedIn Jobs, for job announcements. You may also wish to consult the National Healthcare Foundation Standards, which includes lists of standards that apply to occupations or functions involved in health care, as these will offer you examples of skills related to health care.

2. Identify the skills and traits that will contribute to success in your occupation.

3. Review your work history, externship experience, personal experiences, volunteer activities, and participation in professional organizations.

4. Create three or four headings for clusters that support your job target and give you an opportunity to list your most significant qualifications. The

---

ELIZABETH PEREZ

example@example.com | (555) 555-5555 | Providence. RI

PROFESSIONAL SUMMARY

Committed healthcare professional affering 6 years of demonstrated success in home healthcare. Committed to delivering consistent and focused attention to client safety, comfort and dignity. Well-versed in senior health care with passion for helping others.

SKILLS

- Senior care
- First aid and safety
- Progress documentationipsum

- Medication administration
- Healthy meal preparation
- Feeding assistance

WORK HISTORY

Feb 2016-Current
Home Health Aide
CareLinx Inc. - Providence, RI

- Delivered assistance to an 83 year old elderly client in daily activities including bathing, dressing, physical transfers and care for incontinence.
- Followed nutritional plans set by doctor to prepare optimal meals, including purchasing ingredients from local shops.
- Coordinated daily medicine schedules for and administration to help clients address symptoms and enhance quality of life.

Jul 2014 Jan 2016 Home
Home Health Aide
Bayada Home Health Care-
Providence.RI

- Assisted multiple patients with dressing, grooming and feeding needs, helping to overcome and adapt to mobility restrictions.
- Ensured safety and well-being of each patient in alignment with care plan,
- Completed entries in log books, journals and care plans to document accurately report patient progress.

Aug 2013-Jun 2014
Caregiver
Home Instead Senior Care-North
Kingstown, RI

- Gathered dietary information, assisted with feeding and monitored intake to help patients achieve nutritional objectives and support wellness goals.
- Assisted patients with personal requirements, including keeping spaces clean and helping with grooming.
- Kept close eye on client vital signs, administered medications and tracked behaviors to keep healthcare supervisor well-informed.

EDUCATION

Jun 2012
High School Diploma
North Kingstown Senior High School | North Kingstown, RI

Figure 11.7 Example of a Combination Resume. This type of resume is recommended for applicants who have some experience working in health care but who also want to highlight other skills that support their target job. (Courtesy of Bold Limited.)

following list contains examples of appropriate clusters for health care occupations:

* Communication Skills
* Organizational Skills
* Teamwork Skills
* Interpersonal Relations
* Computer Skills
* Clerical Skills

5. List specific skills under each heading.

Step Four: Choose Which Resume Building Blocks to Use

Your resume should be comprehensive, but it should not repeat information. For example, if you are using a functional format and have listed a special skill in one of your clusters, do not list it again under another heading. When deciding what information should go under which section, think about which items fit together. Each Resume Building Block, or section in your resume, should include several items. If you have only one item in a section, combine it with another section. These are suggestions for how to arrange or combine common items:

1. Licenses and certifications can be placed in their own section, in the Education section, or listed under a Training section.
2. Honors and awards earned in school can be listed under Education. If you have a variety of awards, it might be better to highlight them by listing them in their own section.
3. Memberships can go under Education if they are related to school groups or your health care professional organization. They could go in their own section if you are involved in several organizations. If you have been active in the organizations and want to describe your accomplishments, you could list your role under a Volunteer Experience section.
4. Externship experience can be listed under either Education or Work History. Wherever you place it, include some information about the duties you performed. For career changers and recent graduates, this may be a significant part of your work history. Be sure to indicate clearly that the work was unpaid and part of an educational program.
5. Languages you speak other than English can be listed under the Qualifications, Skills, or Languages sections.

Deciding which headings to use and where to place content depends on the amount of content, how directly it relates to the kind of job you want, and your own organizational preferences. Suppose you speak two languages other than English. If they are spoken by many people in your geographical area, they are likely to be valuable job qualifications and might be listed in a Profile Statement or a Skills section. If they are not commonly spoken in your area, they might best be listed under Languages—skills you want to show but that may not be directly related to the job.

Step Five: Plan the Order of Your Building Blocks

Place the sections that contain your strongest qualifications first. For example, if you are changing careers and recent education is your primary qualification, place this section before Work History.

If your resume is more than one page, try to organize and space your sections so that items in a section do not break across the pages. You would want to avoid, for instance, having a job title, location, and date for a job on one page and your responsibilities and achievements for that job on the next page. It would be preferable in that instance to add space before the job title, so it carries over to the next page.

Before deciding on the order of your sections, you may want to find sample resumes for the type of jobs you are interested in applying for. Seeing examples of how others in your field have organized their resume will help you choose the best format for your needs.

Step Six: Decide If You Want to Add a Personal Statement

Some experts in career planning suggest adding a positive personal statement at the bottom of your resume. This is an opportunity to make a final impression and add an original touch. If you decide to write a personal statement, be sure it is a sincere reflection of you and not just something that sounds good. It should also relate to your job target. Here are some examples:

* "I enjoy being a part of a team where I can make a positive contribution by using my ability to remain calm and work efficiently under stressful conditions."
* "I derive great satisfaction from working with people from a variety of backgrounds who need assistance in resolving their health care problems."

If you decide to include a personal statement, think about your reasons for choosing a career in health care, along with what you believe are your best potential contributions to prospective employers. It would be a good idea to have someone such as your instructor review your statement.

Keep in mind that a cover letter also offers an opportunity to introduce yourself to potential employers and allows you more space to do so. Thus, if the job application allows submission of a cover letter, it would be wise to include one. In the absence of a cover letter, though, a personal statement may help your resume stand out.

Step Seven: Avoid Personal Information

Do not include personal information such as your age, marital status, number of children, and health status. This information should not be disclosed to a future or current employer unless you feel comfortable volunteering it. In fact, it is illegal for an employer to ask you about it during the interview or while you are an employee.

Also, *never* include false statements about your education or experience. If these are discovered later, they can be grounds for dismissal from your job.

Although it is important to have a reference sheet, which is a list of references with their contact information, available for potential employers who request it, it is not necessary to write a statement such as "References Available Upon Request." This may take up valuable room on your resume. You can volunteer to provide the reference sheet or wait for the potential employer to request it from you.

Step Eight: Plan the Layout

Each section of your resume, except the heading at the top and personal statement (optional) at the end, should be labeled: Profile, Education, Work History, and so on. Headings can be flush or aligned with the left margin, with the content set to the right or beneath it:

PROFILE   Obtain an entry-level medical assistant position to provide attentive, highly professional assistance to patients and physicians.

EDUCATION   Medical Assisting, Associate Degree
Advanced Medical College, Atlanta, GA

Alternatively, you can center your headings and list the information beneath and flush left:

PROFILE
Obtain an entry-level medical assistant position to provide attentive, highly professional assistance to patients and physicians.

EDUCATION
Medical Assisting, Associate Degree
Advanced Medical College, Atlanta, GA

The design should be based primarily on whether you need to use or save space on the page. However, you choose to lay out your resume, strive for a balanced, attractive look. See Box 11.5 for examples of various ways to use capitalization and boldface.

Step Nine: Create an Attractive and Professional-Looking Document

Selecting and organizing content can take considerable time and effort, but a poorly laid out resume can belie that effort and give the impression that the applicant does not care about the position. To avoid having your resume tossed aside without even a review, make sure you give due consideration to the overall layout and appearance of your resume.

Your goal should be to create an attractive, easy-to-follow, and organized resume with wording that makes a good first impression concerning your skills, experience, and education. The following tips will help you achieve a professional look:

* Leave enough white space so the page does not look crowded. Double-space between the sections.
* Limit your resume to one page, unless you have 7–10 years of work experience or more. If you do have more than one page, include page numbers on all pages.
* Capitalize headings.
* Use bullets to set off listed items.

BOX 11.5

Using Special Elements

WORK HISTORY	Medical Transcriptionist, 2021–Present
	Hopeful Medical Center, Better Health, NJ
OR	MEDICAL TRANSCRIPTIONIST 2021–Present
	Hopeful Medical Center Better Health, NJ
OR	**Medical Transcriptionist** 2021–Present
	Hopeful Medical Center Better Health, NJ
OR	**Medical Transcriptionist** (2021–Present)
	Hopeful Medical Center, Better Health, NJ

* Try using boldface for emphasis.
* Make sure your spelling and grammar are perfect.
* Leave a 1-inch margin on all sides. If you need more space, you can decrease the top and bottom margins, but it is best to leave the side margins at 1 inch for a well-balanced layout.
* When printing, use good-quality paper in white, ivory, or very light tan or gray.
* Make sure the print is dark and clear.

See Box 11.6 for a resume checklist to ensure you have a comprehensive and quality resume that represents you well.

Step Ten: Use "Power" and Influential Words

It is important to use "power" words in your resume and cover letter when applying for positions. Power words are used to strengthen and highlight duties you have performed in your current or past jobs, as well as your qualifications, skills, or training. Most resumes are fairly standard and often use the same phrases and wording. In fact, many hiring managers tend to quickly skim through resumes and cover letters, especially if there is a high volume of applicants. Using power words effectively will bring positive attention to your resume and cover letter and set you apart from the competition.

Additionally, these power words are often keywords in a company's applicant tracking system (ATS) software. ATS software quickly scans resumes and applications to identify top candidates based on the percentage of keywords that have been identified by the system. Thus, a resume may be eliminated based on not using keywords or not using enough keywords. Keywords usually fall into three categories: skill words, results-oriented words, and achievement words. Examples of keywords for each category are shown in Box 11.7.

Electronic Resumes

Since you are actively seeking new employment, it may be necessary to update your resume. An easy way to make updates and changes is with an electronic resume or e-resume.

Your resume should always reflect your most recent, relevant and valuable skills, experiences, and qualities. Before you apply for new jobs, it is important to review your resume for outdated information and to update each section as necessary. You will need to modify your resume if you are sending it to an employer electronically, if it will be scanned by an ATS, or if you are posting it on an Internet site. This is to ensure that it transmits and scans properly. You will note that some changes require you to do exactly the opposite of the directions given in the previous sections to create an attractive printed resume. It is important to have and keep track of multiple versions of your resume and cover letter.

For a resume to copy and paste into online forms or to post in online resume databases, start by ensuring that your resume is in a readable format. Most online applications can read and convert MS Word or PDF format. Some online applications may require you to convert your resume to a "plain text." If you created your resume using MS Word (on either a PC or a Mac), use the "Save As" command and choose the plain-text format (the ending will be .txt). This format strips your document of all special formatting—things like bullets, bolding, and italics. The instructions embedded to create these formatting options may not

---

BOX 11.6

Resume Checklist

_____ Dates and numbers are complete and accurate
_____ Your phone number(s) and email address are included
_____ The objective is clear
_____ Content supports statements in your cover letter
_____ Content is organized in order of importance
_____ All relevant qualifications are included
_____ Information is not repeated
_____ Spelling is perfect
_____ Grammar is correct
_____ Layout is consistent
_____ The page is attractively laid out and easy to read

BOX 11.7

Categories of Keyword in Resumes

Skill	Results-Oriented	Achievement
Wrote	Increased	Honored
Analyzed	Reduced	Awarded
Quantified	Redesigned	Promoted
Planned	Implemented	Selected
Programmed	Generated	Received a bonus for
Designed	Produced	Recognized
Created	Upgraded	Chosen
Trained	Initiated	Credited

translate well electronically, and your resume can become scrambled or interspersed with odd-looking characters.

Once you have uploaded your resume electronically, perform the following steps:

1. Proofread it for oddly wrapped lines, scrunched-up words, and similar problems that can happen when text is converted.
2. Delete "continued" or "page 2" if these exist.
3. Use caps to emphasize words that otherwise would have been bolded or italicized—your name, for example.
4. Replace bullets with standard keyboard symbols such as * + − ~. (These may have converted to little boxes or other odd characters.)
5. If you need to add spaces, use the space bar, not the Tab key.
6. If you use quotation marks anywhere, these only convert if they are straight, not curly (also called smart). Check your word-processing program to see how to do this.

Just as with the original version of your resume, it is critical that this version be free from errors or irregular formatting. Once sent or posted online, it is there potentially for millions of people to view.

You may also wish to avoid making two different versions of your resume by selecting an ATS-friendly format for your resume. There are many downloadable resume templates available online. However, as plain-text documents and ATS-friendly formats tend to look quite plain, many people prefer two different versions to enable them to use a more attractive layout with more sophisticated formatting than a plain-text format allows.

Introducing Your Resume: Cover Letters

- State the purpose of a cover letter.
- Describe the contents of a cover letter.
- Explain why the cover letter should be customized to a specific employment position.
- List the differences between cover letters for advertised and unadvertised positions.
- Describe the purpose and contents of a letter of inquiry.

The purpose of a cover letter is to provide a brief personal introduction and to highlight your interest, skills, and qualifications for the job. It should be concise, informative, persuasive, and polite. It should demonstrate why and how you meet this employer's qualifications for the position. Whenever possible, send a cover letter with your resume, whether it goes by conventional mail or electronically, as some recruiters and hiring managers may not look at resumes that are not accompanied by a cover letter.

Cover letters should be customized to the position being applied for, but these are guidelines common to all types of cover letters:

1. Use a proper business letter format.
2. Be sure your spelling and grammar are error-free.
3. Address your letter to a specific person whenever possible. Look for a name in the employment ad, ask your contact for the name of the appropriate person, or contact the facility and ask. If you are writing in response to an unadvertised position, having a name on your correspondence is especially important. Letters without names can get misdirected or discarded. Busy facilities do not have time to determine to whom to direct your inquiry. If you cannot locate a name, it is preferable to address your letter to "Hiring Manager" or "Human Resources Manager" rather than "Dear Sir or Madam."
4. Write an introduction. State who you are, why you are writing, who referred you or what ad you are responding to, and what position you are applying for. Employers may have more than one position open so do not assume they will know which job you are applying for.
5. Develop the body of the letter. Explain why you are interested in the position and why the employer should interview you, that is, what you have to offer and how you can benefit the organization. Summarize your qualifications for the job. Do your best to match them with what you believe the employer is seeking. At the same time, do not simply repeat the information that is on your resume or cut and paste the job description. Your cover letter should offer the recruiter or potential employer greater insight into your unique skills and experience and how the position fits into your career goals.
6. Include a closing paragraph. Offer to provide any additional information that would be helpful and conclude with a statement of your interest in the position or a date you will follow up on your application. For instance, you might state that you would appreciate the opportunity to meet with them to discuss how you could add value to their organization.

7. If you are sending your cover letter electronically or having to copy it into an online application, keep the format simple. Some formatting may not transfer. Avoid using bold font, bullets, or other special features and use spaces instead of tabs to indent text.

Letter for an Advertised Position

When you respond to employment ads or job postings, your cover letter should clearly convey how you meet the employer's needs. Use language in your letter that mirrors the words used in the ad or job announcement (Figures 11.8 and 11.9). This is especially important when submitting your application through an online system, as your entire application may be scanned through an ATS that searches for keywords.

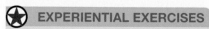
Letter for an Unadvertised Opening

You may learn about unadvertised job openings through your school or from your networking contacts. Before writing the letter, learn as much as possible about the job and the company. Sources of information include the person who told you about the opening, the employer's website, or even a general Internet search. Mention your source of information in the introduction of your cover letter. Be sure to obtain permission from the contact person before using their name.

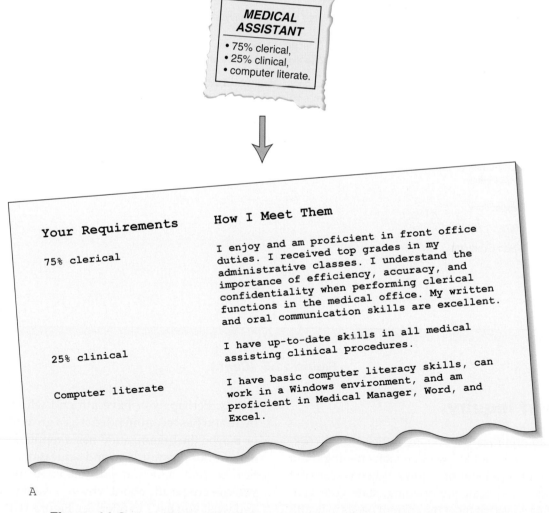

MEDICAL ASSISTANT

- 75% clerical,
- 25% clinical,
- computer literate.

Your Requirements	How I Meet Them
75% clerical	I enjoy and am proficient in front office duties. I received top grades in my administrative classes. I understand the importance of efficiency, accuracy, and confidentiality when performing clerical functions in the medical office. My written and oral communication skills are excellent.
25% clinical	I have up-to-date skills in all medical assisting clinical procedures.
Computer literate	I have basic computer literacy skills, can work in a Windows environment, and am proficient in Medical Manager, Word, and Excel.

A

Figure 11.8 A and **B**, Example of a Direct, Point-by-Point Response to a Job Posting.

1234 Graduate Lane
Collegeville, CA 90123
June 6, 2010

Samantha Ernest, Office Manager
Good Health Clinic
922 Wellness Avenue
Cassidy, CA 91222

Dear Ms. Ernest:

I was excited to see your ad in the Cassidy Times on June 5 for a medical assistant. As a recent graduate of Medical Career College, I believe I can make a positive contribution to your health care team. In addition to submitting my resume for your review, I would like to point out how I believe I meet your needs for this position.

Your requirements:	How I Meet Them:
75% clerical duties	I enjoy and am proficient in front office duties. I received top grades in all my administrative classes. I understand the importance of efficiency, accuracy, and confidentiality when performing clerical functions in the medical office. I have very good written and oral communication skills.
25% clinical duties	I have up-to-date skills in all medical assisting back-office procedures.
Computer literate	I have basic computer literacy skills, can work in a Windows environment, and am proficient in Medical Manager, Word, and Excel.

I am an energetic, detail-oriented person with good interpersonal skills. I understand the need to maintain high-quality patient relations in today's health care environment and know I am capable of providing efficient, caring service.

Good Health Clinic has an excellent reputation in Cassidy and it would be a privilege to have the opportunity to discuss my qualifications with you in person. I will call next week to schedule an appointment or you can contact me at (760)123-4567. Thank you for your time and consideration.

Respectfully,

Gwen Graduate

Gwen Graduate

B

Figure 11.8 (Cont.)

Letter of Inquiry

If there is an organization you are interested in working for, but you do not know of any job openings, you could try sending a letter of inquiry. When you are not responding to a specific job opening, state your general qualifications that meet the current needs in health care. Explain why you are interested in working at the facility. Perhaps you have a friend who is employed there and has recommended it as a great place to work or maybe the organization has a reputation for excellent working conditions and educational opportunities. Learn as much as possible about the facility so you can be specific about why you want to work there and what you have to offer. See Figure 11.10 for a sample letter of inquiry.

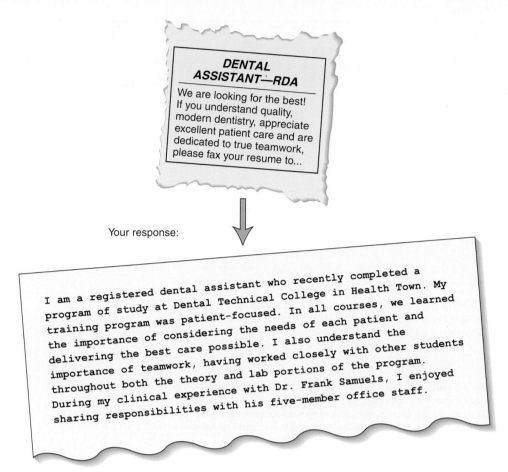

DENTAL ASSISTANT—RDA

We are looking for the best! If you understand quality, modern dentistry, appreciate excellent patient care and are dedicated to true teamwork, please fax your resume to...

Your response:

I am a registered dental assistant who recently completed a program of study at Dental Technical College in Health Town. My training program was patient-focused. In all courses, we learned the importance of considering the needs of each patient and delivering the best care possible. I also understand the importance of teamwork, having worked closely with other students throughout both the theory and lab portions of the program. During my clinical experience with Dr. Frank Samuels, I enjoyed sharing responsibilities with his five-member office staff.

Figure 11.9 Example of a Paragraph That Addresses the Employer's Stated Needs.

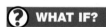 **WHAT IF?**

You want to write cover letters but feel unsure about your grammar and spelling.

Job Applications

LEARNING OBJECTIVE 4: JOB APPLICATIONS

- Explain the purpose of job applications.
- List ways to ensure that you accurately complete job applications.

If you're offered a seat on a rocket ship, don't ask what seat! Just get on.

—Sheryl Sandberg

Most employers require applicants to fill out an online electronic application, even if they have already uploaded a resume. Job applications provide the employer with complete, standardized sources of information. Once you are hired, the completed application is placed in your personnel file and can serve as a legal document and record of information about you and your previous employment.

Read all statements carefully before signing. Applications may contain legal language and unfamiliar words. Do not hesitate to ask for an explanation of anything you do not understand or are unsure about.

Some applications contain important statements you are required to read and sign. For example, employers of home health care workers may protect themselves from liability if employees have an accident when they are driving to and from job assignments. Additionally, most employers have questions on demographic information used to monitor and ensure equal employment opportunity enforcement required by federal and state law. These demographic questions will include your sex, ethnicity and race, disability status, veteran status, and age. Answering these questions is voluntary, and responses will not be shown to the potential employer.

10752 Learning Lane
Silver Stream, NY 10559
July 22, 2010

Ms. Sandra Walters, Manager
Caring Clinic
7992 Oates Road
Greenville, NY 10772

Dear Ms. Walters:

I am writing to inquire about job openings at Caring Clinic. My husband and I are relocating to Greenville in September and I am looking for a position in which I can apply my up-to-date skills as a phlebotomy technician. Caring Clinic has a reputation for excellent service to the health needs of the Greenville community and I would be proud to be a contributing member of your team.

As a recent graduate of Top Skill Institute, I had the opportunity to perform my internship at Goodwell Laboratory Services, an affiliate of Caring Clinic. I understand the importance of combining technical excellence with attention to customer service. While at Goodwell, my technical skills were highly praised by my supervisor, Mr. Jaime Gutierrez. In addition, I consistently received top ratings on patient satisfaction surveys.

My resume is enclosed for your review. I will call you in early September to see if I can set an appointment to meet with you. Thank you for your consideration.

Respectfully,

Carla Martinez
Carla Martinez

Figure 11.10 Example of a Cover Letter of Inquiry.

After the work of creating a resume and cover letter, filling out an application may seem easy. But do not take it for granted. Take time to read the instructions and fill out the application as accurately and meticulously as possible. This is especially important when applying for health care positions because accuracy and being detail-oriented are job requirements. Use this opportunity to demonstrate that you meet these requirements.

Tips for Filling Out Job Applications

Some important tips when completing an application, regardless of the format:
* Read the entire application before you begin to fill it in.
* Fill out all sections completely. Do not leave blanks or write "See resume."

* If it is a paper application, use a black or blue pen, never pencil, and print neatly.
* Proofread what you have written before submitting your application.
* Be honest and accurate when answering questions. Giving false information can be grounds for dismissal if you are hired.
* For questions that do not apply to you, write "N/A" instead of leaving them blank. This way you make it clear that you saw the question and did not accidentally skip over it.
* Many entry-level jobs have a set salary or a salary range. If the job you are applying for does not indicate a salary range, it is best to write "negotiable" in the space asking about salary requirements.
* Be sure to sign and date the application.
* Go to interviews prepared with the completed application, several copies of your resume, and a reference sheet in case they ask you for it.

Electronic Applications

It is very likely that most of your job applications will be done online, which are forms often completed on the company's website. When applying electronically or online, you will need to create an account on the company's or job board's website. Keep a record of the online applications you send, including your username, which is usually your email address; password; and the specific information you have sent, such as the job requisition number.

When applying online, it is especially important to follow the directions and check your entries carefully before pushing the "send" button. Once you submit your online application, you may not be able to make any corrections later. As with traditional written materials, what you submit reflects you as a professional. In fact, some employers use electronic applications to test the computer skills of potential employees. Print your completed application and place it in your job search binder or files.

Distributing Your Resume

> **LEARNING OBJECTIVE 5: DISTRIBUTING YOUR RESUME**

■ Target where you would like to work or who you would like to work with.

■ List the employers and places where you might distribute your resume.

Targeting Your Job Search

Before you begin posting and passing out your resume, consider where and for whom you would like to work. For example, if you want to avoid a long commute, only apply to companies close to where you live. You may want to drive within a certain distance of where you live and make note of the different medical offices, pharmacies, hospitals, and other health care organizations.

Target your job search and application to those employers around you first. Applying to a job that turns out to be too far away is wasting both your time and the hiring manager's time. Keep in mind that if you have only a few health care employers located around you or you have yet to find a job, you may need to expand your search and go farther away from where you live.

In addition to geography, consider the kind of practice, specialty, and workplace setting you may want to work in. Some students may know right away or while they are in school that they want to work with infants, in orthopedic surgery, or in a compounding pharmacy. Some students may also realize they work better in a smaller medical office rather than a high-volume, multispecialty clinic. Focus your job efforts on these kinds of clinics and organizations. However, it is important to remember that more specialized clinics may require more experience; thus, be flexible and open-minded to getting more experience at a general or primary care position first.

Distributing Your Resume

If opportunity doesn't knock, build a door.

—Milton Berle

Make the best use of your resume by distributing it to employers who have or may have job openings and people who might know about available jobs in your field. Here are some suggestions of places to target your search:
* Employers who post job openings on the Internet or elsewhere
* Employers who have unadvertised openings you have heard about from other sources
* Your networking contacts
* Friends and relatives

* Anyone who indicates that they know someone who might be hiring
* Your school's career services department

Although online applications are more common, keep enough copies of your resume on hand to respond to unexpected opportunities. Take copies to interviews (even if you have sent an electronic copy in advance), career fairs, and the Human Resources departments of health care facilities. Have plenty on hand if you decide to drop in on employers.

Networking may be one of your greatest tools when job searching. A large majority of jobs are not advertised, and many people get hired through referrals from friends and acquaintances. Reach out to former classmates and family members who may be able to support your application.

Posting Your Resume on the Internet

There are many types of websites where you can post your resume. Some are general employment sites, such as Monster.com, Indeed.com, or Simplyhired.com, whereas others are specific to health care. All these online employment websites will allow or even require you to apply electronically for specific job openings.

Deciding whether to place your resume on the Internet and which type of website to choose depends on your job target and the kind of employer you are seeking. Although many websites allow job searchers to post their resumes for free, they charge employers to place job ads online and to view the resumes in their databases. Therefore, larger organizations are the ones most likely to pay for this service. A small medical office may not be able to justify the expense for its relatively small staff and its number of hires. In addition to using employment sites, large health care systems and organizations with many employees, such as Kaiser Permanente, often have their own websites and online application capabilities.

Although posting on a large website makes your resume available to millions of viewers, you are also competing with potentially hundreds or even thousands of other job seekers. Experts suggest that posting your resume on a few carefully chosen sites may be more worthwhile.

In general, experts recommend that you should not pay a fee to have your resume distributed. Many of these "services" may indiscriminately send out mass emails containing the resumes of everyone who pays them, regardless of whether they match the jobs posted.

The following suggestions can help you choose an appropriate website:
* Do not use websites that will not allow you to review at least a sample of their job lists before you provide personal information or your resume.
* Read the privacy policy. Some websites sell or give your information to other businesses. Never put your social security number on your resume.
* Check the wording. Do the lists provided include real jobs or are they examples of what the website claims to be trying to fill?
* Verify the timeliness of postings. Are there dates on the jobs listed? Are they recent?
* Look for information about who sponsors the site. Do they have credentials and/or experience in the job search industry?
* If you do not get any responses to your resume within 45 days, remove it. If the job posting is still there, refresh your resume and cover letter and upload them again.

As a courtesy to those who are looking for applicants, remove your posted resume once you become employed. Also, your new employer may see your resume online and wonder if you are looking for another position.

(?) WHAT IF?

You feel shy about handing out your resume. You do not want to "bother" people with it or want to seem too pushy.

References

LEARNING OBJECTIVE 6: REFERENCES

- Give examples of credible references.
- List the characteristics of good references.
- List examples of people who might be good references.
- List the information that should be included on a reference sheet.

Recall that references are people who will vouch for your qualifications and character. Good references can be a key factor in tipping the hiring scales in your favor. Give careful consideration about who you ask to serve as a reference for you. They must be considered credible and must be able to speak to your professional and sometimes personal qualifications. Personal friends and relatives are not generally good choices for work references, but they may be acceptable if you are asked to provide character references.

In addition to being credible, references must:

* Be available and willing to speak on your behalf to potential employers,
* Be able to speak positively about you, and
* Be able to communicate clearly and in an organized way.

The following people are good candidates for work references:

* Instructors
* Program director or supervisor
* Other school personnel
* Externship supervisor(s)
* Current or previous employers
* Supervisors at places where you have done volunteer work
* Professionals who you have worked with on teams or projects

It is recommended to get a variety of references, including instructors and past and current employers. If you have worked at a job for a long time and are a good employee, your current employer may be a good option as a reference even though it may not be in health care.

Contact each person you want to serve as a reference. Do this before you begin your job search. You should always ask for permission before giving out their name and contact information. This can create an awkward situation with your references if they are contacted without their knowledge. Further, the person may not be comfortable serving as your reference. If they agree to be listed as your reference, inform them about the types of jobs you are applying for and what qualifications are important. It is a good idea to provide them with a copy of your resume. This will enable them to be better prepared to answer the potential employer's questions.

Reference Sheet

Create a document listing at least three to five references. Include their names, titles, organization, telephone numbers, and email addresses. You may also want to include their work addresses. It is essential that the telephone numbers be current and accurate. If you list a work number and the person is no longer employed there, this may delay your application process and may suggest that you did not update your reference sheet. Potential employers may not have time to call you back or make numerous calls trying to locate your references, and they may move on to the next candidate. Making it easy for potential employers to contact your references makes it easier for them to hire you.

Organize your reference list in an easy-to-read format and print it on the same kind of paper as your resume. Write "References for [your name]" at the top of the page. The reference sheet should not be mailed with your resume unless it is specifically requested by the employer. If you are asked to interview, take copies with you to the interview to give to potential employers who ask for it. Figure 11.11 shows an example of a reference sheet.

Once you are hired, let your references know. Thank them for their willingness to assist you. Keep them posted on your career progress. You may need to use them again in case you apply for another position at another company.

> ⭐ **EXPERIENTIAL EXERCISES**
>
> 1. Contact at least five people who may serve as good references.
> 2. Once you have their approval, gather the data you need about each person.
> 3. Create your reference sheet.

Letters of Recommendation

> **LEARNING OBJECTIVE 7:**
> **LETTERS OF RECOMMENDATION**

* Explain who should write your letters of recommendation.
* Describe the proper etiquette when asking for letters of recommendation.

Another type of reference is provided through letters of recommendation, sometimes called letters of reference or reference letters. These letters are usually written by supervisors or people in authority, such as instructors, a program director, or an employer, who can attest to your academic or work record, skills, and personal qualities. It is a good idea to request reference letters from employers throughout your career because they can serve as a record of endorsements and achievements over the years. As you leave each job, assuming it was on good terms, ask for a letter of recommendation from your supervisor. Although there is no standard, it is a good idea to keep letters of recommendation current. It is recommended that letters of recommendation be written within 5 years. The most important thing is that you are still in contact and are on good terms with your references.

Make copies of your letters of recommendation to place in your job application files and/or to give to potential employers who request them. It is appropriate at interviews to mention that you have them available.

As with references, ask only those people who you believe can write a positive letter. Also, give potential recommenders adequate notice to compose a strong letter. Finally, let your references know what kind of job you are seeking and what qualities potential employers look for in candidates, so they can phrase their letters appropriately.

Maria Bell, CMA
Email: maria.d.bell@gmail.com
Tel: 555-100-7838

References:

Mark Silverman
Clinical Instructor
Advanced Medical College
Nashville, TN
Tel: 555-333-3344

Carol Coleson
Externship Clinical Coordinator
Advanced Medical College
Nashville, TN
Tel: 255-712-8242

Adrian Whitman, MD
Externship Site
Madison Family Medicine Clinic
Nashville, TN
Tel: 555-205-0402

Figure 11.11 Example of a Reference Letter.

CASE STUDY 11.1
Fish out of Water

Cameron was getting increasingly nervous. He had almost completed his pharmacy technician program and was getting prepared for his externship. As he told his friend, Juan, "School has been okay, but going out after a job—I don't know. It's getting pretty nerve-racking."

Juan tried to reassure him. "You did okay in school. And you liked your classes, right?"

"Yeah," Cameron said. "My pharmacy tech classes are pretty interesting. But after working all those years in masonry, I feel like a fish out of water going in and asking for a job. And now I have to put together a resume for my job search class. I've been putting that off, too. What experience do I have that any employer would want? That I built walls and know how to nail things together for 20 years?"

"That does sound like a challenge. I guess I'm lucky I chose a field I have some experience in," said Juan.

The next day in class, the instructor, Mr. Harmond, asked the students how they were doing on their resumes. "Don't forget," he reminded them. "These are due next week so Ms. Garcia and I can look them over and give you feedback."

Cameron spent the next few days worrying about this assignment. He just did not know how he was going to fill a page when all he had done was graduate from high school, work for 20 years for Cedar Glen Tile and Masonry, and finish a pharmacy technician program. He feared employers would think he did not have much to show for a 40-year-old man.

He finally sat down on Sunday night and put something together. It was not much, but he knew he had to have something to turn in on Monday. After class on Tuesday, Mr. Harmond asked Cameron to wait so they could talk.

"Cameron," said Mr. Harmond, "I reviewed your resume last night and was surprised at how short it was. Did you spend a lot of time on it?"

"Actually," Cameron replied, "I've put *days* of thought into it. Thought and worry. I just couldn't come up with anything."

"That really surprises me," said Mr. Harmond. "From what I know about your experience, you have a lot of experience, and I think you have a lot to offer an employer."

Cameron shook his head and said, "I don't think so, Mr. Harmond, at least not in health care. I've just worked in construction most of my life, mostly in masonry."

"Well, all that counts. Your long work history is important. You're dependable, never late for class, articulate, always ready to help a classmate. Didn't you work for the same employer all that time and move up into a supervisory position?

"Well, yes," said Cameron. "But I don't really understand what all that has to do with applying for a job as a pharmacy tech."

"It has everything to do with it." Mr. Harmond went on to explain how employers were looking for employees with more than just technical skills. "Think about it," he said to Cameron. "You didn't move up with Cedar Glen just because you had good technical skills. You also had good people skills, you were dependable, and you demonstrated strong leadership capabilities. These are all valuable skills. They're examples of the transferable skills we talked about in class."

"I never thought about my masonry and construction experience like that," admitted Cameron.

"Well, let's do this," suggested Mr. Cameron. "Come by my office tomorrow after class, and I'll help you come up with specific transferable skills you can put on your resume. Maybe we'll put together some categories that will supplement your job history section. We can also mention your achievements at Cedar Glen. They may have been in a completely different field, but they show motivation and a good work ethic—all employers want to see those in their employees."

"I'll be there," said Cameron. "Thanks a lot, Mr. Harmond. I really appreciate the extra help."

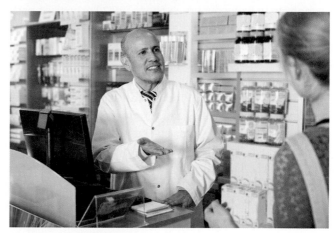
iStock.com/JackF/588595832

QUESTIONS FOR THOUGHT AND CONSIDERATION

1. What was Cameron's challenge in seeing how his past work experience may translate to his current job search as a pharmacy technician?
2. What other skills and characteristics might Cameron have to offer other than those mentioned?
3. Consider your own experience. Identify a job you had that is unrelated to what you are currently studying but may highlight your skill, training, leadership skill, or work ethic.

A Different Path

Steve Bailey is another student in Mr. Harmond's class. He also enrolled in the pharmacy technician program from another occupation—he was a drywaller. Although he did not like his previous occupation and was unable to continue due to the physical demands of the job, Steve did not like the idea of a career where he would have to sit all day or be cooped up in an office, so being a pharmacy tech seemed

like a good compromise. He could stand, walk around, and be in an area that was not too closed in. However, he struggled with some of his courses, especially those that involved math. He got tutoring, passed his classes, and is now near graduation.

Like Cameron, he is struggling with his resume. His spelling and grammar have never been very good, and, although he can use computers for data entry and other simple tasks related to being a pharmacy tech, his word-processing skills are weak. He thinks the school's career services department should be able to take his information and put it together into a resume for him.

"After all," he tells his friend James, "they're the experts. Why should I be tearing out what little hair I have left trying to figure out how to do this?"

"Didn't they give you any help in class?" asks James.

"Some, I guess," replied Steve. "But it seemed complicated. There's this kind of resume and that kind. How am I supposed to figure out which one to use? I'm working part-time. I don't have time to go to class, do my homework, and find a job on top of that. It's too much to do. I have an assignment due on Monday to write a resume. I'm going to ask career services to write one for me."

During their meeting, the career services department informed Steve that they do not create resumes for students, but they provide assistance with all aspects of the career search, including resume writing. They offered to set up an appointment with him to guide him through the process of creating his resume. Steve told them he did not have time to come in for an appointment and decided he just would not turn anything in on Monday. He had passed the technical courses in his program, so he thought it would not matter if he did not have a resume put together on time.

At the class break on Tuesday morning, Mr. Harmond approached him.

"Steve, I noticed that you didn't turn in a draft of your resume," he said.

"Yeah, I just didn't have time, and it's just not something I'm good at. I really think career services should help me out. I'll give you the information about me—lots of it you already have from my school application—and you can put it together. You must have some special software on the computers you have in your office."

Mr. Harmond replied, "Steve, we're here to help you by advising you and giving you the tools you need. But as part of this program and to be prepared as a future professional, you will need to learn how to create a resume. It's a skill that you will most likely need for your entire career in whatever you decide to do. You can set up an appointment, and we will walk you through it, step by step, just like you've been learning in this class."

"I don't know," muttered Steve. "I don't think I have time for that. Maybe I'll find something online and I can get a friend to help me fill it in."

QUESTIONS FOR THOUGHT AND CONSIDERATION

1. Why do you think Steve is so resistant to working on his resume?
2. How do you think his attitude will affect his prospects of getting a job?
3. What do you think about Mr. Harmond's comments to Steve? How else would you advise Steve?
4. Is there anything that Mr. Harmond or the career services department can do to help Steve?

References

Dickel MR. *Guide to Internet job searching 2004-2005*. Columbus, OH: McGraw-Hill; 2004.

Ellis D, Lankowitz S, Stupka E, Toft D. *Career planning*. ed 2. New York, NY: Houghton Mifflin; 1997.

Ireland S. *Susan Ireland's Resume SiteI*. susanireland.com.

The Interview Process

- Effectively Answer Interview Questions
- Demonstrate Behaviors That Create a Positive First Impression
- Communicate Professionally and Effectively During and After the Interview
- Deal Appropriately With Difficult Situations During an Interview
- Develop Criteria for Determining Whether to Accept a Job Offer
- Calculate the Total Value of a Compensation Package
- Know How To Properly Accept or Decline Job Offers
- Describe How to Deal With and Learn From Not Being Offered a Job

Preparing for the Interview

LEARNING OBJECTIVE 1: INTERVIEWING TO MARKET YOURSELF

- Discuss a positive approach to interviewing for jobs.
- Understand the importance of preparing for job interviews.
- Give an example of each type of interview questions.
- Understand how to use the STAR approach when answering behavioral questions.
- Getting organized before the interview.
- List the items the applicant should take to a job interview.
- Explain the importance of first impressions.

In the previous chapter, we learned about the beginning of the job search process, including getting the most out of your training and education, identifying your skills, locating health care jobs, networking, learning how to write an effective resume and cover letter, and securing professional references. The purpose of this chapter is to guide you through the next important step in the job search process: the interview. We will cover all aspects of a successful interview to secure a job—from preparation for and fielding questions during the interview to negotiating and accepting or declining a job offer.

If you received an offer to interview for a job, congratulations! That means that your resume, cover letter, and job application were effective in describing that you are qualified for the position you applied for. Now that you have gotten your foot in the door, the next step is the interview process, which will be one of the most critical steps to landing the job.

Receiving an invitation for an interview can be both exciting and nerve-racking. Your job search efforts are beginning to pay off, but there remains a good deal of work to do before securing a job offer. Obtaining an interview means you meet the minimum qualifications for the position, but the interviewer will want to see whether you can communicate well and learn more about how your experience and skills could contribute to the organization.

The interview often represents a source of anxiety for many candidates, who worry about saying the right thing during the interview and whether they have the skills employers are looking for. However, with adequate preparation, the interviewing process can offer an excellent opportunity to market your skills to potential employers and show them how you can meet their needs. By learning what will be expected of you at an interview and practicing your presentation skills, you can interview with confidence.

Understanding the Employer's Needs

You don't have to be perfect. Just be the best for the job.
—Rick Baird

A common reason for not being hired is lack of preparation for the interview. In addition to practicing by talking about your skills and experience and being ready to answer common interview questions, your interview preparation should include learning about the company and the employer's needs. To ensure a successful interview, complete the following in advance:

* Identify possible needs of the employer. The job posting is a good place to start, but you can also search for the job title to find common tasks and responsibilities in that profession.
* Think of ways you might meet those needs as an employee. If you do not have direct experience in that field, focus on your transferable skills and your education and training.
* Anticipate what types of questions might be asked and practice answering them. There will be several sets of practice questions in the next section.
* Create examples to demonstrate your qualifications. For instance, if the job you are applying for requires you to supervise the work of others, think of examples of when you took a leadership role. Try to focus on the results of your work, rather than the tasks you completed.
* Prepare appropriate questions to ask the interviewers. Avoid asking obvious questions that can be

answered by looking at the company's website. In the initial interview, it is not recommended to ask about compensation during the interview because it may give the interviewer the sense that you may be more focused on making money, which is certainly a reality, than learning about the position. Learning when to discuss compensation and how to negotiate will be discussed later in this chapter.

Individual employers have specific requirements based on factors, such as patient population, services offered, size of the facility, and budgets. Learn as much as possible before attending the interview. Here is a list of information sources:

* Direct contact by phone or in person: ask questions, request a job description, observe the facility
* Brochures produced by the organization
* People who work there, such as friends, classmates, or networking contacts
* The local newspaper: large facilities are sometimes the subject of news articles
* The employer's website
* Your school's career services department
* The local chamber of commerce and other organizations that have information about large employers
* The local chapter of your professional organization
* Information gathered at career fairs and employer orientation meetings
* Job posting if the position was advertised

At a minimum, you should try to learn how many health care providers are in the facility, who they are, the type of specialty that is practiced, and the patient population served. If you are unable to learn very much about the employer before the interview, it is especially important that you listen carefully to the interviewer and ask good questions. Understanding the needs and concerns of the interviewer helps an applicant navigate the interview process (Figure 12.1).

⭐ EXPERIENTIAL EXERCISES

1. Select a health care facility where you might want to work.
2. Learn as much as possible about the facility: type of work they do, patient or client population, size of the staff, jobs for which you might qualify, mission of the organization.

Knowing What to Expect

Some interviews are highly structured, meaning that each candidate is asked the same set of prepared questions. Others are more conversational, with topics and questions generated freely and based on the direction

At the Interview:
How to Show You've Got What It Takes

Employers want to hire someone who is:	How to show that you are that someone:
Qualified to perform the job	1. Be familiar with and able to document all your skills 2. Create a portfolio that contains evidence of your qualifications
Reliable	1. Arrive on time to the interview 2. Send any requested follow-up materials
Trustworthy	1. Have a good handshake 2. Maintain appropriate eye contact 3. Include only accurate information on your resume and job application 4. Do not lie during your interview 5. Avoid saying anything negative about a previous employer 6. Do not engage in any type of gossip
Professional	1. Dress appropriately 2. Be clean and well groomed 3. Bring needed materials to interview
Motivated and willing to learn	1. Know something about the facility and why you want to work there 2. Ask questions about the job 3. Inquire about learning opportunities on the job 4. Have a plan for professional development
A good communicator and able to work well with others	1. Show consideration for everyone at the interview site 2. Introduce yourself 3. Behave courteously 4. Listen actively throughout the interview 5. Use feedback appropriately to check your understanding of the speaker's message 6. Answer all questions completely but concisely 7. Speak clearly and with proper expression
Likable	1. Smile 2. Be enthusiastic 3. Have a sense of humor 4. Show interest in job 5. Express interest in employer's needs 6. Be comfortable with yourself 7. Show respect for interviewer 8. Avoid showing impatience, annoyance
A problem-solver	1. Describe examples of problems solved in the past 2. Be prepared and willing to participate in any problem-solving exercises given 3. Suggest specific ways you can help the employer

Figure 12.1 Understanding the needs and concerns of the interviewer helps an applicant navigate the interview process. (Copyright © istock.com.)

of the conversation. Most interviews fall somewhere between these patterns, with interviewers preparing at least a few questions in advance and asking follow-up questions based on candidates' answers. The style of the interview and types of questions most likely depend on the size of the organization and the preference of the hiring manager.

Large health care systems, hospitals, and clinics usually have dedicated personnel to conduct initial interviews. As human resource professionals, they

have the time and expertise to study the latest hiring practices and develop their interviewing skills. A physician who has a single practice is more likely to focus on what skills you have acquired through your education and experience—the specific skills they need, for example, in a clinical medical assistant or receptionist. Regardless of who is interviewing you and the type of interview, you need to be prepared.

There are different types of interview questions: traditional, behavioral, and situational. These questions will focus on different areas of your qualifications and will evaluate how you respond.

Traditional Interview Questions

There are many standard questions that interviewers use. Here are a few common examples:

1. Could you tell us a little about yourself?
2. What are your long-range career objectives? Or, where do you see yourself in 5 years?
3. Why did you choose this career? Or, why do you want this job?
4. Why did you leave your last position? Or, why did you change career paths?
5. Can you explain this gap in your resume?
6. How well do you work on a team? Individually?
7. What type of work environment do you prefer?
8. What do you consider your greatest strengths?
9. What do you think are your weaknesses?
10. Tell me about a time you faced a challenge at work and how you dealt with it.
11. What makes you qualified for this position? Or, why should I hire you?
12. Do you have any questions for us?

You can see that these questions are very open-ended. As you can answer them in many ways, it is important to make sure your answers are clear, specific, and relate to the job you are interviewing for. Employers want to know how your answer applies to *them*; they do not want canned responses. For example, in explaining why you chose a career in health care, focus on the aspects that connect to the position for which you are being considered. You would not want to talk about how you prefer to work alone or independently if you are interviewing for a job that requires you to work in a team setting.

Further, be specific in your answers. Saying, "I've always been a people person" does not give the interviewer much insight into your interests or how you approach challenges. Instead, you might say, "I've been interested in health care since I was 11, when I spent time playing chess with my grandfather after he had a stroke. I noticed how he really perked up when he played, and I became fascinated by how the brain works better when stimulated by an enjoyable activity. This led me to exploring a career in occupational therapy. I really enjoy interacting with people in my work, and helping patients regain or develop their skills is so rewarding." This more specific answer gives the interviewer more insight into who you are and why you are applying for the position.

When answering "Why should I hire you?," mention specific skills and professional qualities that will make a positive contribution to the health care organization, department's success, patient satisfaction, and so on. Also, remember that "soft skills," such as communication and time management, are often strong assets to the organization. When explaining what your unique qualifications are, be sure to connect them to the job requirements and the organization's needs. You must demonstrate that you will be a good fit for the organization and that you will succeed in the position. To do this, focus on the impact of your skills and strengths. For instance, dependability and time management ensure that a medical practice runs smoothly; attention to detail reduces errors in medical coding or patient files; and strong communication and interpersonal skills encourage good rapport with patients and promote successful collaboration between co-workers. Think about the daily tasks and challenges of the job you are interviewing for, and then highlight how your skills and expertise would help you succeed in that role and benefit the organization.

⭐ **EXPERIENTIAL EXERCISES**

1. Review your skills and qualities.
2. Create examples from your experience that demonstrate these.
3. Practice answering traditional interview questions using your examples.

Behavioral Interview Questions

Behavioral interviews have been part of the hiring process in many large organizations since the 1970s, including the health care industry. Using these types of interview questions, applicants are asked questions about their past performance and how they handled specific situations. Behavioral interviews are based on the premise that past performance is a good indicator of future performance. Behavioral interviewing has been found to be 55% predictive of future behavior on the job compared with traditional interviewing, which is 10% predictive.

Interviewers prepare in advance by listing the key qualifications for the jobs they post. They then develop questions to help determine whether applicants possess the desired characteristics. For example, suppose that getting along with others is very important in the position. A question might be "Describe a time when you had to work with someone who you felt was difficult to get along with." As you tell your story, the interviewer may follow up with additional questions, such as:

* "In what ways was this person difficult?"
* "What did you need to do together?"
* "What did you say to this person?"
* "Did you get the job done despite the difficulties?"
* "How did you feel about this situation?"
* "What did you learn from this?"

Table 12.1 contains examples of behavioral interview questions.

When preparing for behavioral questions, you should practice explaining your examples in a way that emphasizes positive outcomes and your strengths rather than dwelling on the bad behavior of others or the negative aspects of a previous work environment. Remember to never speak badly about a former employer or co-workers.

Preparing to answer behavioral questions usually takes more preparation than traditional questions. Some of the preparation is similar, as you will

TABLE 12.1
Behavioral Interview Questions

Qualifications	Sample Questions
Interpersonal skills	Tell me about a time when someone disagreed with you about a major decision. What did you say or do? How was the decision ultimately made? Describe a situation in which you were able to use persuasion to successfully convince someone to consider your ideas.
Flexibility	Describe a situation in which you were required to conform to a work policy you did not really agree with. What was the policy? Why did you disagree with it? How did you feel about the situation? Give me an example of a job in which your working conditions frequently changed. How did you adapt to these changes? Tell me about a time when you had to reorganize your schedule in order to help a co-worker meet a deadline. How did you help? What was the result?
Communication	Give me a specific example that shows how you typically deal with conflict. Describe a time when you had to communicate something difficult to your supervisor. What was the situation? How did you plan your communication? What did you say? What was the result? Describe a situation in which you felt you did not communicate well. How did you follow up? What did you learn?
Customer service skills	Tell me about a time when you had to deal with a very upset customer/patient. How did you handle the situation? What was the result? Give me a few examples of what you have said to customers/patients who have approached you for help. How did you decide the appropriate way to work with each one? Describe something you did to help another employee improve their customer service.
Stress management	Describe a stressful situation in which you applied your coping skills. What specifically caused the stress? How were you feeling at the time? What techniques did you use? How was the situation resolved?
Problem solving	Describe a time when you anticipated a potential problem(s) and developed preventive measures. How did you identify the problem? What were the signs? How did you determine ways to prevent it? How did others feel about your actions? What was the final result? Describe a time when you were asked or assigned to do a task you did not feel qualified to handle. What did you do?
Integrity	Describe an incident in which you made a serious mistake. How did you handle this with your supervisor and/or co-workers? Tell me about a time when you had to make an unpopular decision. What were the circumstances? Why were others unhappy with the decision? Why did you believe you were making the right decision?

collect examples of your skills and qualifications for both types of interview questions. The key is to anticipate the kinds of knowledge, skills, and abilities an employer wants and then search your inventory for experiences you have had that illustrate those qualifications. Examples can come from any area of your life. You may never have worked in health care and may have limited work experience of any kind. If so, you can draw from experiences in your externships, volunteer opportunities, or personal life. For instance, your experience raising children may help you answer questions about making unpopular decisions. These were likely based on good judgment, time management, and even your values and ethics. Other experiences you can draw from include previous jobs, even if they were not in the health care industry; schoolwork, such as classes, labs, and extra activities; and community or service work.

In a behavioral interview, it is essential to *listen carefully*. Not only must you understand the question but you also need to understand *what the interviewer wants to know*. That is, what qualification is important for this job, and how can you demonstrate that you have that qualification? For example, if the interviewer asks a lot of questions on how you manage conflict or how you address angry patients, the position you are applying for most likely must address many stressful situations.

Do not hesitate to ask for clarification if you do not understand the question. It is better to ask questions than to provide an inappropriate or incomplete answer. It is completely acceptable to take a few moments to think about an answer. If the question asks about an experience you have never had before, for example, "Tell me about a time when you had to fire a friend," admit that this has never happened to you. Do not try to make up an answer. If you can think of a related experience, you could describe that instead. You might respond, for instance, "I've never had to fire a friend, but I could tell you about a time when I had to give critical feedback to a friend at work."

Interviewers may also ask you to describe failures and how you handled them, so it is a good idea to be prepared with some examples. Reflect on what you learned from experiences that did not turn out as you hoped they would or how you overcame challenges.

Many job search experts recommend using the **STAR** approach when answering a behavioral question. The STAR approach is effective in helping you organize your responses:

1. **S** and **T**: Choose and describe a **Situation** or **Task** that enables you to best demonstrate that you have the desired qualifications. What did you need to accomplish? What goal were you working toward?

2. **A**: Explain the **Actions** you took in dealing with the situation. Give enough details to show your skills but take care not to ramble or give unnecessary information.

3. **R**: Describe the **Results**. Explain what happened, what you learned, and how the outcome of your actions made a difference. Give numbers and percentages when possible.

Although it is advisable to have examples in mind and practice telling your "stories," be careful not to overly memorize what to say. You want to avoid giving a canned or overly practiced response that may not apply to the question.

⭐ **EXPERIENTIAL EXERCISES**

1. Review your skills and abilities.
2. Create examples from your experience that demonstrate these.
3. Practice answering behavioral interview questions using your examples.

Situational Questions

Situational questions present situations or problems you might encounter on the job. You are asked to explain how you would respond to and/or handle the problem. Box 12.1 provides examples of situational questions.

BOX 12.1

Examples of Situational Questions

What Would You Do?
- You see a co-worker who does not have the authority to administer medications taking some from a locked cabinet.
- You disagree with your supervisor about how to handle a problem.
- You hear a co-worker discussing confidential patient information with their friend, who is not involved in the patient's care.
- You are not sure how to prioritize your work, and no one is available to discuss it with you.
- You are working with an angry patient who insists on seeing the physician—who is not available—immediately.
- You have a problem to solve. What steps would you take?
- You offer ideas at staff meetings, but no one seems to take them seriously.

As with behavioral questions, you need to practice in advance to be prepared for situation questions by:

* Learning as much as possible about the organization and the specific job. If possible, read the mission statement and goals of the organization.
* Thinking about your own values and mission statement. These may provide guidelines for answering questions that do not have easy answers but can be based on ethical standards.
* Reviewing your personal inventory of skills and qualifications.
* Recalling hypothetical situations you learned about in your classes. Use those to guide your answers to questions about similar situations. For instance, perhaps you learned about dealing with difficult patients in your phlebotomy course. You could apply the techniques you learned to a scenario about dealing with a patient who fears the dentist or receiving an injection.

 EXPERIENTIAL EXERCISES

1. Review your skills and qualities.
2. Create examples from your experience that demonstrate these.
3. Practice answering situational interview questions using your examples.

Occupation-Specific Questions

Questions in this category explore your specific knowledge, skill mastery, willingness to learn new procedures, and the general content of your training. The type of question will vary but may include the following:

* Describe how to perform a specific procedure.
* Explain how to operate certain equipment.
* Describe appropriate action to take in a given situation that directly relates to this job.
* Suggest how to solve a health care problem.
* Explain how you plan to keep your skills updated.
* What do you know about (a theory, new procedure, etc.)?
* Why do you want to work in pediatrics/dermatology/children's dentistry, etc.?

Some employers give practical skill tests or ask you to demonstrate your knowledge and skill. Examples of these tests include a typing speed test, filing or recordkeeping exercise, spelling test, calculation of drug dosages, or demonstration of a procedure. If you are asked to perform a practical test that is appropriate for your level of training, use the exercise as an opportunity to show that you have confidence in your

abilities and can handle stress. If the task is something you have not been trained to do but is required for the job, tell the interviewer you would welcome the opportunity to learn.

Practice Interviewing

Successful interviews usually depend on good preparation.

—John D. Drake

Of course, you cannot anticipate the exact questions interviewers will ask. What you can do is prepare yourself to answer a variety of questions. Here are some things you should be prepared to do at an interview:

* Listen carefully.
* Ask for clarification when necessary.
* Think through your "inventory" of capabilities and characteristics that you can apply when answering questions.
* Think of examples to back-up your answers.
* Project self-confidence.

Preparation entails practice-answering questions, aloud, under conditions as close to those of an actual interview as possible. The best way to practice is to role-play with someone who acts as the interviewer. This can be an instructor, classmate, mentor, networking contact, friend, or family member. Many schools require mock (practice) interviews as part of professional development classes. Take advantage of these opportunities, and do your best to conduct yourself as if you were at a real interview. Videotaping or having an observer take notes can be helpful, even if it feels a little intimidating. It is better to make a few mistakes now, in front of a supportive audience, so you can avoid them at interviews.

If you believe you might be asked to demonstrate skills or react to a scenario in your interviews, include them in your practice sessions. The career services personnel at your school may be familiar with the interviewing practices of facilities in your area and can give you additional information about what to expect and how to best prepare.

The goal of mock interviews is not to memorize answers you can repeat. It is to develop a level of comfort about the interviewing process and have examples fresh in your mind so you can call on them as needed and respond to questions intelligently and confidently.

 EXPERIENTIAL EXERCISES

1. Prepare a variety of interview questions.
2. Choose a partner who will read the questions for you to practice answering.

Before the Interview

Having everything you might need at the interview will help you feel organized and confident. It also demonstrates to employers that you are organized and think ahead—valuable qualities for health care professionals. Although your list will be different, here are some suggestions for what to take along:

* Extra copies of your resume
* Copies of licenses, certifications, and other documentation
* Proof of immunizations and results of health tests
* Reference sheet
* Any documentation of skills and experience requested by the employer
* Pens
* Notepad
* Your list of questions (discussed later in this chapter)
* Appointment calendar/planner/electronic organizer/phone (Make sure to silence your phone during the interview.)
* Personal items, such as breath mints, medications, or other "emergency supplies"

A small case or large handbag is a convenient and professional way to carry your papers and supplies. It can be inexpensive, but it should be a conservative color, in good repair, and neatly organized so you can quickly find what you need.

Making the First Impression Count

The way in which we think of ourselves has everything to do with how our world sees us.

—Arlene Raven

Just 60 seconds: That is how long you have to make a positive first impression. Although it is possible to eventually reverse a negative first impression, it is a lot easier to make a first good one than fight to try to make a good second one. This is why maintaining a professional appearance both during the job search and on the job is so important. An appropriate appearance and professional demeanor communicate to the interviewer that you:

* Are able to professionally represent the clinic or organization.
* Understand what is appropriate appearance for the job.
* Practice good hygiene.
* Respect both yourself and the interviewer.
* Take the interview seriously.

Although the standard for interview attire is a matching two-piece suit, there is some flexibility when applying for health care jobs. Some schools and employers encourage their students and applicants to wear a clean, pressed uniform since that is what they will be wearing on the job. Other schools still advise students to wear standard business attire. It is important to pay attention to the professional advice of the career services staff at your school. The best choices for clothing are generally conservative colors and simple styles. When in doubt, wear a suit. It is better to be overdressed for an interview than underdressed. Jeans, t-shirts, tennis shoes, or anything remotely similar are not appropriate for an interview. Keep in mind that "nice" clothes, such as those for going to a party, a restaurant, or a club, may not be professional and appropriate for an interview.

If you are not sure about what to wear, ask your instructor or someone in your school's career service department for help. If money for buying interview clothes is a problem, ask if your school has a clothes-lending program or knows of an organization that donates suits to job applicants. Almost every town has excellent thrift shops that sell nice clothes at reasonable prices, although it may take some time and effort to find the right size and style. Some even specialize in helping people dress for job interviews.

First Contacts

Many job applicants fail to realize that the interview actually starts before they sit down with the person asking the questions. From the time you first inquired about a job opening or scheduled the appointment, you began making an impression. If you arrive for the interview and are rude to the receptionist, you may have already failed in your bid for the job. Make sure that you are polite and professional in every encounter you have with staff or employees. You cannot know what information is shared with the hiring manager. Keep in mind that these may be your future co-workers.

Learn the name of the person who will be conducting the interview. Be sure you have the correct spelling (for the thank-you letter, discussed later in this chapter) and pronunciation. This information should be provided to you in the informational email about the interview. If not, call the receptionist and ask.

When you first arrive, show courtesy and confidence. Make eye contact and offer a firm—not weak or too strong—handshake to exhibit warmth, confidence, and professionalism. See Box 12.2 for ways to express courtesy and self-confidence when meeting the interviewer.

Appearance Dos and Don'ts

Here are some additional guidelines that apply to all health care job applicants:

* **Be squeaky clean**. Take a bath or shower, wash your hair, scrub your fingernails, and use a deodorant or antiperspirant. If you smoke, do not smoke on the way to the interview. Strong fragrances in perfumes or colognes and other personal products should also be avoided, because many patients find them disagreeable or have allergic reactions. Men who have facial hair should groom it neatly (Figure 12.2).

* **Save the fashion trends for later**. Hair and nails should be natural colors, tattoos should be covered up, and visible rings and studs from piercings should be removed. Limit earrings to one set. Those who wear makeup should opt for a lightly applied, natural look over a dramatic look. Do not wear a hat or sunglasses during the interview.

* **Be a health care professional**. Long fingernails can scratch patients and harbor germs and dirt under them; thus fingernails should be short and polish-free. Free-flowing hair and dangling accessories can be grabbed by patients or caught in machinery. Hair should be neat or tied back. Wear closed-toe shoes.

Punctuality

Being late is a sure way to make a poor impression. Nothing ruins an interview faster than being late. Time management is an essential health care job skill, and you will have failed your first opportunity to demonstrate that you have mastered it. Arriving late gives the impression of a lack of preparedness and not being serious about the interview and job. The interviewer may also find it to be rude and inconsiderate. To avoid this, make a few advance preparations to ensure that you arrive on time for your interview:

* Write down the date and exact time of the appointment.
* Verify the address and ask for directions, if necessary.
* If the office is in a large building or complex, get additional instructions about how to find it.
* Inquire about parking, bus stops, or subway stops.
* Even if you think you know where it is, practice going there a couple of days before the interview to be sure you can find it. This will also allow you to account for traffic and possible construction.
* Allow extra time to arrive, park, or walk from the bus stop, find the front desk or reception area, and plan to be there about 10–15 minutes before the appointed time.
* If there is an emergency that cannot be avoided (i.e., a flat tire or unexpected snowstorm), call as soon as possible to offer an explanation and reschedule the interview.

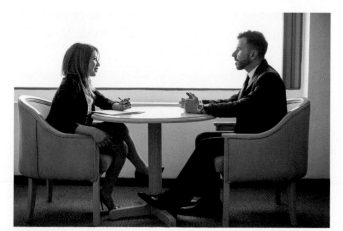

Figure 12.2 Making a good first impression is critical during an interview. (iStock.com/Antonio-Diaz/592682082.)

The Interview

- Discuss best practices for during the interview.
- Explain the role of active listening, mirroring, and body language in the job interview.
- List behaviors that should be avoided at interviews.
- Give examples of difficult interviewer behaviors and how to best respond to each.
- List information that employers cannot legally use when making hiring decisions.
- Describe the different types of interviewing styles and interview settings.
- Give examples of appropriate questions to ask.

Professional Conduct

Maintaining eye contact while the other person is speaking conveys that you are interested in what they are saying. When you are speaking, it is natural to look away occasionally. Most of the time, however, you should look at the listener. This is a sign of openness and sincerity. If there is more than one person interviewing you, try to make eye contact with everyone in the room, not just the person who asked the question.

The following is a summary of behaviors to avoid even if the interviewer engages in them:

* Interrupting
* Cursing
* Using poor grammar or slang words
* Gossiping, such as commenting on the weaknesses of other facilities, professionals, or your previous employer
* Telling off-color jokes
* Putting yourself down
* Chewing gum
* Discussing personal problems, such as transportation or childcare issues or issues you had while you were in school.

While you do not want to come across as stiff or impersonal, you do want to give the impression that you will work well in a team. Try to be relaxed and act natural while maintaining a professional demeanor.

Apply Your Communication Skills

A successful job interview depends on effective communication. An interview is essentially a conversation between two or more people who are trying to determine whether they fit each other's employment needs. You must express yourself clearly so the interviewer can gain an understanding of what you offer as a candidate and a positive impression of you as a person. You can improve your ability to communicate effectively by using the techniques discussed in the next sections.

Active Listening

Understanding begins by listening actively. Active listening consists of paying attention, focusing on the speaker's words, and thinking about the meaning of what they say. This takes practice. During an interview, focus on listening carefully to the questions and then formulating an appropriate response. It is okay to pause for a moment to think before you answer. You will be evaluated on the quality of your answer, not on how quickly you gave it.

The importance of listening carefully to the interviewer cannot be overstated. Often, we become so caught up in thinking about what we are going to say next that we fail to fully hear, let alone actively listen to, the other person. This is especially true in an interview when we are nervous and worried about whether we will say the right thing. This, however, is the very situation in which we can most benefit from listening carefully, so we can base what we say on what we hear.

Mirroring

An effective communication technique for interviews is known as mirroring, which entails observing the communication style of the interviewer and then matching it as closely as possible. This does not mean mimicking, so be cautious it does not appear as if you are making fun of the other person. It does mean adapting a style that will be most comfortable for the interviewer and help to build trust. Table 12.2 provides examples of mirroring.

Feedback

Whatever the style of the interviewer, use feedback when necessary to ensure that you understand the message. Feedback is a communication technique used to check your understanding of the speaker's intended message. It is not necessary—or even desirable—to repeat everything the speaker says, because this can be annoying to speakers. Used when needed, however, feedback can help ensure you understand the other person, so you can respond appropriately and

TABLE 12.2
Examples of Mirroring at the Job Interview

If the Interviewer Is:	It Is Best To:
Very businesslike. Direct and to the point.	Answer questions concisely, quickly getting to the point. Avoid long introductions, wordiness, and unnecessary details.
Warm and friendly. Conversational tone.	Reflect the interviewer's warmth without becoming too casual. Include human interest and details, when appropriate, in your answers.
Seemingly unhurried. Spends time describing the job in detail.	Include details to support your answers without giving unnecessary or unrelated information.

TABLE 12.3
Examples of Feedback

Paraphrasing
Saying what you heard the speaker say in your own words.

	What the Speaker Says	Feedback
Job Search	We really need employees we can rely on to be here on time every day. It is also essential they can get along with their co-workers.	It sounds like two of the most important characteristics you are looking for are punctuality and the ability to work well with others.
Career	It really hurts most when I get up in the mornings. I feel a little better as the day goes by.	It sounds like the pain is much worse when you first wake up in the morning but decreases during the day.

Reflecting
Repeating what the speaker said.

	What the Speaker Says	Feedback
Job Search	Here is a copy of the job description. It has most of the duties required for this position, although there are some others.	The job description has most of the duties required, but there are a few others. (The interviewer has given the impression that more may be expected than just what is listed on the job description.)
Career	I have not lost any weight because the diet the doctor gave me is not working.	You have not lost any weight because the diet is not working. (There may be other reasons, such as not following the diet exactly, lack of exercise, and so on.)

Clarifying
Asking the speaker to explain or give examples.

	What the Speaker Says	Feedback
Job Search	It is easy to find. We are really close to the Cross Town Shopping Center.	You said you are close to the Cross Town Shopping Center. Can you tell me about how many blocks that is?
Career	I give him the medication on schedule, but ever since he has been taking it, his behavior has been kind of strange.	Can you explain what you mean when you say your son has been acting "strangely" since he started taking the medication?

intelligently. See Table 12.3 for examples of feedback, such as the use of paraphrasing, reflecting, and clarifying.

Organization

When speaking, do your best to present your ideas in an organized manner so they are easy for the listener to follow. This can be difficult when you are nervous, so take your time to think before you speak. Recall the STAR technique described earlier in this chapter.

You can also jot down notes in your notepad if that will help you organize your thoughts. Silence can feel uncomfortable but taking a few moments to consider what you are going to say will result in better answers. Saying something meaningful after a pause is more important than simply responding quickly.

 EXPERIENTIAL EXERCISES

For the next week, take every opportunity to practice your communication skills by actively listening, mirroring, and using feedback.

Nonverbal Communication: It Can Make You or Break You

If you want a quality, act as if you already have it.

—**William James**

You can eloquently speak and correctly answer questions and yet fail in your communication efforts if your actions do not match your words. What you *do* communicates as much as what you say. More than half the meaning of our messages is communicated nonverbally based on our movements, posture, gestures, and facial expressions. You can enthusiastically claim that you would love the challenge of working in a fast-paced, think-on-your-feet clinical environment. But, if your face and body language reflect fear, anxiety, or subtle expressions of disdain, your verbal message will not ring true.

Videotaping yourself or rehearsing in front of a mirror can be very helpful when practicing interviewing skills, as it allows you to observe your body language and nonverbal cues. You can catch inappropriate facial expressions and other behaviors that might betray your words. If you do mock interviews, you could also ask the other person to give you feedback on your nonverbal communication. The career service at your school may offer opportunities for mock interviews.

Developing a positive attitude about the interviewing process and having confidence in your abilities will help ensure that your body language communicates the appropriate positive messages. At the same time, developing the body language of a positive, confident person will help you become that person. Table 12.4 lists ways to communicate self-confidence and respect for the other person. Figure 12.3 illustrates positive body language.

 EXPERIENTIAL EXERCISES

1. Choose a day to observe other people as they communicate. Look for examples of body language. What do they communicate to you?
2. Describe actions you observe that communicate positive messages.
3. Pay attention to your own body language. What do you think you are communicating to others?

TABLE 12.4
Positive Body Language

What You Do	The Message You Send
Stand up straight, with head held up and shoulders back	I am a candidate worthy of your consideration.
Maintain eye contact	I am sincere in what I am saying.
Avoid nervous action such as jiggling a leg	I want to be here.
Lean forward slightly toward the other person	I am interested in what you are saying.

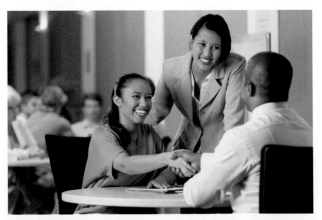

Figure 12.3 Use body language that communicates respect for the interviewer and confidence in yourself. (Copyright © istock.com.)

TABLE 12.5
Handling Difficult Interview Situations

If the Interviewer	What You Can Do
Keeps you waiting a long time	If you are interested in the job, do not show annoyance or anger. It is best not to schedule interviews when you have a very limited amount of time. Remember, this person may be overworked and overscheduled, and that is exactly why there is a potential position for you! Keep in mind that health care work does not always proceed at our convenience. A patient with an emergency, for example, will certainly have priority over an interviewee.
Allows constant interruptions with phone calls and/or people coming in	Again, do not show that you are irritated. This person may be very busy, disorganized, or simply having a difficult day. (This could be another good sign that this employer really needs your help.)
Does most of the talking and does not give you an opportunity to say much about yourself	Listen carefully and try to determine how your qualifications relate to what you are hearing. Being a good listener in itself may be the most important quality you can demonstrate.
Seems to simply make conversation Does not discuss the job or ask you questions	Try to move the discussion to the job by asking questions: "Can you tell me about what you are looking for in a candidate?" "What are the principal duties that this person would perform?" It is possible that this is a test to see your reaction, so take care to be courteous.
Tries to engage you in gossip about school, personnel, and so on	Say you do not really know about the person or other professionals, facilities, or situations and cannot comment. Ask a question about the job to redirect the conversation.
Allows long periods of silence	This may be a test to see how you react under pressure. Do not feel that you have to speak, and do your best to remain comfortable. (Say to yourself, "This is just a test, and I am doing fine.") If it goes on too long, you can ask, "Is there something you would like me to tell you more about or discuss further?"
Does not seem to understand your training or qualifications	Explain as clearly as possible. Use examples, as appropriate, to illustrate your skills.
Makes inappropriate comments about your appearance, gender, ethnicity, and so on	Depending on the nature of the comment and your interpretation of the situation, it may be best to excuse yourself from the interview. For example, comments of a sexual nature or racial slurs should not be tolerated. You should discuss this situation with your instructor or career services department for advice on how to proceed.
Is very friendly, chatty, and complimentary about you	This may not be a problem, but be careful not to get so comfortable that you share personal problems and other information that may disqualify you from the job.

Handling Difficult Interview Situations

Despite your best efforts, some interviews can be more demanding and challenging than others. Table 12.5 contains difficult situations and suggestions for managing them.

Keep in mind that the questions reveal something about the interviewer and possibly about the organization, so consider them when deciding whether you would enjoy that job and working for that organization.

As much as you need to be a good fit for the employer, your employer also needs to be a good fit for you.

Illegal Questions

There are several topics and questions that interviewers are not permitted to ask applicants, based on guidelines from the US Equal Employment Opportunity Commission (EEOC). Asking questions on these topics can result in charges of discrimination and potentially a lawsuit if the issue cannot be resolved. According to the EEOC, it is illegal to ask a candidate questions about the following:

* Age (assuming the applicant is of legal age to work)
* Criminal background, specifically having no conviction or being found guilty
* Disability
* Citizenship
* Ethnic background
* Financial status
* Marital status and children
* Pregnancy status
* Physical condition (as long as the applicant can perform the job tasks)
* Race or national origin
* Religion
* Sexual orientation or gender identity

Although questions that require the applicant to reveal information about these factors are illegal, they are sometimes asked anyway. In some cases, the interview may take a more casual tone and the interviewer may inadvertently share information or ask an illegal question, such as "Oh, I went to Grady High School, too. What year did you graduate?" It may not be obvious from the question that answering them will, in fact, reveal information that should not be considered when hiring, such as your age. The basic rule of thumb for knowing whether a question is appropriate or not is: Does the question have anything to do with your work skills or experience for the job you are applying for? Table 12.6 contains examples of seemingly innocent questions but may be illegal for the employer to ask. Thus, it will be your responsibility to be aware of and navigate potentially illegal questions.

Responding to Illegal Questions

Responding or not responding to illegal or inappropriate interview questions can be tricky and requires some navigating. Answering the question may hurt your chances of being hired but not answering may do that as well since you may seem defensive or unfriendly.

Illegal questions put you in a difficult situation, and there are no easy formulas for handling them. In deciding what to do, you need to ask yourself several questions:

* Is the subject of the question of concern to me?
* Do I find the question offensive?
* Does the interviewer appear to be unaware that the question is illegal?
* What is my overall impression of the interviewer and the facility?
* Would I want to work here?
* How badly do I want this particular job?
* If this person is to be my immediate supervisor, is the question an indication that this is not a person I would want to work with?
* What do I think the interviewer's real concern is? Is it valid?

Based on your answers to those questions, there are several ways you can respond to the interviewer:

1. Avoid the question and steer the conversation to a different topic. ("What a coincidence that we went to the same high school. I heard that they have made a lot of renovations to the building.")
2. Ask the interviewer to explain how the question relates to the job requirements. ("Is there a reason you asked about the year I graduated from high school?")
3. Respond to the interviewer's apparent concern rather than to the exact question.
4. Decline to answer or state what you would rather not say.
5. Keep the answers short, broad, and general.
6. Redirect a question to your interviewer.

If the interviewer is persistent and it is apparent that asking illegal questions is deliberate, try to end the interview as soon as you can. Afterward, you may want to report the incident to the Civil Rights Commission or EEOC. Even if you are given a job offer from this employer, you may want to reconsider. Intentionally violating federal laws may be the first sign and indication that there may be other compliance or safety issues by the employer.

Legal Versus Illegal

Employers, however, have the right and the responsibility to make sure that applicants can both physically

TABLE 12.6
Questions Requesting Information That Cannot Be Used for Hiring

Question	What It Can Reveal
Do you own your home?	Financial status
Where are your parents from?	Ethnic background
How do you think our current president is doing?	Political affiliation
Are you planning on having a family?	Pregnancy
When did you graduate from high school?	Age
What does your husband/wife do?	Marital status
Where do your children go to school?	Family status

and legally perform the job requirements. Sometimes there is a fine line between a question that is legal versus illegal, as in the following examples:

Illegal Questions	Legal Questions
How old are you?	Are you over 18?
Where were you born?	Do you have the legal right to work in the United States?
What is your maiden name?	Would your work records be listed under another name?
Have you ever been arrested?	Have you ever been convicted of a crime?
How healthy are you?	Are you able to lift 50 pounds as required by this position?

As these examples demonstrate, it can be easy for employers to mistakenly ask illegal questions. So, if you are asked an illegal question, an effective method is to reword the question in a legal way. For example, if you are asked what neighborhood you live in, which illegally questions your financial status, you can respond by saying, "I am local and should not have any issue arriving on time to work." This indirectly and professionally answers the question without addressing the legality of it and reminds the interviewer of your qualifications for the job.

Responding to Employer Concerns

Many employment experts recommend that you respond to the employer's concerns rather than the questions. This requires that you determine what the concerns are. See Table 12.7 for examples.

One strategy for handling common employer concerns is to bring them up before the interviewer does. This gives you the opportunity to present them in a positive light. Employers may be uncomfortable addressing certain issues and instead may simply drop you from the "possible hire" list. For example, if questions are asked about where you live or if you have a car, the employer may be asking you about your ability to arrive to work on time or your dependability. To better address that, you can tell the employer, "Unless it's something unforeseeable, I'm never late for work. In fact, I've won the Perfect Attendance award at my school for the last 3 years." By taking the initiative, you gain the opportunity to explain your situation and remain under consideration for the job.

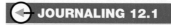 **JOURNALING 12.1**

Is there anything you think employers might see as an obstacle to hiring you? How can you turn the obstacle into a positive characteristic?

Stay Focused on the Positive

To win big, you sometimes have to take big risks.
—Bill Gates

It is important to maintain a positive attitude throughout the interview process. An interview is not the place to bring up problems or what you believe you cannot or do not want to do. Remain positive and future-oriented and arrive prepared to emphasize the following:
* What you can do
* How you can help
* Ways you can apply what you have learned

Never criticize a previous employer, instructor, classmate, or anyone else. It reflects poorly on you. Additionally, potential employers realize they may someday be your previous employer and do not want to be the subject of your comments to others in the profession. The health care community where you live may be small, and it is also possible that the interviewer is a friend of the person you are criticizing.

TABLE 12.7
Addressing Employer Concerns

Questions	Possible Concerns	Possible Responses
Do you have young children?	Your attendance and dependability	Explain your child care arrangements, good attendance in school and at other jobs, and your understanding of the importance of good attendance.
Where do you live?	Reliable transportation and punctuality	Describe your transportation and previous good attendance.
Which religious holidays are you unable to work?	Scheduling problems	Explain that you are a team player and understand that all workdays must be covered. You are willing to cover when co-workers have a holiday you do not observe.

Keep in mind that every interview is a like a marketing presentation. Emphasize the positive aspects of your skills and character (Figure 12.4). However, if you sincerely feel that you are not qualified for a job (and this is an important consideration in health care), you should never pretend that you are. Lacking needed skills is not a negative reflection on you as a person. It simply means that this job is not appropriate for you. Other jobs will be. In fact, there may be many reasons why jobs and applicants do not match. After all, that is the whole purpose of job interviews: for you and the employer to make that determination. Table 12.8 contains suggestions for showing the employer the positive aspects of various employment concerns.

Subjects to Avoid

There are several subjects to avoid during the interview, at least during the early stages of the interview process. You are there to help solve the employer's problems, not necessarily find solutions to your own. Employers are looking for independent problem solvers.

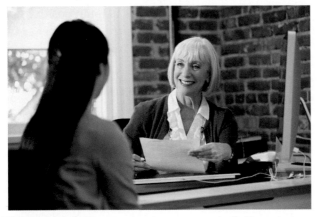

Figure 12.4 The interview is your opportunity to market yourself.

Giving the impression that you are more concerned with what you can get from the job than what you can contribute is a sure way to get nothing at all. Do not mention your personal problems. Avoid asking about the interviewer's background. Do not ask if the job details and duties or the schedule can change. The following questions may send the message "What's in it for me?" and should be avoided until you receive an offer and can negotiate:

* How much does the job pay?
* What are the other benefits?
* How many paid holidays will I get?
* Is Friday a casual day?
* Can I leave early if I finish my work?
* When will I get a raise?

Even though the time to negotiate specific conditions, including your salary and benefits, is after you have been offered the job, it is acceptable to inquire about the work schedule, duties, and other expectations. How to negotiate salary, benefits, and schedule will be discussed later in this chapter.

Different Types of Interviews and Interview Settings

Interviews can take many different forms other than the more traditional in-person, one-on-one interviews. An in-person interview is time consuming for both the applicant and interviewer. As a time- and cost-effective measure, there are often several rounds of interviews to narrow the applicant pool down to just a few before the in-person interview.

Employers are also using a variety of technologies and software systems to attract, assess, and hire candidates and to help make the hiring process more efficient and effective. While one-on-one, in-person

TABLE 12.8
Addressing Concerns as a Job Candidate

Concerns	How to Manage
You are young and have little work experience.	You are energetic, eager to learn, "trainable," and looking for long-term employment.
You have a criminal record.[a]	You have learned from your mistakes and are eager to have an opportunity to work and serve others.
You are over age 40.	You are experienced, have good work habits, and are patient.
You have had many jobs, none for very long.	You have a variety of experiences, are flexible, can adjust to the working environment, and have now found a career to which you want to dedicate your efforts.

[a]Some states do not allow individuals who have been convicted of specific crimes to work in certain health care occupations. In some cases, these individuals are not even allowed to take certification examinations.

interviews are still common, employers are using a variety of other methods to assess candidates.

Computer-Assisted Job Interviews

Some employers conduct interviews with the help of a computer. The advantage for the employer, in addition to saving time, is to prepare a set of questions, often up to 100, to ask of every applicant. Most interview programs consist of multiple-choice questions with several answers to choose from. This enables the employer to compare "apples to apples" when deciding whom to interview in person. The advantage for you is that you have more time to think about your answers and can, through the types of questions asked, learn a little about the organization before you have the face-to-face interview.

Answer the questions carefully and honestly. Computers report inconsistencies in your answers. At the same time, take care not to give unnecessary information that may harm your chance of getting hired. Studies have shown that people are more likely to "tell" a computer information they would never tell a human being. Also, be aware that most computer-assisted interviews must be completed within a certain amount of time, so make sure you know how much time you have and keep track of it as you move through the questions.

Another way computers are used in the hiring process involves presenting scenarios to applicants and asking them what they would do in that situation. Computers also administer skills tests, integrity tests, and personality tests. Some organizations administer computerized interviews and tests on their own computers at their facility; others make them available on the Internet and give applicants a password to gain access to testing websites.

Personality Tests

You may be asked to take a personality test as part of the interviewing process. Personality assessment tests are increasingly used in the candidate selection process, especially in larger organizations. As many as 30% of all companies now use personality tests. These tests involve answering a series of questions on paper or on the computer, and they measure qualities, such as conscientiousness and if a person is an extrovert or introvert. Studies suggest that organizations find better matches for positions when applicants take these tests. This is because certain jobs require specific characteristics, and these are more reliably determined by tests than by interviews. The research also claims that

the individuals hired tend to have greater satisfaction with their jobs when employers use these tests in the matching process.

The best advice for taking a personality test is to answer the questions honestly. The tests contain a variety of questions to assess each trait. Answering as you think you should or randomly selecting answers could have negative results. If you are offered a position based on inaccurate answers, it is very possible you would not enjoy either the work or the setting. You are more likely to find a job that suits your abilities, traits, and work preferences if you answer questions honestly. This has been one of the reported benefits of personality assessments: less turnover among employees who, with traditional hiring methods, end up deciding the job is just not for them. Box 12.3 provides examples of questions on personality tests.

Phone Interviews

In most cases, the phone interview is the first round of interviews. You should prepare for a phone interview just as you would an in-person interview. Here are several important things to consider:

* Be sure to clarify the day and time of the phone call, especially if one of you will be in a different time zone.
* Make sure to have all your documents in front of you. This will be one of the advantages of doing a phone interview—you will be able to look at your resume or the job application or take notes without the interviewer watching you.
* Make sure you are in a quiet place where you will not be disturbed.

BOX 12.3

Examples of Questions on Personality Tests

- Do you like meeting new people?
- How long does it take you to calm down when you've been angry?
- Are you easily disappointed?
- Are you considerate of other people's feelings?
- Are you always busy?
- Do you like solving complex problems?
- Do you make people feel welcome?
- Do you feel overwhelmed often?
- Do you prefer familiarity over unfamiliarity?
- Do you tend to always see the good in people, no matter what the circumstance is?

* Even though you will not be seen, it is still helpful to "feel" the part by dressing the part. This is a mental tactic that will help you get into the right mindset.

The benefit of a phone interview is that you can have your notes in front of you to help you answer questions. A challenge is that you will not be able to see the interviewer and must rely on paying attention to the tone and word selections. Not performing well on the phone interview will most likely mean not advancing to the next round of interviews.

Video Interviews

If an applicant makes it past the phone interview, the video interview, sometimes called the virtual interview, is often the next round in the interview process. In fact, a majority of employers are now using video interviews as part of their hiring process.

There are many different video-conferencing programs that can be used for video interviews, such as Skype, Good Hangout, WhatsApp, Facetime, and Zoom. Like an in-person interview, both the applicant and the interviewer can see and interact with each other, but there are fewer logistical issues in arranging a meeting.

Preparing for a video interview is similar to an in-person interview, including dressing for the interview. When you get dressed for a video interview, you want to be just as formal as you would be for an in-person interview at the same company. This should be from head to toe.

These are some additional best practices for video interviews:

* Do a trial run with whichever video-conferencing program you will use to prevent any technical difficulties.
* Set up the shot to make sure it is not too bright or too dark, that there is no glare, and that the background is appropriate.
* Try to minimize interruptions but take them in stride if they happen.
* Maintain good eye contact, although this is somewhat harder to do in video.
* Make sure to smile and act confident and at ease.
* Pay attention to your posture and the positioning of the camera. Try not to sit too far or too close.

If you are new to video conferencing and meetings, it would be a good idea to practice your video interview skills ahead of time. Setting up a mock video interview with a friend or career service staff member can help you identify anything you need to watch out for, such as looking away from the camera, hand gestures, bad posture, or fiddling with your hair. Once

you see them, you can adjust your mannerisms and behaviors accordingly.

Panel or Group Interviews

Instead of the standard one-on-one conversation with a single person, a panel interview is with several people, all at the same time. Panel interviews are common in many industries, including health care and medicine and government positions, especially for positions with a lot of demands and responsibilities. Each member of the group of interviewers may come from different parts of the company and will have their own questions about your credentials, experience, and skills.

Interviewing with multiple people at once can be intimidating and, for some employers, panel interviews are beneficial as being more efficient and practical but also a way to preview how you will perform under a stressful situation.

Preparing for a panel interview is not so different from getting ready for a standard interview. You should do your homework on the company, carefully review the job posting, and practice answers to common interview questions and position-specific questions. Ask the scheduler or recruiter for the names of the panel attendees, so you can research their positions and background. Knowing which people are in the interview room, and what their job titles and responsibilities are can provide a sense of where the job you are interviewing for fits within the company.

A panel interview may be in-person or virtual (Figure 12.5). If you are interviewing in person, make sure you have a copy of your resume for everyone who will be at the panel interview. During the interview, engage with the entire room and avoid overly focusing on one or two individuals. You may not know who

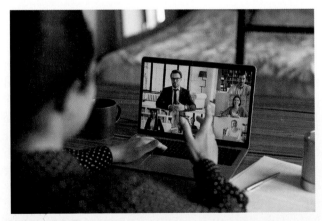

Figure 12.5 Virtual panel interviews are increasingly common in multiple settings, including health care. (iStock.com/fizkes/1331487210.)

has the most decision-making power about hiring, so aim to respond to everyone who asks you a question with a thorough and thoughtful answer, regardless of job title or the way people present themselves. When answering questions, look at everyone as you answer questions, instead of focusing solely on the person who asked the question.

Similar to panel interviews, some employers may use group interviews, where one interviewer may speak to several candidates at once, or several interviewers may interview a group of candidates. Group interviews are common in many industries and help employers save time when searching for new hires. They can be structured in different ways.

Companies may conduct group interviews because they can show which candidates work well with others. A group interview may also show an employer which candidates fit well with the company culture. For example, positions involving high-stress, fast-paced work or patient or customer interaction commonly require group interviews. If you perform well during a stressful interview, you may be more apt to perform well in a challenging job.

While this can be efficient and time saving for the employer, these types of interviews demand confidence and self-assertion. However, your preparation and the skills you will need for the interview will not change. Be prepared by reviewing a variety of interview questions and practicing them. Be a good listener and carefully listen to what both the interviewer(s) and other candidates are saying. When you answer a question, refer to what another person said, which shows that you were listening. You may also be able to tell which candidate responses are resonating well with the interviewers and which are not.

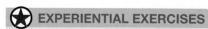 **EXPERIENTIAL EXERCISES**

Select one of the video-conferencing tools, and practice answering interview questions. Pay attention to the positioning of the camera—not too close and not too far away from you. Listen to the volume of your voice and where you look while you are answering questions.

Asking Your Interviewer Questions

You have the right and the responsibility to ask questions about the job you are applying for, so you can fully evaluate the opportunity presented. Remember that this job must fit your needs as much as you need to fit the employer's needs. In addition, well-stated and thought-out questions about the job communicate

motivation and interest and help promote positive dialogue. It also gives both the applicant and the employer a chance to get to know one another better and see what it could be like to work with one another.

Ask Questions

When you are in class, it may be true that "there are no stupid questions." However, at a job interview, the quality of your questions does count. Avoid asking questions that you could have found on the company's website or job description. The questions you ask during an interview should show that you:

* Have a sincere interest in the job.
* Want to understand the employer's needs.
* Understand the nature of health care work.
* Have thought about your career goal.
* Want information that will enable you to do your best.

It is a good idea to prepare, in advance, a list of general questions, along with a few that are specific to the job and the facility. Not everyone is skilled at thinking on the spot, particularly in a high-pressure situation like a job interview. Here are some questions to get you started:

1. How could I best contribute to the success of this facility?
2. What are the most important qualities needed to succeed in this position?
3. What is the mission of this organization/facility? (However, do not ask this question if this information is listed on the organization's website.)
4. What are the major challenges faced by this organization/facility?
5. How is the organization structured? To whom would I be reporting? Whom would I work with on a regular basis?
6. What values are most important to the organization?
7. I want to continue learning and updating my skills. What opportunities would I have to do that here?
8. How will I be evaluated and learn what I need to improve?
9. What does success look like in this position?
10. Are there opportunities for advancement for employees who perform well?

It is perfectly acceptable to ask questions throughout the interview where they are logical. This will be more natural and lead to a smoother interview than asking a long list at the end. You do not have to wait until you are invited to ask them. You should also feel free to take notes on the answers to your questions.

In addition to asking questions, observe the facility and the people who work there. Does this feel like a place you would want to work? Is it clean? Organized? Does it appear that safety precautions are followed? What is the pace of work? Are the people who work there courteous and helpful? What is the mood of the other employees? How do they interact with patients and with one another? If your interview is with the person who would be your supervisor, do you think you would get along? Do you believe you would fit in?

It may not be possible for you to see anything other than the interviewer's office. In fact, at a large facility, your first interview may take place in a conference room or in a recruiter's office. You might not see the area where you would work. If this is the case, you may want to ask for a tour if you are offered a job.

Work Preference Questions

You may be asked about your job preferences. Be prepared to answer questions such as:
* Whether you are looking for a full-time or part-time position if there is an option for either
* The hours you are willing to work
* The length of shift you prefer
* The days and time of day you can work
* When you will be able to start

Remember to be realistic when applying for jobs. However, avoid being overly specific or demanding, which may result in you not being offered the job.

 EXPERIENTIAL EXERCISES

1. Review your work preferences and needs.
2. Practice answering questions about your preferences and needs.

Ending the Interview

The end of the interview provides you with an opportunity to make a positive final impression. If you are interested in the job, say so in the wrap-up statement. Tell the interviewer, for example, why you believe you will be an asset to the organization, that you are impressed with the organization, and that your qualifications fit the position.

Express your enthusiasm about working there, and state that you hope you are chosen for the position. You may also ask about what the next steps are and when they think a decision will be made. Ask if there is anything you need to do to follow up. If requested, give the interviewer your reference sheet. Be sure to get the interviewer's last name, title, and email address, if possible. An easy way to do this is to ask for their business card. And be sure that you provided your contact information. Then smile, give a firm handshake, and leave as confidently as you entered. Whether you want the job or not, always thank the interviewers for their time. This applies even if the interview did not go well. Even if you are not offered the job or do not accept, which will be discussed later in this chapter, consider all interviews as an opportunity to practice your interviewing skills and to learn more about your industry and profession.

 EXPERIENTIAL EXERCISES

1. Create several short summaries that express your interest in various jobs.
2. Create statements about why you should be hired.
3. Practice your statements aloud until you are comfortable saying them.

CASE STUDY 12.1

Emily, the medical administrative assistant student, was interviewed by Mr. Bard, the director of human resources at St. Francis Clinic, where she was doing her externship. She had learned a lot from the information he gave her about electronic applications and what he looks for in a resume when he is hiring.

Emily shared what she learned with the class. Her instructor, Ms. Harris, wondered if Mr. Bard would be willing to come to BeWell College and talk to the class about interviewing for jobs.

Ms. Harris called St. Francis Clinic the next day, and Mr. Bard agreed to come talk to her class. After giving a brief overview of what he looks for in candidates and the interview process at his clinic, he invited students to ask questions.

Student: What advice would you give applicants who are interviewing for a job at your clinic?

Mr. Bard: First, I would say they should use common sense. I might add here that common sense is not always so common! What I mean is, they need to think about the impression they are giving the employer. If applicants are not at their very best at an interview, what is the employer going to expect from them once they are on the job?

Student: Can you say a little more about what you mean by applicants being "at their very best"?

Mr. Bard: Sure. Good candidates for jobs in health care are friendly, engaged, and respectful. They show this in the way they interact with the interviewer. For example, they are on time, showing they respect the other person's schedule. Health care today is a high–customer service environment, and we are looking for employees who take this seriously. After all, we have patients' health in our hands. Our work can have profound effects on people's lives.

Student: You mentioned the impression that applicants give the employer. How important do you think appearance is in today's health care facilities?

Mr. Bard: Well, what we're looking for are "reasonable" standards; that is, we want an employee's appearance to convey professionalism. But, as we all know, styles and trends change. For example, multiple piercings and tattoos used to be deal breakers, but now they're becoming more acceptable, but within limits. They can't be too excessive or too outlandish. Also related to appearance is language. Communication and the impressions given to patients are important, so inappropriate language is absolutely not okay. Anything off-color or offensive—that kind of thing.

Student: What kinds of questions should interviewees be prepared for?

Mr. Bard: Patients today are considered to be *customers*, so I'm interested in knowing what an applicant can do that will help us make our patients satisfied with our service. How will they make our patients feel important? Those are questions I would ask. The bottom line is that I'm looking for

people who want to help make this place better. And I want to know *how* they're going to do it. What specific steps will they take?

We sometimes give behavioral or situational interviews. This means we give applicants scenarios of typical work situations and ask for examples of how they have handled them in the past or how they would handle them in the future. What we are looking for is caring—respect for people—their general approach to work. Sometimes we require a demonstration of a skill related to the job.

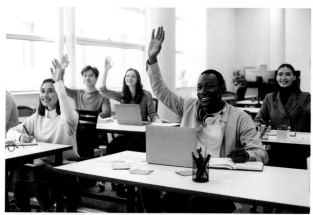
iStock.com/Prostock-Studio/1342228491

QUESTIONS FOR THOUGHT AND REFLECTION

1. What does Mr. Bard mean by common sense?
2. Why are health care providers today thinking of their patients as customers?
3. According to Mr. Bard, what are the most important personal characteristics employers want their employees to have?

A Different Path

Abrianna has about had it with the job search. She graduated from her medical assisting program over 3 months ago and still cannot find a job. She knows it is not her fault. After all, the career services people at her school just are not giving her good leads. She has tried to tell them that the employers they have sent her to are really not interested in hiring a recent graduate. But they just keep encouraging her to keep the appointments and interview.

As she told her friend Denise, "Last Thursday was a waste of time. I went to an interview, but how was I supposed to act enthusiastic about a job in a little office working with an old doctor? It didn't look like it would be a fun place to work. So, I answered his questions, but I really couldn't pretend I was interested."

"So, what did he say when you finished the interview?" asked Denise.

"He thanked me for coming in and just said good-bye," answered Abrianna.

"That was all?"

"Yeah, can you believe that?" Abrianna complained. "After I went to the trouble of getting dressed up and going in. Even if I didn't want the job, he could have said he would call me back or something."

Abrianna believes that she has bad luck with interviews. Sometimes she was late because the office was hard to find or they did not give her good directions. Other times, career services called her at the last minute, and she did not have time to get her clothes ready, her car gassed up, or her resume copied. As she told Denise, "What is that school thinking? That I'm just waiting around for them to call me about an interview?"

Later that week, Mr. Craig called from her school. "Abrianna, I'd like you to come in so we can talk about your job search and the interviews you've been on, so we can see how we can better help you."

Abrianna responded, "That sounds like a good idea, because I need to talk to *you* about these employers you've sent me to. They've all been a waste of time."

Mr. Craig replied, "Can you be here at 2:00?"

Abrianna arrived at Mr. Craig's office at 2:15. He looked at his watch. "Abrianna, our appointment was at 2:00."

"The babysitter arrived late, and I had to stop and get gas," explained Abrianna.

"I understand that, but you knew when our meeting would be, and you needed to prepare for it just like an interview. Punctuality is very important. Employers expect their employees to be on time. And if you can't get to an interview on time, why would they think you will be on time for work?" Mr. Craig asked.

"Work is different. I can be on time. And even if I can't, you know, if there's some kind of emergency, there are co-workers who can cover me for a few minutes. It won't kill them," said Abrianna.

"I'm afraid that's not a good approach to interviewing or a job, Abrianna. But I really wanted to talk to you about some of the past interviews you've gone on. I called a few of the employers who have interviewed you to see if they can provide any feedback," he said.

Abrianna was surprised but couldn't imagine any of them would have anything really negative to say about her.

Mr. Craig continued, "You seem to have a problem showing interest in the employers or their needs or even showing professionalism. One employer told me you actually answered your cell phone during the interview! That is simply not acceptable. It's unprofessional and shows a lack of regard for the employer and a lack of interest in the interview or the job."

"Well," she interrupted, "that was an important call. I didn't think they would mind and that employers expected me to put my life on hold during an interview."

"The fact is, they want your full attention—just like they want it when you are working for them. The interview is like a test: Are you the kind of person they want as an employee? And unfortunately, the behaviors you're demonstrating to me and to them are not going to get you employed."

QUESTIONS FOR THOUGHT AND REFLECTION

1. Why do you think Abrianna believes her actions are acceptable?
2. What other feedback could Mr. Craig give her?
3. What do you think should happen next after the meeting with Mr. Craig?

After the Interview

Nothing is a waste of time if you use the experience wisely.

—Auguste Rodin

LEARNING OBJECTIVE 3: AFTER THE INTERVIEW

- Explain why it is important to conduct a post-interview evaluation.
- Explain the importance of sending thank-you letters.
- Describe the recommended strategy for contacting an employer after an interview.
- List the information you should have when making a decision about accepting a job.
- List the types of benefits offered by some employers.
- List the questions you should ask yourself when deciding whether to accept a job.
- Explain how to correctly decline a job offer.

Being invited to interview is an accomplishment, whether or not you are hired for a particular job. You have qualifications that were worthy of the interviewer's time, you prepared well, and you met the challenge of presenting yourself to potential employers. Take a moment to reward yourself for completing this important step.

Make the most of every interview by viewing each one as an opportunity to improve your presentation skills and learn more about the health care world. This knowledge can help you in future interviews and other work-related situations, such as performance evaluations. When you leave the interviewer's office, your reaction may be "Whew! That's over!" and the last thing you want to do is spend more time thinking about it. This is especially true if you feel the interview did not go well. But this is precisely when you need to spend some time thinking about and evaluating the experience and your performance. Box 12.4 contains questions to ask yourself.

You may want to discuss your self-evaluation with someone you trust, such as your instructor, career services personnel, or a mentor. Friends and family members may also be able to provide insight and support. Use their feedback to create an improvement plan and practice, so you will feel more confident at the next interview.

When seeking help or discussing interviews with others, it is best not to make negative remarks about the interviewer or the facility. A friend may have a friend who works there, and your words, said in confidence, may be passed along to the wrong party.

If you are seeking advice about whether to accept a job you have doubts about, it is okay to discuss your concerns with someone you trust, but take care again not to disparage any individuals or the organization. Even if you believe you will receive a job offer, it is wise not to cancel or turn down other interviews until you are formally hired. Even if you did very well in your interview, things can happen that are beyond your control. For instance, the facility may plan to hire you, but the next day, your soon-to-be supervisor is informed of a company hiring freeze. You also never know what other candidates you are competing with. So, until you have a written offer, you should stay actively involved in the job search.

Thank-You Letter or Email

Whether the interview went like a dream or a nightmare, you should send a thank-you letter or email. Too many job seekers neglect this common courtesy, but it is a simple action that can set you apart from others and will keep you in the employer's mind when considering candidates. Suppose the employer interviewed nine people in two days. Your interviewer(s) may not be able to clearly remember each candidate and recall who said what. Receiving a thank-you email from you will leave an impression on them and potentially at a pivotal time when they are deciding on who to hire.

Thank-you letters or emails should be sent within 24 hours of the interview. Interviewers will be impressed when they receive your letter the very next day when your interview is still fresh in their minds.

In many cases, thank-you notes sent as an email are appropriate and becoming increasingly common. Take the same care you would with a written letter: include a salutation, write complete sentences, use correct grammar, spell all words correctly, and use a proper closing. Regardless of how you send the thank you, be sure the name and title of the person(s) who interviewed you are correct. Make sure you include every person who interviewed you if you did a panel interview.

If you know for sure that you do not want the job, send a thank-you letter anyway. Keep it simple, say something positive about the interview, and express your appreciation for the time taken to meet with you. Figure 12.6 is an example of a thank-you letter. In your thank-you letter, do not say that you are not interested in the job because you never know if you will change your mind or will apply for another job with them in the future. Additionally, the employer may know someone else who is hiring. Impressed by your follow-up, they may recommend you to a colleague or another clinic. Or another opening for a job that you do want may become available with the same employer.

Thank-You-Plus Letter

If you are truly interested in the job, take the time to write a thank-you-plus letter. The "plus" refers to a paragraph or two in which you do at least one of the following:

* Briefly summarize your qualifications in relation to the job as it was discussed in the interview.
* Point out specifically how you can make a positive contribution—again, based on the details you learned.

Let the employer know you want the job and hope to be the candidate selected. Include your full name and telephone number. Figure 12.7 shows an example of a thank-you-plus letter.

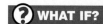 **WHAT IF?**

You just left an interview for a job you want. What might you say in your thank-you letter?

When to Follow Up

Following up after an interview is a kind of balancing act: you do not want to be considered a pest by calling too soon and too frequently. On the other hand, you took the time to attend the interview and you are eager to know when the hiring decision is made. Plus, following up may communicate interest in the job and perseverance, which are not bad things to convey to an employer.

1642 Windhill Way
San Antonio, TX 78220
October 18, 2010

Nancy Henderson, Office Manager
Craigmore Pediatric Clinic
4979 Coffee Road
San Antonio, TX 78229

Dear Ms. Henderson:

Thank you so much for the time you spent with me yesterday. You have a busy schedule, and I appreciate the time you took to describe the opening for a medical assistant at Craigmore Pediatric. The Clinic enjoys a good reputation in San Antonio for the services it provides children in the community, and it was a pleasure to learn more about it.

Sincerely,

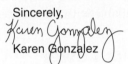

Karen Gonzalez

Figure 12.6 Simple Thank-You Letter.

The best strategy is to wait until the day after you were told a decision would be made. Call or send an email and inquire about the decision. If none has been made, ask when you might expect to hear. Be courteous and not pushy. Remember that every contact you have with the employer is part of the interview process, and courtesy counts. Never express impatience about a delay. You want to show interest but not pressure the employer for a decision they may not be ready to make. Sometimes the interviewer is deciding between two candidates, and the decision may be influenced by your follow-up.

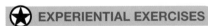 **EXPERIENTIAL EXERCISES**

1. Read the following articles, available online:
   - "How to Follow Up After a Job Interview" https://www.thebalancecareers.com/how-to-follow-up-after-a-job-interview-2061333
   - "Job Interview Follow-Up Do's and Don'ts" https://www.livecareer.com/interview/questions/interview-follow-up-dos-donts
   - "The Art of the Follow-Up After Job Interviews" https://www.livecareer.com/career/advice/interview/job-interview-follow-up
2. List what you think are the five most important actions to take following an interview.

1642 Windhill Way
San Antonio, TX 78220
October 18, 2010

Nancy Henderson, Office Manager
Craigmore Pediatric Clinic
4979 Coffee Road
San Antonio, TX 78229

Dear Ms. Henderson:

Thank you so much for the time you spent with me yesterday. You have a busy schedule, and I appreciate the time you took to describe the opening for a medical assistant at Craigmore Pediatric. The Clinic enjoys a good reputation in San Antonio for the services it provides children in the community, and it was a pleasure to learn more about it.

After visiting your facility and meeting the health professionals who work there, I sincerely believe I could make a positive contribution to your facility. My ability to communicate in both English and Spanish would allow me to work with patients from various cultural backgrounds. My previous experience working in a day care facility gave me a love for and understanding of children that enables me to work effectively with them. Finally, my organizational skills and knowledge of current insurance requirements would be of benefit in helping to develop the new billing system you described.

I am interested in this position and enthusiastic about working at Craigmore Pediatric. Please let me know if you need anything further from me. I can be reached at (210) 123-4567. I look forward to hearing from you.

Sincerely,

Karen Gonzalez

Karen Gonzalez

Figure 12.7 **Thank-You-Plus Letter.**

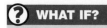
Considering a Job Offer

A job offer may be extended in a telephone call or at a second or even third interview. A job offer should never be considered official unless it is sent in a letter or email. The job offer should include the compensation amount, amount of vacation days and sick days, any benefits, and a start date.

Even if you feel quite sure that this is the right job, you still need to be sure that you have all the information needed to make a final decision. It is essential that you understand the following:

* The duties you will be required to perform. If you have not seen a written job description, ask for it now. If there is no written description, ask for a detailed oral explanation if this was not provided in the interview.
* The exact date and time you are to report for work.
* The days and hours you will work. Ask about the likelihood of required overtime and any change of hours or days that might take place in the future.
* Your salary. Earnings are expressed in various ways: hourly, weekly, biweekly, monthly, or annual rates. If you are quoted a rate that you are not familiar with, you might want to convert it to one you know. For example, if you are accustomed to thinking in terms of the amount per hour but are given a monthly salary, you may want to calculate the hourly equivalent. Annual bonuses are another form of remuneration that should be considered.
* Orientation and/or training given. This is especially important for recent graduates. Learning the customs and practices of the facility can make a big difference in your success.

You may have received all this information in the interview(s). Do not hesitate, however, to ask about anything you do not fully understand. It is far better to take the time now than to discover later that the job or working conditions are not what you expected. If you did not have an opportunity to see beyond the interviewer's office, you may want to ask for a tour of the facility and your potential workspace before deciding whether to accept the job.

Negotiating Salary

If you are offered the job, you will now need to evaluate the job offer, the amount of compensation, and any benefits that come with the position. Most career experts recommend that you not discuss salary with a potential employer until you have been offered the job. In many cases, this will not be an issue because salaries are often predetermined by the company and may not be negotiable. Some occupations, such as nursing, have labor unions, and the employer cannot change agreed-upon salaries for specific positions. In other cases, there may be a specified salary range for the position, and you can negotiate your pay within that range.

Doing your research before you attend an interview may provide you with this information. If a salary range for a position is given, the amount offered to you will most likely depend on the experience you bring to the job. Recent graduates tend to start at the lower end of a range, earning more as they gain experience. However, if you have experience or special skills that you think make you eligible for the higher end of the range, it does not hurt to negotiate.

When negotiating for a higher salary or hourly rate, be realistic. Keep in mind that, as a new graduate, you will most likely be starting in an entry-level position and the compensation may start in the lower pay range. This may be particularly difficult for students who have worked in other industries for many years, such as retail or food service, and are paid more. Often, changing to a new industry may require you to start over and build experience over time in order to make more money.

If you do not feel the pay aligns with your education, career level, skill set, and experience, you may choose to negotiate for more money. In general, there is no harm in asking as long as you are respectful and are prepared to accept a no. When negotiating, research industry salary or hourly rates for your profession and consider geographic location, education, years of experience, and certification when forming a response. It might also be helpful to answer the following question as a framework for your request: *Why do I feel I deserve a higher salary than the one the employer is offering?*

Once you have compiled all the support facts, you can either email the employer stating why you should receive a higher salary or schedule a time to speak with the employer on the phone. Do not be insulted or dejected if your request for higher compensation is denied. In many cases, an employer has a strict budget to maintain and may not have the flexibility to increase salaries. You must now make the decision if you should accept the job offer or not.

Understanding Benefits

Benefits can represent a significant portion of your compensation. Health insurance, for example, can cost hundreds of dollars per month for an individual and even more for a family. If full family coverage is offered by the employer, this may be worth thousands of dollars each year. Find out if you must pay part of the cost of the premiums and what type of coverage is provided. Health insurance for individuals (or families) is often more expensive than the group rates available through an employer. Health insurance is becoming an increasingly important benefit to consider when choosing where to work. There are other types of insurance, too, that can add value to the benefits package, including dental, vision, life, disability, and life insurance.

If you are planning to continue your education, tuition benefits might be important to you. Some employers cover all or part of educational expenses if the studies are related to your work and you receive a grade of C or better. Time off to take classes and workshops is an additional advantage. This benefit is especially helpful for health care professionals who are required to earn continuing education units on a regular basis. Some employers also offer student loan repayment benefits. Related professional expenses that some employers cover are the dues for professional organizations and required uniforms.

Other benefits to consider when calculating your overall compensation include the number of paid vacation, holiday, and personal or sick days offered and whether there is a retirement plan, such as a 401(k) plan. With an employer retirement plan, you choose an amount to be deducted from your earnings each pay period. You typically pay no taxes on this money until you withdraw it, usually after you reach the age of 59½. The money is invested, often in mutual funds. Some employers match the money you save up to a certain percentage. For example, an employer may match up to 6% of your earnings but allow you to contribute up to 50% of your salary. It is beneficial to, at least, contribute as much of your salary to match your employer's contribution.

When considering the compensation offered by an employer, think in terms of the total package. One job may offer a higher hourly rate but require you to pay part of your health insurance premium. You may end up financially ahead by accepting the lower salary if benefits are included, such as health insurance. On the other hand, if you are included in your spouse's group insurance plan, this might not be significant. Thus, salary should not be the sole factor for evaluating compensation, especially when comparing job offers.

Consider the following example of an entry-level job. Suppose you are offered Job A, which pays $30,000 and includes health insurance, for which the employer pays $7,000. The total value of this package then is $37,000. Another employer offers you Job B at $34,000 in salary with no insurance benefits. You need insurance and plan to pay for it yourself with the extra salary you will earn. If everything else about the two jobs is equal, which job would benefit you more financially? Although paid less, it is Job A, because:

1. You will pay less taxes since you will be taxed on wages of $30,000 rather than $34,000. (Health insurance benefits are not taxed.)
2. The $7,000 for medical insurance is the cost paid by the employer for a member of a group plan. If you buy insurance as an individual and not as a part of an employer-sponsored plan, it will likely cost you even more, with the average annual cost of almost $8,000 for individual coverage.

Job A

$30,000 − $12,000 (standard tax deduction and single exemption)	= $18,000 (taxable income)
$18,000 × 15%	= $2,700 (taxes)
$30,000 − $2,700	= **$27,300** (amount of money you keep)

Job B

$34,000 − $12,000	= $22,000 (taxable income)
$22,000 × 15%	= $3,300 (taxes)
$34,000 − $3,300	= $30,700
$30,700 − $8,000 (amount spent on health insurance)	= **$22,700** (amount of money you keep)

Note: This is only a basic example. The numbers are based on estimated insurance costs and simplified tax rates, as rates vary by state and income level.

Although this is a simplified example and not based on current tax rates and insurance costs and subsidies, it shows how important it is to thoroughly evaluate and do the math when comparing job offers. The lesson here is to collect as much information as you can and consider all aspects of the compensation plan for each offer you receive.

Is This the Job for You?

Jobs are usually not offered on the spot during the first interview. If this does happen to you, it is a good idea to ask when a decision is needed and say that you are very interested but need time to make a decision. You may also want time to negotiate salary and benefits. You should not feel pressured to immediately accept a job.

Interviewers will usually give you a time range during which a hiring decision will be made. You, too, need to make a decision—is this the job for me? Many factors will influence your decision. Box 12.5 contains questions to help you select an appropriate job.

Although you should consider these questions carefully, remember that a perfect job that has everything you want is rare for your first job. Finding the right job for you is a matter of finding a close match on the most important elements, which may include the commute to and from your home, flexible schedule, and career advancement opportunities. You are starting a new career, and there are certain factors that will help your long-term success. Working with someone who is interested in teaching you, for example, may be a better choice than choosing a slightly higher-paying position that offers no opportunities for acquiring new skills. Many health care facilities make it a practice to promote from within. If there is a facility where you want to work, consider taking a job that gets you in the door.

BOX 12.5

Questions to Guide Your Job-Selection Process

Here are some questions to guide your thinking about the specific job and facility in which you will be working:

1. Do the job duties match my skills and interests?
2. How closely do the job and facility match my work preferences?
3. Does the facility appear to follow safe and ethical practices?
4. Do I agree with the mission and values of the organization?
5. Could I make a positive contribution?
6. Who are the clients/patients? Will I enjoy working with them?
7. How well do I think I would fit in?
8. Are there opportunities to learn?
9. Will there be opportunities for advancement?
10. Can I commit to the required schedule?
11. Is the management style compatible with my work style?
12. How did the facility "feel"?

As a new graduate, it is important to not wait too long before accepting a job. The longer you wait, the more you may need to explain to a potential employer why you waited so long. Employers may also worry that your skills may not be honed and that you will be out of practice if you wait too long. Even if you are offered a job that is less than ideal, getting experience is critical at this stage.

The Job Offer

When you accept a job, express your appreciation and enthusiasm. In addition to responding orally, write a letter of acceptance. The letter should include a summary of what you understand to be the terms of employment.

When speaking with the employer, inquire about any necessary follow-up activities. It is also a good idea to disclose any future commitments or other factors that will affect your work. For example, if your son is scheduled for surgery next month or you have a planned vacation, this is the time to disclose it. You may need to request that your start date is later. However, you should be prepared for the chance that the employer may rescind the job offer if they need someone to start soon.

You may want the job but still need to negotiate some conditions. For example, suppose the work hours are 8:00 a.m. to 5:00 p.m. You have a 3-year-old child who cannot be left at day care before 7:45 a.m., and it takes at least 25 minutes to drive to work. It is better to ask if you can work from 8:30 a.m. to 5:30 p.m. than to take the position and arrive late every day. Many problems on the job can be avoided by discussing them openly and in advance. However, accommodations like this are not always possible if they disrupt the facility's schedule and patient flow. You may want to have a "Plan B" that will enable you to meet the employer's needs and your own, such as having someone reliable who can take your child to day care.

Turning Down a Job Offer

After careful consideration, you may decide not to accept a job offer. It may be because you decided to accept another job offer or the conditions of employment were not right for you. Regardless, there is a proper method to declining a job offer. If you end up declining the offer, it is important to do so in a friendly and professional manner. After all, you never know what opportunities they may have available for you in the future.

It is not necessary to explain your reasons to the employer. But do express your appreciation and thank them for the opportunity to interview with them. This will leave a positive impression on employers. You may want to work at this facility in the future, or the employer may have connections with other facilities or organizations you wish to apply to. Additionally, most health care communities are tight-knit, and they will likely know each other. So, you do not want to get a bad reputation in the community or burn any bridges, as the expression goes.

What to Expect

Once you are hired, employers can ask questions that were previously unacceptable during the interview process. Information that cannot be used to make hiring decisions is often necessary to complete personnel requirements. Examples include the following:

1. Provide proof of your age (to ensure you are of legal age to work).
2. Provide verification that you can work legally in the United States.
3. Identify your race (for affirmative action statistics, if applicable in your state).
4. Supply a photograph (for identification).
5. State your marital status and the number and ages of your children (for insurance).
6. Give the name and address of a relative (for notification in case of emergency).
7. Provide your Social Security number (for tax purposes).

There may be mandatory health tests and immunizations. In addition, some employers may require drug tests and criminal background checks for all employees.

If you are asked to sign an employment contract, read it carefully first. As with all other employment issues, ask about anything you do not understand. Ask for a copy of anything you sign, and keep it in your personal files.

If You Do Not Get the Job

The secret of life is to fall seven times and to get up eight times.

—Paulo Coelho

It can be disappointing when you are not selected for a job you really want. Although it may feel like a personal rejection, there are many reasons why applicants do not get hired. Some are beyond your control, such as:

* Another applicant had more experience or skills that more closely met the employer's current needs.
* An employee in the organization decided to apply for the job. Internal hires, or hiring a current employee, are often preferred over external hires.
* Budget cuts or other unexpected events prevented anyone from being hired at this time.

On the other hand, you may have lost this opportunity for reasons you can change. How do you know? First, do an honest and objective evaluation of your interview. Are you presenting yourself in the best possible way? Second, look over the list in Box 12.6. Health care employers and career services personnel name these as major reasons why job applicants fail to get hired. Do you recognize anything that might apply to you? Third, ask the interviewer for feedback. This may be difficult to ask for and to hear, but it may be the best assessment of your performance during the interview. In some cases, your career services personnel may be able to contact the employers on your behalf to find out how you might improve on future interviews. Employers are sometimes more willing to share reasons with school personnel than candidates so that school staff can better assist their students. Be willing to listen to any constructive criticism offered and make any needed changes.

You must be honest with yourself and commit to improving your attitude and/or job search skills. If necessary, seek advice from your instructor, career services personnel, or a mentor. The job search process can be discouraging at times but remember that your education and training have equipped you with the necessary qualifications to find employment in the health care field. It is common for people to interview

---

BOX 12.6

Why Job Applicants Fail to Get Hired

1. Failure to sell themselves by clearly presenting their skills and qualifications
2. Too much interest in what is in it for them rather than what they can contribute
3. Unprofessional behavior or lack of courtesy
4. Lack of enthusiasm and interest in the job
5. Poor appearance
6. Poor communication skills
7. Unrealistic job expectations
8. Negative or critical attitude
9. Arriving late, bringing children or the person who provided transportation, or demonstrating poor organizational skills

multiple times before receiving a job offer. Also, remember that interviewing is just like any other skill. Practice, evaluate, and practice some more. Try to stay positive and seek support from friends and family members if you are feeling down.

Although you may not feel enthusiastic about writing a letter to an employer who chooses another applicant, consider this: you may have come in close second. The next opening may be yours. In fact, the employer may contact you again with the same or another job opportunity. So, take a few moments and demonstrate your high level of professionalism by thanking the employer and letting them know that you are still interested in working for the organization in the future if another opportunity becomes available.

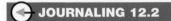

JOURNALING 12.2

If I do not get the job I want, what can I learn from the experience?

CASE STUDY 12.2

Jessica was really excited when she received the phone call yesterday from Blaine Clinic asking her to come in for an interview. This clinic had a reputation as a great place to work, and she had dropped off her resume there last week. She had learned through doing research on the clinic that it had several specialties and that there were advancement opportunities for employees.

She was surprised, then, by what happened at her interview. After arriving a few minutes early for her 10:30 appointment, she had to wait until almost 11:00 before Dr. Spader, the director of the department who is looking to hire a medical administrative assistant, asked her into his office. As soon as she had introduced herself and sat down, the phone rang. Dr. Spader took the call and was brief, but this was only the beginning of many interruptions to their interview. The phone rang several more times, staff members knocked on the door, and some employees just walked into Dr. Spader's office without knocking.

Jessica could see that Dr. Spader was stressed. He looked harried and apologized many times for the interruptions. Jessica tried her best to stay calm and answer his questions in ways that presented her as a good candidate for the job. Sometimes, she lost her train of thought when an interruption occurred, but she would smile, take a breath, and continue. Dr. Spader seemed to understand that this was difficult for her.

That evening, Jessica thought about the interview and the clinic. It looked very busy with patients and staff coming and going, especially in the department where she interviewed. She was still interested in working there, despite the interview not going as smoothly as she expected. She spent some time thinking about Dr. Spader and how stressed and apologetic he was. She did not know whether to be annoyed or sympathetic.

The next day, she remembered what she had learned in her job search class: focus on the employer's *needs*. Obviously, there were problems in the department resulting in his not having the time to interview job candidates in a quiet environment. Jessica decided she really had nothing to lose and decided to write a thank-you letter that included her observations and how she could help. She had always been an organized person, and she mentioned this in her letter. Of course, she did not say she thought the department was disorganized, but she did mention how busy Dr. Spader seemed to be and that she knew her organizational skills could be a great help with his obviously heavy workload. Wording her letter carefully, Jessica included a couple of specific suggestions based on what she saw and heard during the interview.

QUESTIONS FOR THOUGHT AND REFLECTION

1. What do you think of Jessica's strategy in writing a thank-you-plus letter?
2. How would you have handled the situation during the interview?

Sarah and Jessica were classmates and graduated together. Sarah did well in the medical administrative assistant program, and she prides herself on being punctual and organized. She and Jessica both received interviews with Dr. Spader at Blaine Clinic. Like Jessica's, Sarah's interview was interrupted by constant phone calls and staff asking Dr. Spader questions. Despite Dr. Spader's apologies for the interruptions, Sarah believes he was being inconsiderate and rude by not focusing his time on the interview. She finally tells Dr. Spader that she is finding it difficult to concentrate, saying, "Wow! It's really crazy here. Is it always this disorganized? The staff doesn't seem to know what they're doing."

The situation does not improve, however, and by the time Sarah leaves, she is truly annoyed. "What a madhouse," she tells her boyfriend, Mike, after the interview. "They could really use my organizational skills. Maybe Dr. Spader heard enough of what I said about myself to realize what a good employee I'd be."

"You're kidding, right?" asked Mike incredulously. "Why would you want to work in a place like that? Wouldn't it drive you crazy?"

"Probably. But that's only one department. The clinic has a good reputation, and they do pay well. I'm thinking if I just got my foot in the door, I could get to know people in the other departments and just get a transfer as soon as possible," Sarah explained.

"That's smart," said Mike. "You're always thinking ahead. So, are you going to drop him a note and thank him for the so-called interview?"

"That would be a waste of time. He'd probably just lose it!" she laughed. "Besides, it's not like I have anything to thank him for. That interview was awful."

QUESTIONS FOR THOUGHT AND REFLECTION

1. Do you think Sarah's feelings are valid? How about her reaction?
2. What do you think of Sarah's reasons for wanting the job?
3. How do you think Dr. Spader and his staff interpreted Sarah's behavior and comments during the interview?

References

Anderson R, Barbara A, Feldman S. *What patients want: a content analysis of key qualities that influence patient satisfaction.* 2009. Retrieved July 28, 2015, from www.drscore.com/press/papers/whatpatientswant.pdf.

Cha AE. Employers relying on personality tests to screen applicants. *Washington Post.* March 27, 2005. Page A01. http://www.washingtonpost.com/wpdyn/content/article/2005/03/26/AR2005032605181.html (accessed July 28, 2015).

Graber S. *The everything online job search book.* Holbrook, MA: Adams Media; 2000.

Hansen K. *Behavioral interviewing strategies for job-seekers.* www.quintcareers.com/behavioral_interviewing.html (accessed July 28, 2015).

Lock RD. *Job search: career planning guide, book II.* ed 3. Pacific Grove, CA: Brooks/Cole; 1996.

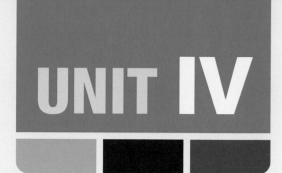

UNIT **IV**

PROFESSIONAL SKILLS AND DEVELOPMENT

Ready for Work

BY THE END OF THIS CHAPTER, YOU WILL BE ABLE TO	
	■ Explain the Different Members on a Health Care Team
	■ Discuss How Scope of Practice Relates to Each Health Care Provider and Professional
	■ Understand the Behavioral Skills of a Health Care Professional
	■ Understand How Your Appearance Affects Your Success
	■ Know How to Represent Your Employer to Customers and Patients
	■ Demonstrate Good Grooming and Personal Hygiene

The Health Care Team

No one can whistle a symphony. It takes a whole orchestra to play it.

—H. E. Luccock

LEARNING OBJECTIVE 1: THE HEALTH CARE TEAM

■ Explain the title of "doctor" and which professions can use that title.
■ Define what other professionals may be a part of the health care team.
■ Discuss how scope of practice relates to being a health care professional.

As there are many different types of health care settings and facilities, there are even more different functions and roles on a health care team. Depending on the size of the practice or organization, a variety of qualified and trained professionals are needed to fill both clinical and nonclinical staff roles and duties. The clinical side of health care is involved in diagnosing and treating patients. The administrative or nonclinical staff is instrumental in receiving and scheduling patients, coordinating the practice's daily activities and operations, and billing for visits.

As you prepare for your new profession, it will be helpful for you to understand the different members on a health care team. You may work with many of them or even report to some of them. Being able to understand the different positions and roles and their functions will help you perform your job better in your future profession.

Physicians

Physicians are the primary providers of medical care to patients. Becoming a physician requires advanced education or a doctorate degree as a Medical Doctor

(MD) or Doctor of Osteopathic Medicine (DO); as a result, they are commonly referred to as "doctor." Less common than a Medical Doctor, a Doctor of Osteopathic Medicine, or an osteopathic doctor, has educational requirements similar to those of a Medical Doctor. Both MDs and DOs are licensed physicians and must pass state board examinations to become licensed to practice medicine in their state. Additionally, DOs learn the skill of manipulation therapy as part of their training.

Physicians diagnose illnesses and prescribe and administer treatment for people suffering from injury or disease. They examine patients; obtain medical histories; and order, perform, and interpret diagnostic tests. They counsel patients on diet, hygiene, and preventive health care (Figure. 13.1).

An important role of the physician is to create an individualized care plan for the patient. In general, the patient's care plan includes an accurate and comprehensive assessment of the patient's health status, a problems list of the medical diagnoses, and the treatment plan. The purpose of the care plan is to guide all who are involved in the care of the patient—other physicians, nurses, or medical assistants—through a plan to appropriately care and treat the patient to ensure that the patient's continuity of care is complete. This care plan will be included in the patient's medical records for proper documentation, which will also be necessary for insurance and medical billing for services rendered.

Additionally, physicians can specialize in different fields of medicine, such as cardiology, dermatology, or surgery. Becoming a specialist requires additional education and training. All types of health care professionals will work with physicians in some capacity.

Surgeons

Surgeons are specialized types of physicians who treat injuries and diseases through operations, although they often perform many of the same duties as other physicians. Using invasive surgical procedures, surgeons are able to correct physical deformities, repair bone and tissue after injuries, and perform preventive surgeries on patients with debilitating diseases or disorders. Additionally, some surgeons may choose to specialize in a specific area of surgery, such as orthopedic surgery or plastic or reconstructive surgery.

Other Doctors

In addition to doctors with MDs and DOs, there are several other health care professionals who are designated as "doctors." In general, any person who has a doctorate degree is addressed as "doctor" in a professional setting, such as a hospital, medical office, or college. The abbreviation for doctor is "Dr." In the health care field, the title of "Dr." indicates a person who is qualified to practice medicine. In other fields, the title of "Dr." means that a person has completed the highest education degree in their field. Table 13.1 lists examples of other types of doctors.

A Doctor of Chiropractic (DC), commonly called a chiropractor, is trained in the manipulation of the spinal column and other areas of the body (Figure 13.2). Becoming a DC requires 2 years of premedical studies and 4 years of training in a licensed chiropractic school.

A Naturopathic Medical Doctor (ND or NMD) focuses on holistic and preventative health care. A naturopathic doctor is a licensed primary care physician, who is trained to diagnose and prescribe

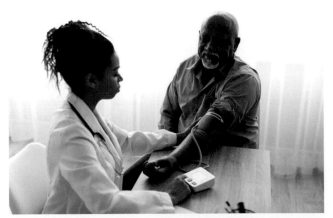

Figure 13.1 A physician plays an important role in managing patient's health. (Stock photo ID: 1374577605.)

TABLE 13.1
Examples of Different Types of Doctors

Degrees	Abbreviations
Doctor of Chiropractic	DC
Doctor of Dental Medicine	DMD
Doctor of Dental Surgery	DDS
Doctor of Education	EdD
Doctor of Medicine	MD
Doctor of Naturopathy	ND
Doctor of Optometry	OD
Doctor of Osteopathy	DO
Doctor of Philosophy	PhD
Doctor of Podiatric Medicine	DPM

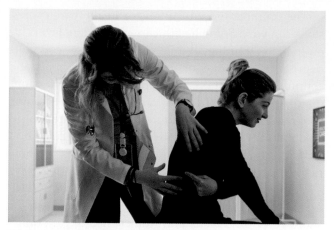

Figure 13.2 A doctor of chiropractic performing a spinal adjustment. (Stock photo ID:1070099076.)

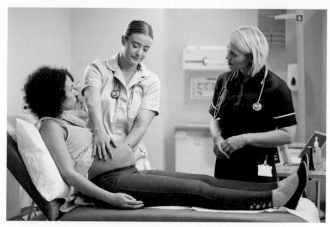

Figure 13.3 Nurses may specialize in many different fields. (Stock photo ID:1056977996.)

treatment, as with other physicians, but emphasizes naturopathic medicine and the use of natural healing agents, such as food, herbs, and water. Some states currently do not regulate naturopathic medicine as a medical profession.

Nurses

A nurse is a health care professional who provides care to patients. The nurse's responsibilities and duties are extensive and include performing physical examinations and health histories; providing health promotion, counseling, and education; administering medications; wound care; and numerous other medical interventions.

Nurses may also coordinate care, based on the care plan created by the physician, and direct and supervise care delivered by other health care staff. Although nurses may share similar duties to a physician, nurses, in general, do not require as much education and do not receive as extensive medical education or training. As a result, nurses have a more limited scope of practice, authority, and responsibility in patient care compared with physicians. However, some nurses with advanced training may be able to interpret patient information, diagnose illnesses and diseases, prescribe medication, and make critical decisions about patient care.

As the demand for patient care expands, this has allowed the nursing profession to expand and specialize in different fields, such as critical care, anesthesiology, pain management, and midwifery (Figure. 13.3).

Although most nurses work in hospitals, a large number of nurses work in different settings and fields, such as schools or hospices. Other nonhospital nursing careers include nurse-midwife, forensic nurse, nurse educator, school nurse, academic nurse writer, and legal nurse consultant. Some nurses may even

travel around the United States as traveling nurses or travel to the patient's home to provide health care.

Other Health Care Professionals

Health care professionals, sometime called allied health professionals, include jobs that fall outside the traditional health care professions, such as physician, nurses, pharmacists, and dentists. Health care professionals is a broad term and defined as a large cluster of health care–related professions and personnel whose functions include assisting, facilitating, or complementing the work of physicians and other health care providers in the health care system.

According to the Association of Schools of Allied Health Professions, there are more than 100 different types of health care professions comprising 5 million or approximately 60% of all health care professionals (Figure. 13.4). Careers in the health care field involve many types of duties and responsibilities.

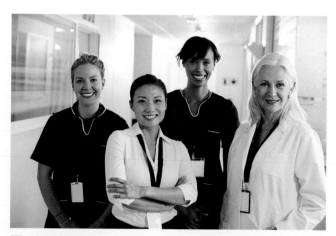

Figure 13.4 There are more than 100 different health care professions. (Stock photo ID:1147980009.)

The most common method of categorizing the many different health care professions is based on the National Career Clusters Framework, created by the Career and Technical Education (CTE), which is a national nonprofit that represents secondary, post-secondary, and adult career education. This framework was developed to define the body of knowledge and specific skills health care workers are expected to possess for entry-level and technical-level positions. These core standards are used by schools, colleges, and health care facilities to establish curriculum and competencies for a wide variety of professions. The National Career Clusters Framework describes 16 Career Clusters and represents more than 79 different Career Pathways with similar knowledge and skill sets.

The Health Science Career Cluster outlines the knowledge and skills necessary for a career that promotes health, wellness, and diagnosis, and treats injuries and diseases. Some careers involve working directly with people, while others involve research into diseases or collecting and formatting data and information. The health care career may allow a person to work in hospitals, medical or dental offices, laboratories, communities, or medivac units.

The Health Sciences Career Cluster focuses on planning, managing, and providing therapeutic services, diagnostic services, health informatics, support services, and biotechnology research and development. There five different pathways under the Health Sciences Career Cluster are described in Table 13.2. Figure. 13.5 provides examples of careers for each pathway.

The training and education for health care professions can vary. Some health care professionals receive on-the-job training, while others must complete degrees or diplomas or get certified credentials and continuing education. Most health care professions may require completion of an education or training program that is several months to 2 or 4 years long at a community, career, vocational, or 4-year college. A growing number of health care professions are now requiring a bachelor-level or graduate-level degree.

Employment in the health care industry is estimated to grow due to a variety of reasons. With the shortage of physicians and nurses, health care delivery will rely more heavily on health care professionals providing medical care and services. In addition, the demand for many of these professions is expected to increase as hospitals and clinics adopt more innovative health care delivery models that depend on health care staff to help coordinate care and to be compliant in the use of electronic medical records and health information exchange, particularly for medical assistants, physician assistants, health information technology staff, physical therapist, nursing assistants, and home health and personal care aides.

Scope of Practice

As a result, many stakeholders, including state legislators, are looking to broaden the roles of some licensed health care professionals to meet the demand for health services. By expanding the authority or "scope of practice," many health care professionals may be able to perform additional procedures and treatments

TABLE 13.2
National Career Clusters Framework – Five Career Pathways

Pathways	Categories
Therapeutic Services Pathway	Provides treatment over time and includes such providers as physicians, dentists, veterinarians, nurses, pharmacologists, and emergency personnel
Diagnostic Services	Provides a picture of the patient's health status and includes technicians in radiology, medical, dental laboratory, and cardiography
Health Informatics	Processes data and provides documents; these include administration, secretaries, and medical records personnel
Support Services	Provides a supportive environment for the patient and includes nutrition services, central supply, and facility management personnel
Biotechnology Research & Development	Provide research in bioscience to develop new treatments, medications, and tests. These professionals include biochemists, bioinformatics scientists, cell biologists, and pharmaceutical scientists

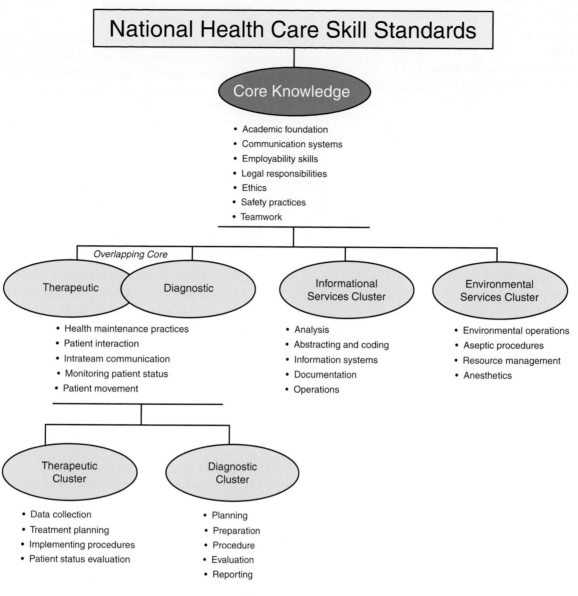

National Health Care Skill Standards

Core Knowledge

- Academic foundation
- Communication systems
- Employability skills
- Legal responsibilities
- Ethics
- Safety practices
- Teamwork

Overlapping Core

Therapeutic **Diagnostic** **Informational Services Cluster** **Environmental Services Cluster**

- Health maintenance practices
- Patient interaction
- Intrateam communication
- Monitoring patient status
- Patient movement

- Analysis
- Abstracting and coding
- Information systems
- Documentation
- Operations

- Environmental operations
- Aseptic procedures
- Resource management
- Anesthetics

Therapeutic Cluster **Diagnostic Cluster**

- Data collection
- Treatment planning
- Implementing procedures
- Patient status evaluation

- Planning
- Preparation
- Procedure
- Evaluation
- Reporting

Courtesy WestEd, SanFranciso, Calif.

Figure 13.5 The Health Sciences Career Cluster from the National Career Clusters Framework. (From National Health Care Skill Standards (1995) by Sri Ananda and Joan DaVanzo. Used by permission from WestEd.)

to help alleviate shortages of other health professionals and providers, including physicians. For example, several states have passed legislation for physician assistants to provide care without a physician being present and for nurse practitioners to practice without physician oversight.

Proponents of expanding the "scope of practice" argue that these licensed health care professionals can be trained quicker and less expensively than physicians without compromising safety and quality. However, some physicians' groups disagree, arguing that the more intensive and extensive physician training better equips them to diagnose more accurately and treat patients more safely.

Modeling Professional Behavior

Sticks and stones may break our bones, but words will break our hearts.

—**Robert Fulghum**

LEARNING OBJECTIVE 2: MODELING PROFESSIONAL BEHAVIOR

- Understand your role in the support and success of the organization where you work.
- Identify behavioral clues of your co-workers.

- Make introductions easily and smoothly.
- Understand the importance of titles and positions.
- Build your conversation skills.
- Learn to be on time and to be discreet.
- Practice the little courtesies that make a big difference.
- Create a positive reputation for yourself.

Professional behavior is the actions and conduct that support and build positive relationships with others. Professional behavior has many important purposes. The first purpose of professional behavior and conduct is customer care and service. To each client, patient, or family member you interact with, you *are* the company you work for. In many cases, you may be the first, last, or the only employee a patient or client meets from your organization. As a result, much of your customers' judgment about your employer will be based on their judgment of *you*.

The second purpose of professional behavior is to create a positive work environment for you and your colleagues. Each employee must be accountable for maintaining a professional workplace. A sense of professional behavior contributes to the smooth flow of operations in a work environment. This is especially important in a health care setting, which is often stressful and chaotic. Professional behavior and conduct contribute to clear and respectful communication, mutual support, and, ultimately, the delivery of quality patient care. This also requires flexibility and open-mindedness and contributes to a work environment that is safe, accepting of cultural differences, and free from inappropriate and abusive behavior. For example, today's workplace is incredibly diverse and comprises four generations of workers, due to people living and working longer. You must be able to step outside of your generation and interact professionally with people of all ages. What used to be "appropriate" or the norm 30 years ago may not be appropriate professional behavior now. In addition to working alongside people of different ages, you will likely encounter clients and colleagues from different ethnic, national, cultural, and socioeconomic backgrounds. Regardless of their backgrounds, you must conduct yourself at all times in a professional manner and treat each person with respect.

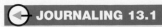

Recall the last time you sought health care, whether at a walk-in clinic, a dentist's office, or a physical therapy appointment. Describe your impression of the facility. Recall the employees you interacted with. How were you treated? How did these interactions contribute to the overall impression you have of the facility?

Skills to Improve Your Professional Behavior

Professional Conversations at Work

The "rules" of professional conversation should generally be the same regardless of where you work. How you conduct workplace conversations can set the tone for professional relationships. In the health care setting where people work closely together, conversations about nonwork topics are not only common but also practical and beneficial, as long as the topics are appropriate. Conversation builds relationships and comradery between co-workers and makes work more enjoyable and rewarding. Much of the richness in life has to do with the quantity and quality of friendships you have in your life, and conversation leads to the creation and maintenance of friendship.

Many people are natural conversationalists, whereas others struggle with feeling like they lack good conversation skills. However, like any skills, conversation skills can be developed. Virtually anybody can become a better conversationalist by mindfully following a few strategies and techniques. For instance, avoid debating or arguing and, instead, focus on positive topics. Try not to dominate the conversation but ensure that you are actively contributing to the conversation. Conversation will be easiest when you are genuinely interested in the other person or topic. Who is this person and what can I learn about them?

I keep six honest serving-men
(They taught me all I knew);
Their names are What and Why and When
and How and Where and Who.

—Rudyard Kipling

Interestingly, the best conversationalists are often the ones who speak the least and are good listeners. People generally like to talk about themselves, especially if they have an interested listener (Figure. 13.6). Try to give the other person your full attention during

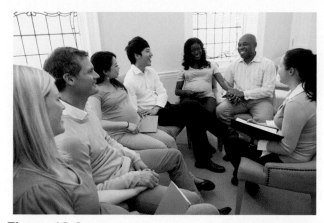

Figure 13.6 The best conversationalist includes being a good listener. (Copyright © istock.com.)

the conversation. It works the other way around, as well. When you are asked an open-ended question, which is a question that requires more than a short "yes" or "no" answer, you will generally be able to create a back-and-forth exchange that will go beyond simple pleasantries. When you feel comfortable, do not be afraid to reveal something about yourself. When you share something about yourself, trust develops, and friendships can form.

You should try to discuss topics you are familiar with. Common conversation topics include books, movies, sports, travel, food, music, and hobbies. However, try to avoid discussing controversial issues at work, such as politics, religion, immigration, abortion, or overly personal matters. For example, regardless of how close you are to your co-worker, it is always inappropriate to discuss your or your co-worker's sex life. Confiding too much may compromise not only your confidentiality but also your spouse's or partner's. Further, this type of conversation may cross the line into sexual harassment, which may result in legal issues for the company and the employee involved. It is also recommended to not discuss pay, how much you are paid, or your financial situation.

Respecting Professional and Personal Titles

In a health care setting, it is important to understand and acknowledge your co-workers' positions and accomplishments by using professional titles. This is most apparently demonstrated when using introductions. It is important to know how to properly introduce people to one another using proper salutations and their appropriate titles, to show respect and professionalism.

Professional Titles

As discussed earlier, physicians should generally be addressed and introduced as "doctor," often abbreviated with "Dr." Even if you are on a first-name basis with a physician, you should still refer to this person as "doctor," especially in front of patients and other physicians.

In fact, any health professional who has earned a doctorate degree in their profession should be addressed as Doctor. Thus, an audiologist with a PhD or AuD, a nurse with a PhD or DNSc, and a pharmacist with a PharmD should be called Doctor. The title often refers to a physician, and some patients may be confused by that. You can always clarify the role or title of the health professional to a patient by explaining the person's title or role. For example, you can say, "Dr. Appleton is the Assistant Director of Nursing here." Or "Dr. Harris manages the Speech Therapy Department."

Needless to say, when you are introduced to someone with a "Dr." in their name, whether the person is a physician or any other health care professional with a doctorate degree, they may use their first name in their response. This is not usually an invitation to call the doctor by their first name. For example, if you are introduced like this: "Dr. Tolland, this is Jim Holtz, the new medical assistant," and she says, "Hi Jim, I'm Monica Tolland. Welcome aboard," this may be her warm greeting and not necessarily an invitation for you to call her by her first name, unless she specifically says so. You should reply, "Thank you, Dr. Tolland. It's nice to meet you." Even if the physician encourages the usage of her first name, it is recommended that you still refer to the physician as "Dr." in the presence of patients, unless specifically told otherwise.

For nonphysicians and other health care providers or professionals, depending on your clinic, you may use the title of "Mr.," "Mrs.," or "Ms." followed by their last name or even first name. For example, you may introduce the registered nurse to a patient as "Ms. Tammy, the nurse, should be in shortly to talk to you about your medication." Figure. 13.7 provides a helpful diagram of appropriate uses of titles in the health care setting. Protocols for making proper introductions are summarized in Box 13.1.

Personal Titles

How do you know which feminine title to use when addressing women in the workplace? Women without doctoral degrees should be addressed as "Ms." unless you are specifically told otherwise. The use of "Miss"

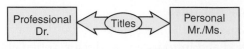

Figure 13.7 Professional and personal titles.

Doctors and health professionals with doctorate degrees. Refer to these professionals using their title and last name.

Health professionals without doctorate degrees. The use of Miss or Mrs. to indicate relationship status is outdated unless specified by your practice.

Figure 13.7 Professional and personal titles.

BOX 13.1

Protocols for Introductions

- As the customer, the client or patient is *always* the most important person, so they should be introduced first.
- Every health care professional with a doctorate degree should be introduced with the title *Doctor*.
- You can clarify the introduction by explaining the roles of the people you are introducing. This can be especially important in clarifying the role of a health care professional who has a doctoral degree but is not a physician.
- Never address, refer to, or introduce a doctor by their first name, unless you are specifically told to do so.

and "Mrs." to indicate whether a woman is married is somewhat antiquated, and it makes assumptions about a female colleague's marital status. The marital status or relationship status of any colleague—male or female—is irrelevant at work and not something that needs to be disclosed or known for an effective working relationship to take place.

This should generally be the case when you are addressing or introducing a patient; "Mr." and "Ms." should be used. However, some patients, particularly older patients, may find it offensive to be referred to as "Ms." Since marital status is documented in the patients' medical records, use "Mrs." when you know the patient is married. When in doubt, you can ask the patient what she prefers to be called.

Examples of introduction are:

"Mr. Adler, this is Dr. Berthold, the physician on duty today. Dr. Berthold, this is Saul Adler."

"Ms. Christy, this is Ms. Izzo, the Radiological Technician. Ms. Izzo, this is Callie Christy."

Introductions can be confusing at times, and mistakes will occur. For some health care professionals and patients who identify as nonbinary or gender fluid, where they do not identify as male or female, using these terms may cause some discomfort,

confusion, and misunderstandings. For patients, these situations can be avoided by checking the patient's chart. Many electronic health records systems now include a self-identification approach to better capture patient information (Box 13.2). In addition to collecting gender identity data, asking patients to include the name they want the health care team to use as well as the correct pronouns to use is also recommended. Collecting accurate gender identity data in electronic health records is essential to providing high-quality, patient-centered care and is recommended by both

BOX 13.2

Collecting Sexual Orientation and Gender Identity Information

Sexual Orientation

Do you think of yourself as:
- Straight or heterosexual
- Lesbian or gay
- Bisexual
- Queer, pansexual, and/or questioning
- Something else, please specify: _____
- Don't know
- Decline to answer

Gender Identity

Do you think of yourself as:
- Male
- Female
- Transgender man/transman/female-to-male (FTM)
- Transgender woman/transwoman/male-to-female (MTF)
- Genderqueer/gender nonconforming (neither exclusively male nor female)
- Additional gender category (or other); please specify: _____
- Decline to answer

What sex was originally listed on your birth certificate?
- Male
- Female
- Decline to answer

Name and Pronouns

What is your name as you would like it to appear on your health records?

What are your pronouns?
- He/him
- She/her
- They/them
- Other:_____

the National Academy of Medicine and The Joint Commission.

? WHAT IF?

1. *What if you have to introduce someone, but you are not sure of this person's title or role?*
2. *What if you have to make an introduction, but you forgot the name of someone you are supposed to know?*
3. *What if you need to introduce a colleague but this person's name is difficult to pronounce?*

Reliability in the Workplace

Reliability is essential to your performance as an employee, as well as to your ability to maintain your job. Reliability is the ability of an employee to show up to work on time and be prepared to complete work in a timely manner. Ask yourself: Can people count on me? Can I accomplish tasks on time and discreetly?

For one thing, punctuality is absolutely essential in health care. An efficient and effective patient workflow depends on each team member arriving as scheduled and getting things done on time. Health care professionals and patients usually work on an appointment basis, and co-workers who have put in a full shift expect to be relieved on time. Thus, not arriving on time or not performing your duties negatively affects everyone around you. For example, many tasks have to be performed on a strict schedule. Vital signs may need to be taken at precise intervals. Input and output charts must be performed and accurately documented in a timely basis. Meals are usually served at specific times. Breaks are scheduled at specific times to ensure a smooth workflow, while giving every employee a break from their routine.

The reliability of individual workers has a tremendous effect on the performance of the entire health care team and affects patient outcomes. Ensuring that you are doing your job in a timely manner reduces the potential for harmful mistakes in patient care. For example, Dr. Sanders asks you to renew the prescription for Mr. Tang's antihypertensive medication, and you forget to add it to his medical records. What are the repercussions from that?

Politeness and Courtesies

The simplest acts of courtesy can create a positive impression and attract people to you with very little effort. For example, a smile and looking directly at the person are among the most open and welcoming gestures you can make to create a positive environment (Figure. 13.8). Similarly, saying *please* when you ask for something, whether it be information, some help with a task, advice, or some teaching, is all it usually takes to get positive results. Afterward, thanking people for their help makes them glad they gave it, strengthens the relationships, and paves the way for future assistance.

Another easy gesture of courtesy that can go a long way is addressing people by their names occasionally when you are speaking with them. Dale Carnegie, who wrote *How to Make Friends and Influence People*, said that no sound is more pleasing to a person than the sound of one's own name.

> *Practice random acts of kindness and senseless acts of beauty.*
>
> —Anne Herbert

"Practicing random acts of kindness" and "paying it forward" are two concepts from popular culture that express the idea that if you do something nice for someone with no expectation of ever being repaid for it, two things will happen. First, the world will be a better place. Second, good things will come back to you. At work, your kindnesses will make your workplace a better place for everyone, and your reputation for kindness will be noticed and most likely returned to you.

Tackling Bad Days at Work

Some days will be tougher than others. However, regardless of what is causing the bad day, whether it is a personal problem or a troubling issue at work, how you respond to it with professional behavior will determine what kind of employee you will be.

> *A smooth sea never made a skilled sailor.*
>
> —Franklin D. Roosevelt

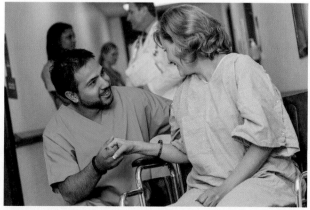

Figure 13.8 A nurse greets a patient with a smile. (Copyright © istock.com.)

Tackling Your Own Bad Days

If *you* are experiencing a bad day, you can try several strategies for maintaining a positive and professional approach at work:

* **Let work be therapeutic for you.** Even on the worst day, there are many positive aspects of work, such as the people you enjoy seeing or specific activities you like performing. Consider focusing on your work as a means of pushing your other problems and concerns to the back of your mind.
* **Act "as if..."** Even if you don't feel like it, sometimes you have to act the way you wish you felt. Act *as if* you are happy to be at work. Act *as if* you are enthusiastic. Force yourself to smile. Chances are that your actions will start affecting your mood, and your day will improve.
* **Stop and reframe.** Cognitive psychologists urge people to reframe their outlook to gain a new perspective. Can you reframe your perspective on your problems by imagining how much worse they could be? Can you make a problem smaller in your mind by telling yourself that you will deal with it little by little until it's solved, just like the vast majority of problems you have ever encountered? Can you put the problem out of your mind by telling yourself that there is nothing you can do about it while you are at work and that you will confront the problem later at an appropriate time? If the problem is a work-related conflict, try simply resolving to take the high road rather than engage in disputes that are likely to be both petty and temporary.
* **Practice mindfulness and relaxation techniques.** Every time you have a quiet moment, close your eyes and take some deep breaths to clear your mind. If you are feeling irritable, pause before you respond to someone and carefully and thoughtfully choose your responses.

If all else fails, without sharing too many details, explain to your co-workers that you are having a bad day and that you would appreciate their understanding. Finally, realize that bad times do not last forever and resolve to make the next day better.

Helping a Co-Worker Experiencing a Bad Day

If one of your co-workers is having a bad day, try to be understanding and helpful by following these tips:

* **Make reasonable allowances.** Most people have good intentions, so a bad day should be tolerated now and then.
* **Be willing to listen.** If you are close to the person, you can offer to listen to them. Ask them if there is anything you can do to help.

* **Know when to step aside.** Naturally, if someone else's bad days are extensive enough to be chronic behavior problems, they are beyond your capacity to help. These are matters for supervisors and your organization's human resource department. If someone else's behavior becomes problematic for you, discuss the issue privately with your supervisor.

JOURNALING 13.2

Reflect on your personality. Are you naturally friendly and outgoing, or are you more of an introvert who has to make a conscious effort to be friendly? Were you raised to be polite, or is politeness a skill you still have to develop? Once you have thought about your traits and characteristics, describe any challenges you may face when adopting a positive attitude toward professional behavior and conduct.

Social Networking and Professional Behavior

In this age of hackers and security breaches, many companies find it necessary to employ filters and monitors that help ensure responsible Internet use at work. Familiarize yourself with your company's written policies about Internet use, email, and professional social media. If no written policy exists, ask your supervisor what the acceptable practices are at your place of work.

Use your computer and Internet access at work only for business purposes. It might be permissible to check your personal email while on a break, but you should not be spending time on social networking sites. Using the Internet and social networking sites for your own interests while at work is contrary to the professionalism you are trying to build (Figure. 13.9).

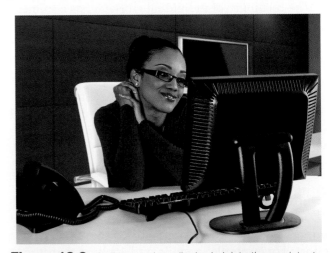

Figure 13.9 A distracted medical administrative assistant uses the company computer for her own interests. (Copyright © istock.com.)

Additionally, you most likely have a work-related email account and are expected to communicate via email promptly and professionally. Your employer may even have a presence on such sites as LinkedIn, Facebook, and Twitter (now X). Be cautious about posting or transmitting inappropriate photographs or videos and messages that include drinking or using drugs, discriminatory comments, or negative comments about a previous company or co-worker. Keep in mind that your work email account is not private and may be monitored and viewed by your employer.

What You Can Expect From Your Workplace

What you can expect from your employer is usually codified by labor law. What you can expect from your co-workers is determined more by general behavior expectations. However, this distinction is not absolute.

Your employer must avoid all discriminatory actions by either co-workers or supervisors. You cannot be sexually harassed or treated unfairly because of your gender, race, ethnicity, age, sexual orientation, disability, or religion and beliefs. You do not have to tolerate physical or verbal threats, coarse language, bullying, or intimidation. Box 13.3 lists employee rights according to the US Equal Employment Opportunity Commission (EEOC).

Depending on your position, your employer must also provide fair compensation and adequate benefits, including personal time off. You have a right to a safe and drug-free work environment, and your personal information should remain confidential. Any criticism of you or your work should be delivered in a private and appropriate setting. Your employer's human resource department should ensure compliance with employee and occupational laws and can serve as a mediator when disputes or conflicts arise, in order to protect both you and your employer.

BOX 13.3

Employee Rights

Employees have a right to:
- Not be harassed or discriminated against (treated less favorably) because of race, color, religion, sex (including pregnancy, sexual orientation, or gender identity), national origin, disability, age (40 or older), or genetic information (including family medical history).
- Receive equal pay for equal work.
- Receive reasonable accommodations (changes to the way things are normally done at work) that are needed because of their medical condition or religious beliefs, if required by law.
- Expect that any medical information or genetic information that they share with their employer will be kept confidential.
- Report discrimination, participate in a discrimination investigation or lawsuit, or oppose discrimination (e.g., threatening to file a discrimination complaint), without being retaliated against (punished) for doing so.

These rights are based on federal employment discrimination laws. Other federal, state, or local laws may also apply to your business. Federal, state, and local government websites may have additional information about these laws.

(Source: U.S. Equal Employment Opportunity Commission.)

JOURNALING 13.3

Think about people you know at school or at work whom you would never want to offend, not because they are powerful or intimidating but because they are decent people who try to do their best. Describe the behavior and traits of these people to illustrate why they command such respect.

CASE STUDY 13.1
Rookie

Stuart was the latest hire as a drug counselor in a drug treatment clinic in Madison, Wisconsin. He had been the first new hire for quite a long time. The rest of the staff had been at the clinic for more than 5 years and had a strong

bond with one another. Stuart learned all this on his first day when everyone started calling him "Rookie."

The title was fine at first, but it began to annoy him after a few weeks. He actually had more education than many of the other counselors and had worked with addiction cases for many years. He did not see himself as a rookie. Further, he would notice that they would joke with one another and have conversations in small groups that did not include him.

After a few months, he found himself pacing around his living room as he talked to his wife, Antonia. "I can't seem to connect with these people," he was saying. "They're nice enough to me, but I'm not part of the group. It's like they speak in code about experiences they've all shared, and I'm on the outside." He shook his head.

"Well, it does take time. Who do you think should break the ice?" asked Antonia. "Who should make the first move, you or them?"

"Well, I think both of us. They have a responsibility, too."

"You're right, but you're not them. You can only be in charge of your actions."

On Monday, Stuart decided to take his wife's advice and be more proactive. He volunteered to run an activity group when one of their co-workers became ill. He also decided to clean up the staff room, which seemed to be in a perpetual state of disarray. A couple of his co-workers noticed the cleaned staff room. "It's good to have a rookie around," one person told him.

That night, Antonia asked how his day was and if anything improved. He relayed his day and the compliment he received to her. But he was still referred to as "rookie" and he was not included in any group conversation. Antonia listened and then asked who the leader was in the group.

"The leader?" he replied.

"Yes, the person everyone else looks up to. The one whose opinion seems to matter more than others."

"That would be Schechter," he said. At work, he noticed that she was quiet, but she commanded respect.

"Break the ice and get to know her. Getting her on your side may help you with the rest of the group," Antonia recommended.

The next day Stuart took an opportunity to sit down next to her while she was taking a break in the day room.

"What's up, Rookie," she said in her gruff way.

"Not much," said Stuart, "but I thought you could explain something to me."

She looked at him without responding, so he forged ahead.

"We have a lot of tough clients around here. Some are hard and kind of unapproachable, but you don't seem to care. You just go up to anybody and start talking, and pretty soon there's a good exchange going on. How do you do that and make it look so natural?"

Schechter proved for the first time that she could smile. "I don't care how hard they are. Everyone can be approachable. Neil Young said, 'Every junkie is a setting sun'. They're not going to get much farther down the road if they're just hard and unapproachable. That's not an option for me."

"For you?"

"Look, Rookie, I lost my brother when I was 15. He was my only brother, and he was the only one who cared about me. He was hard and unapproachable. I knew him though. Underneath. I knew that's not the way he really was. But he didn't get any help, and he was dead before he was 19. I'm not giving these guys here a pass just because they're unapproachable."

Stuart told her he was sorry about her brother, that he appreciated her advice, and that he would try to follow her lead.

Later that day, she called him "Rook."

On Friday morning, he found Schechter again on a break in the day room.

"Hey Schechter," he said, sitting down. "Do you actually have a first name?"

"Yeah," she said.

"My first name is Deborah, but you can call me Shecky. That's what they called my brother. I can see you know what you're doing, and you'll do great here. Keep it up and everyone else will see it, too."

"Thanks, Shecky. You can call me Stuart."

QUESTIONS FOR THOUGHT AND REFLECTION

1. What would have happened to Stuart if he had not been proactive in changing the staff's initial perception of him?
2. What actions did Stuart take to establish himself as a member of the team?
3. Why was it so important for Stuart to feel like a part of the group?
4. Why do you think Stuart was so offended by being called "Rookie"? Would you be offended if you were in his place?
5. What would you have done to get to know your co-workers better?

Marianne was having a bad day at the job that she just started 2 months ago. First, her sister, who watches her young son during the day, was late. Then, the traffic was bad on her way to work. She arrived at the hospital 15 minutes late, and the administrative medical assistant who was waiting to be relieved yelled at Marianne, telling her she better "get it together" and "maybe you shouldn't be working at a place that expects you to be *on time!*"

Marianne's heart was pounding in her chest while she waited for her angry co-worker to leave. "Give it a rest, Grandma," she said under her breath, while the nurses in the nursing station tried to pretend that they did not witness the scene.

A little while later, one of the medical residents came in to enter some prescriptions and orders at the computer. All the terminals were busy, so he said brusquely to Marianne, "Do you mind?" She rolled her chair a minimal distance away and glared at him while he logged into his account.

After that, someone from Medical Records came up with an armload of files. "Give it to the new girl," said the charge nurse.

"I've got a name," said Marianne replied. When she started, she noticed that none of her co-workers asked her what it was.

The next day, Marianne was on time for work, but the administrative medical assistant she relieved was not any friendlier. After she left, Marianne said in a loud voice, "I can see why she works nights." Everyone in the nursing station looked up. "She's not fit to be around people in the daytime," she added. Again, the other staff members ignored her comments and continued with their work.

That afternoon, after getting home from her shift, Marianne told her sister, "I don't think this job is working out. These people are jerks."

"Why are they jerks? What are they doing?"

"They're unfriendly. Like hostile. Nobody talks to me, except to tell me to do this and do that."

"Well, you do have a job there, Marianne, and you are new. You may have to try harder."

"Yeah, thanks for the show of support," Marianne says sarcastically. "You made me late for work too. How do you think *that* made me look?"

QUESTIONS FOR THOUGHT AND REFLECTION

1. List the professional behavior mistakes that Marianne made.
2. What could she have done better to handle being late?
3. If you were Marianne's sister, how would you respond to making her late for work?
4. What can Marianne do to redeem herself at this point?

 EXPERIENTIAL EXERCISES

1. Practice introducing people.
2. Initiate a conversation with a smile and a compliment. What response did you get?
3. Learn something new about a good friend today by asking her an open-ended question.
4. Create a LinkedIn profile for yourself that reflects your professionalism.

 CROSS CURRENTS WITH OTHER SOFT SKILLS

LISTENING ACTIVELY: If you learn to listen actively, you will learn a lot and base your behavioral decisions on solid information (Chapter 6).

DRESSING FOR SUCCESS: Ralph Waldo Emerson once said to someone, "*Who* you are is speaking so loudly that I can't hear what you're saying." You should know what your appearance is saying about you and make sure the message is what you want it to be (Chapter 12).

PROFESSIONAL PHONE TECHNIQUE: Speaking with customers and clients on the phone is a special case for business etiquette, with its own challenges (Chapter 4).

AIMING TO BE ADAPTABLE AND FLEXIBLE: It is hard to model proper business etiquette without a foundation of adaptability (Chapter 1).

MAINTAINING CONFIDENTIALITY AND DISCRETION: Every business benefits from discretion. Health care businesses demand it (Chapter 14).

Dressing for Everyday Success

What a strange power there is in clothing.

—Isaac Bashevis Singer

- Review the written dress code of your employer.
- Understand appropriate and professional clothing for your workplace, including scrubs.
- Familiarize yourself with universal precautions and wear protective garments when needed.

You can have anything you want in life if you dress for it.
—**Edith Head**

Dressing well is one of the best things you can do to establish professional behavior and immediate credibility at work, whether in the eyes of your co-workers, your manager, or your patients and clients. Patients want to encounter health care professionals whose appearance reflects professionalism and competence.

❓ WHAT IF?

What if a friend or colleague of yours showed up for work in an inappropriate outfit? How would you bring this to their attention? What reasons would you give on why appropriate attire is necessary in your workplace setting?

Everyday Professional Dress

In many health care facilities, employees who have direct patient interactions are often expected to wear medical uniforms, such as scrubs. Scrubs are intended to protect your personal clothing from being contaminated while at work. They should not be tight and should allow you free movement. They should not be baggy or loose either, causing safety and sanitation problems, such as being caught on an object. Another alternative is a laboratory coat worn over regular clothing (Figure. 13.10). Depending on the facility, you may or may not wear a laboratory coat, and you may be required to wear a specific color of scrubs.

Scrubs and similar uniforms must always be freshly laundered and ironed, so change your scrubs or laboratory coat if they become soiled on the job. In addition to uniform policies, many facilities require badges for security purposes, identifying you as an employee with access to specific areas. In many health care facilities, it is mandatory to always have your badge on while at work and with your name and photo visible to everyone.

Depending on your facility, there may be specific days when you are allowed to wear your own clothes at work. Your clothing should still be conservative and

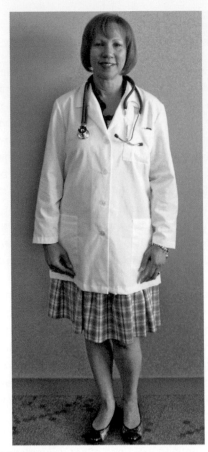

Figure 13.10 Work clothes should be conservative and tasteful.

BOX 13.4

Considerations for Selecting Work Clothes

- Choose fabrics that resist stains, shrinkage, fading, and wrinkling.
- Select colors and patterns that aren't distracting.
- For women, dresses and skirts should fall around the knee level. Pants or pantsuits may be appropriate.
- For men, trousers and shirts should be clean, pressed, and subdued in color.
- Avoid any clothes that are frayed, worn, ripped, or sloppy.
- Know the difference between your professional work clothes and your casual clothes.

tasteful. Clearly, there is nothing in these guidelines that says you cannot be stylish, fashionable, or consistent with your gender, culture, or religion. Box 13.4 offers some considerations when choosing clothing appropriate for work.

Footwear

Health care professionals are often on their feet for many hours during the workday. Comfort is certainly a primary consideration in choosing footwear. Other considerations include cleanliness, safety, and style. Many health care facilities encourage their staff to choose athletic-style shoes designed specifically for health care professionals because they are comfortable, easy to clean, and have rubber soles and traction for safety. Floors in health care workplaces can be slippery, and the pace is often hurried and hectic. If your employer allows ordinary street shoes, keep qualities such as comfort and traction at the top of your mind. Avoid open-toed shoes, high heels, straps, buckles, and ornaments that can be difficult to keep clean. Some traditional worksites encourage wearing white shoes, which require extra care to keep them clean and white.

If you work in a surgical center or in a profession where you are likely to be exposed to blood or other potentially infectious materials, you may be required to wear more protective equipment, such as shoe covers. You may also be required to wear footwear that will protect you from spilled blood and that is thick enough to prevent puncture in case of an accidental needlestick injury.

Jewelry and Body Adornments

Minimal jewelry, such as a wedding band or a simple watch, is fine. But most jewelry detracts from your professionalism and may even create a safety or health hazard. Jewelry may harbor dirt and microorganisms; it may puncture gloves and scratch patients, for example, if there are jewels on a ring or bracelet. Even tasteful jewelry can scratch, snag, or distract a client or patient. Children and patients with dementia may snatch dangling earrings or necklaces. Thus, small earrings are permissible, as long as they are professional looking and not dangling.

Visible tattoos and body piercings, such as eyebrow and nose piercings, might not represent your employer well to some patients. In fact, some patients may even find them offensive. Since they are becoming more common, particularly tattoos, many health care facilities include a section regarding tattoos and body piercings in their employee handbooks. In a few cases, some employers require their employees to have no visible tattoos or piercings. Some employees may even resort to using makeup to hide tattoos that may be visible on their hands or neck. If tattoos are on your arms, you may want to consider wearing long sleeves, including under your scrubs, or a laboratory coat. Most medical offices are intentionally maintained at a cool temperature, usually between 68°F and 76°F, so having that extra layer of clothing may be helpful. Other employers may permit tattoos and/or body piercings as long as they are not excessive or offensive.

According to the US Equal Employment Opportunity Commission (EEOC), the federal agency that administers and enforces civil rights in the workplace, employers can establish policies for dress code and appearance as long as they do not discriminate based on race, color, religion, sex, national origin, age, disability, or genetic information. Thus, make every effort to remove visible piercing jewelry and cover your tattoos at work.

> **JOURNALING 13.4**
>
> Write down your thoughts about tattoos. Why do you think people get tattoos? What messages are they trying to send? How might patients react to seeing tattoos on their health care provider?

Special Situations

Specialized Attire to Reduce Risk of Infection

As discussed earlier, for health care professionals who work in a surgical center or in a facility with a high risk of exposure to bloodborne pathogens or other potentially infectious materials specific attire may be required. Some infections can be transmitted through contact with blood and body fluids, including HIV and hepatitis A, B, and C. Thus, working with patients with infectious diseases will require the practice of universal precautions.

Universal precautions are a standard set of guidelines to prevent the transmission of bloodborne pathogens from exposure to blood and other potentially infectious materials. Universal precautions affect the way you dress as a health care professional. With even the slightest risk of being exposed to blood or any body fluids, you are likely to have to use gloves, masks, surgical booties, and a disposable gown, which are often situated in the nurses' station or outside of a patient's room or a quarantined area. Your employer will also be required to provide you with these protective clothing items to ensure your safety. Your clothing choices should make it easy for you to put on these additional safety garments. Universal precautions include:

* Using disposable gloves and other protective barriers while examining all patients and while handling needles, scalpels, and other sharp instruments.
* Washing hands and other skin surfaces that are contaminated with blood or body fluids immediately after a procedure or examination.

* Changing gloves between patients and never reusing gloves.

The health care worker in Figure 13.11 is outfitted to protect themself and their patients from infections.

Casual Fridays

Many workplaces may specify a preference for daily casual dress. For example, many medical offices designate each Fridays as "casual Fridays" and an administrative day when no patients are seen. As a result, scrubs or medical uniforms are not required to be worn, and more casual wear is permitted. However, an understanding of what constitutes casual work attire can be tricky. Should you play it safe and wear khakis and a polo shirt? Or, are blue jeans and leggings appropriate?

No matter how casual the dress code, there is such a thing as *too* casual. Certainly, you should never wear shorts, a tank top, or a tube top to work. Health care professionals should be careful not to wear anything too revealing. Carefully investigate the guidelines where you work. When in doubt, ask your co-workers or supervisor what appropriate attire is. The people depicted in Figure. 13.12 display appropriate work attire.

JOURNALING 13.5

Describe your style of dress. Differentiate between your weekend and the workweek style. What influences have contributed to your style? Do you need to make any changes for work? How will you come to terms with these changes?

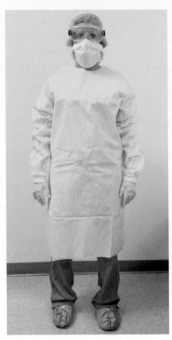

Figure 13.11 A health care professional in a mask, disposable gown, and surgical booties. (From Proctor DB, Adams AP: *Kinn's the medical assistant: an applied learning approach*, ed 12, St. Louis, 2014, Elsevier.)

I base most of my fashion sense on what doesn't itch.

—Gilda Radner

First Impressions Last

On your first day at work, your co-workers will formulate an impression of you in 7 seconds. Every day, the process repeats as you meet clients or patients.

Figure 13.12 **A**, Proper business casual attire. **B**, Proper scrub attire.

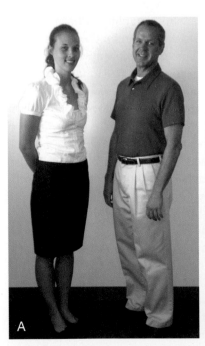 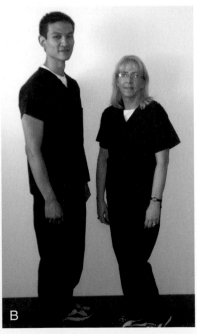

Negative first impressions are difficult to overcome. Fortunately, dressing for a good first impression is something you can control.

Seldom do people discern eloquence under a threadbare cloak.

—Juvenal

CASE STUDY 13.2
A Difficult Conversation

Bill, a practice manager at a Village Family Clinic, was very happy with Mary, the medical assistant he inherited from his predecessor. She was efficient and friendly. She answered patients' calls with professionalism and a cheerful note in her voice. One day, Bill stopped to talk with Helen, the vice president of Human Resources, in the hallway. She said, "Bill, did you see the announcement about the new dress code we're implementing?"

"Yes, I did," he said, thinking to himself that he did not like the new dress code policy.

"What do you think of it?"

"It seems fine. But why do you think we need a dress code?"

"Because of your medical assistant!" she said.

"Mary? What did she do?"

"Yes! She wears those hip-hugger, capri pants and I've even seen her in a tank top! My recommendation is for you to meet with her about it."

Bill knew that Mary's apparel was overly casual, but he had not given much thought to it because she mostly worked at the back office, processing reimbursement claims, and checking out patients as they completed their medical visit. He did not think she interacted with patients that much. He felt somewhat annoyed at himself for not noticing and intervening earlier to avoid this problem.

Bill became concerned that Mary's unprofessional dress could limit her opportunities. Apparently, it had already been noticed by some important people in the company. He decided to talk to Mary about her appearance.

"First, I wanted to tell you I think you are an excellent medical assistant, Mary. I really value you as an employee here," he said to Mary in the privacy of a small conference room, "But I'm concerned about your attire at work."

"A concern?"

"Yes," he said. "For one thing, it's not in compliance with the new dress code policy that will be announced soon. In fact, it's one of the reasons we have a new dress code."

Mary blushed with embarrassment and rising indignation. "Nobody's said anything to me before."

"You're right and that's my fault. I should've talked to you about this sooner."

"You know, I don't make much money here. I can't afford to buy fancy outfits." Mary was becoming defensive, probably without realizing it.

Bill decided to do a little reality testing with Mary. "You know," he said, "appropriate clothes don't cost any more than inappropriate clothes. It's all a matter of the choices you make when you shop. Your attire is certainly stylish. It's just not right for work."

At this point, Mary couldn't hide her anguish anymore, and she covered her face.

After a moment, he said, "Mary, you're excellent at your job and I'm very happy with your work. I'm having this conversation with you because I want you to be successful here and I don't want anything to stop it. I know this is hard to hear, but this has nothing to do with your performance here."

Mary looked up and nodded.

The next day, Mary arrived wearing a white blouse and a pencil skirt. That afternoon, a young mother and her two small children were sitting in the waiting room. The mother's arm was in a sling and she seemed to be in pain. Mary introduced herself to the patient and asked her if she could help her by taking the children to play. The patient happily agreed, and Mary took the girls to a conference room with a big white board and lots of dry-erase markers. They played a few games of tic-tac-toe and then drew pictures. Mary transferred her calls to the phone in the conference room until the patient's appointment was over.

Shortly before the office closed, Bill called the medical assistants together and praised Mary for thinking on her feet and showing initiative in helping the patient and her family. A week later, Bill posted a handwritten letter from the patient, thanking Mary for her customer service and professionalism. There were also two "portraits" of Mary drawn from crayons enclosed in the envelope.

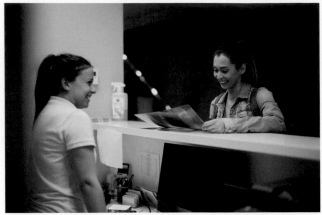

iStock.com/Drazen Zigic/1393284394 Filio Marineli, Gregory Tsoucalas, Marianna Karamanou, George Androutsos, Mary Mallon (1869-1938) and the history of typhoid fever. Annals of Gastroenterology, Vol. 26, issue 2, page 132-134, 2013

Filio Marineli, Gregory Tsoucalas, Marianna Karamanou, George Androutsos, Mary Mallon (1869-1938) and the history of typhoid fever. Annals of Gastroenterology, Vol. 26, issue 2, page 132-134, 2013

QUESTIONS FOR THOUGHT AND REFLECTION

1. What could Mary have done to better familiarize herself with professional dress attire at her clinic?
2. How would you have handled this difficult conversation? What would be the same or different from the way Bill handled it?
3. What should Bill do moving forward to prevent another situation like this?

A Different Path

Lucy was a very competent medical assistant at a large medical clinic. Along with being a certified medical assistant, she has training in medical insurance and coding and is a good resource for answering the staff's questions on any reimbursement and billing issues. Lucy also has a natural ability with patients, and her smile and warm personality put patients at ease. However, her appearance and hygiene were becoming problems for her supervisors.

Lucy predominantly works the front office and is often the first staff member that patients meet. One day, she would wear a red skirt straight out of the 1940s, short in the front and long in the back. The next day, she would wear a blouse with a shaggy fur collar. She would always have bright red lipstick on and garish blue eyeshadow. Her co-workers would occasionally make subtle comments and light jokes about her appearance. Lucy would just roll her eyes and brush off any discussion of her odd clothing style and loud makeup. But the physician in charge of the medical clinic, Dr. Arthur, had lost patience with Lucy's unprofessional appearance.

"Please talk to her about it," he told her supervisor. "It's an embarrassment."

Natalie, the clinic manager, and Lucy's supervisor had tried to broach the topic with Lucy before. She would become sullen and would begrudgingly agree but her appearance showed little improvement. Lucy knew that everyone valued her abilities, but she was unaware that her dress had become an issue.

The next day, Natalie arranged a meeting with Lucy. "We need to talk again about your appearance." Natalie told her, "You are an excellent employee. But your dress and makeup are becoming more of a distraction and issue to our staff and patients. I need you to be more mindful about the way you dress and how you represent the clinic."

Lucy scowled and reluctantly nodded. "I understand."

The next day, Lucy showed up in a pair of black slacks with a satin stripe down the sides, and a yellow cotton jersey with a smiley face pattern. Her makeup still included bright red lipstick and blue eyeshadow.

Natalie pulled Lucy into her office as soon as she noticed and said, "Lucy, I want to remind you of our conversation we had yesterday about your appearance. You said you understood but I'm not sure you do. You are a great medical assistant, but you do not look professional."

"What?" said Lucy. "What are you talking about? That's not true!"

Ignoring her reaction, Natalie pressed on. "We've talked several times about this before and you seem to refuse to do anything about it. Your clothing contradicts the professionalism we're trying to convey in this clinic. Everyone likes and respects you, Lucy. I need you to dress more professionally. You can even wear scrubs if you prefer."

"Well, I've got a right to my personal style," she said. "I'm not some carbon copy of what you think I should be. I do my job very well, and that's all you should be concerned with. When you have a complaint about my clinical skills, let me know." With that, she got up and stormed out of the room.

Later, Dr. Arthur asked Natalie about how the meeting with Lucy went.

"Well, let's document the meeting and contact HR to see what our next steps are, then," he said.

1. Why do you think Lucy has been so reluctant and defensive in changing her appearance?

2. How do you think Natalie handled the discussion with Lucy? Would you have handled anything differently?

3. Is there anything Natalie or Dr. Arthur can do before contacting Human Resources?

⊛ EXPERIENTIAL EXERCISES

1. Spend a half-hour in a hospital lobby or medical office. It is easy to identify the staff? Are there staff members who, in your opinion, are particularly well dressed? Are there others who, in your perception, dress poorly or inappropriately?

2. Visit a local uniform store. Introduce yourself to the manager or owner, who can be a very knowledgeable resource to you, and discuss appropriate clothing options at health care facilities in your area. Examine the uniforms in the store and the various options. Learn about pricing, styles, colors, fabrics, and procedures for laundering and ironing.

3. What have you learned about professional attire while you have been a student? Are the school's dress code guidelines consistent with dress codes at local employers?

4. Prepare a checklist and a weekly schedule that details which day you will do laundry and iron your uniform.

⊘ CROSS CURRENTS WITH OTHER SOFT SKILLS

ADOPTING A POSITIVE MENTAL ATTITUDE: Your clothing can reflect your attitude, positive or negative (Chapter 12).

DISPLAYING GOOD GROOMING, PERSONAL HYGIENE, AND CLEANLINESS: These are as important to your appearance and professionalism as *dressing for success* (Chapter 9).

READING AND SPEAKING BODY LANGUAGE: Your dress is part of your body language, and your body language can dress up your clothing, appearance, and professionalism (Chapter 6).

FOLLOWING RULES AND REGULATIONS: You want your appearance to be within the range of appropriate guidelines at your place of employment (Chapter 14).

EXUDING OPTIMISM, ENTHUSIASM, AND POSITIVITY: Appropriate dress enhances your positivity; let your dress help your enthusiasm shine through (Chapter 11)!

Grooming and Personal Hygiene

People often say that motivation doesn't last. Well, neither does bathing—that's why we recommend it daily.

—Zig Ziglar

LEARNING OBJECTIVE 4: DISPLAYING GOOD GROOMING AND PERSONAL HYGIENE

- Review any written procedures pertaining to personal hygiene and grooming at your school or place of employment.
- List five solid strategies for maintaining sanitary hands.
- Explain ways in which pathogens can be spread at work.
- Explain proper hand hygiene.

Because there is a direct correlation between poor personal hygiene and transmissible diseases, it is critical that health care professionals understand and practice good basic hygiene habits, including proper hand washing, on a regular basis. Additionally, your clean and healthy appearance projects competency and professionalism to your patients and clients.

Checklist for Personal Work Hygiene

Depending on the volume of your facility, you may interact and be exposed to dozens of people every single day. As a result, you will most likely face constant exposure to germs, odors, and dirt. Over the course of a day, you may be accumulating bacteria, viruses, skin cells, and dirt on your skin and under your nails. Box 13.5 lists common ways germs can spread in a health care setting. Thus, practicing good hygiene will ensure that you are clean and pathogen-free throughout the day and as you provide care to each patient and client.

Common Transmission of Germs

- Sick employees
- Unwashed hands or contaminated gloves
- Employees with open cuts and scrapes
- Employees who touch their faces and mouths with their hands
- Improperly disposed hygienic items (e.g., toilet paper, paper towels)
- Employees who do not wash their hands after using the restroom
- Unwashed and poorly sanitized preparation surfaces, utensils, and preparation areas
- Soiled wiping cloths and cleaning items

What separates two people most profoundly is a different sense and degree of cleanliness.

—Friedrich Nietzsche

 JOURNALING 13.6

Talk with a physician, nurse, or staff member at the hospital or medical office and ask about their hygiene practices. How do they prepare for a day at work? What do they do during the day to ensure their personal hygiene is clean and professional?

The following checklist is a good basic guideline for daily personal hygiene for health care professionals:

* **Shower or bathe daily.** Both before and after work, if possible. Remember that you will also be bringing home germs and dirt from your job, and you want to avoid exposure to you and your family.

* **Use deodorant** after showering, especially unscented or lightly scented products. You may want to refresh your deodorant in the middle of the day depending on your perspiration and odor level.

* **Avoid strong fragrances at work.** Avoid wearing strong perfumes or aftershave because some of your co-workers and patients may be allergic or sensitive to strong scents. Remember that you will often be working in small and confined spaces at work, which may amplify the smell of your perfume or aftershave.

* **Choose an appropriate hair style.** Touch up your hair as needed during the day; wear longer hair back or up so it does not hang in your face, impair your vision, or touch a patient. In the health care setting, avoid hair that is dyed an unnatural color or that may be too trendy or unprofessional, such as a mohawk.

* **Apply makeup modestly.** If you wear makeup, use it sparingly. Follow the general rule: less is often more.

* **Keep your fingernails clean and short.** Fingernails should be trimmed straight across and rounded at the corners. Keeping your nails trimmed will reduce the amount of germs and dirt collected underneath them. Long nails not only will collect more germs and dirt but may also scratch a patient, resulting in an infection. Fingernails should be polish-free to avoid any flaking or chipping. Keep your nails clean; patients should not see dirt underneath your nails. A nail brush is a useful tool, and the stiff bristles are able to scrub dirt and germs away.

* **Practice daily oral and dental hygiene.** Brush your teeth, and floss at least twice daily. It is also recommended to brush after lunch. When brushing, remember to brush your gums as well to prevent gum disease (gingivitis). Box 13.6 lists tips on how to maintain oral hygiene. There are a host of benefits to good oral and dental health. It can help prevent bad breath, tooth decay, and the development

Practicing Good Oral Hygiene

- Brush your teeth twice a day with toothpaste and a toothbrush bought within the last 3 months.
- Consider brushing your teeth after lunch, especially when you are working, because certain spices and foods can cause lasting bad breath.
- Brush for at least 2 minutes, paying attention to both the inside and outside surfaces of your teeth, all four quarters of your mouth, and molars in the back, which can be hard to reach but are just as susceptible to decay as any other teeth.
- Use an antimicrobial mouthwash for good gum health and fresh breath.
- Floss your teeth twice a day. This is the only way to effectively clean between your teeth and under your gum line for good gum health.
- Scrape your tongue to remove bacteria that cause bad breath.
- Drink lots of water and use it to flush food particles away from your teeth.

of other diseases, such as diabetes and cardiovascular infection.

* **Smoking.** Employers can refuse to let you smoke on company premises or on company time, with some states and cities banning smoking on public property. Just as with perfume and aftershave, the smell of cigarette smoke on your clothing, hair, or breath can be unpleasant for patients and clients. Some patients and clients may even be allergic to the nicotine in tobacco smoke.

For that reason, you must make every effort to eliminate the smell of tobacco smoke if you do smoke. Be mindful that the smell of smoke can be absorbed in your clothing, fingers, and hair.

Be mindful that some employers, especially in health care, may require job applicants to take and pass a preemployment drug screen before they are hired. These drug screens, which usually test urine samples, can include testing for nicotine. The drug test for nicotine will test positive for the presence of nicotine, regardless of how it was consumed, including cigarettes, smokeless tobacco, and even patches.

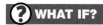**WHAT IF?**

You have a classmate or co-worker who has very strong body odor. What could you say to them about this problem?

Proper Hand Hygiene

One of the most important practices as a health care professional is practicing good hand hygiene. As a health care professional, you will most likely be working with patients and clients all day long and using your hands. Make sure that you begin each patient encounter with freshly cleaned hands to prevent the transmission of germs.

Pathogens, or agents that can cause disease, include different types of bacteria, viruses, toxins, parasites, chemicals, and even metals. They can be harbored in the hair, skin, nails, nose, eyes, blood, feces, mucus, saliva, lymph, and urine of an infected person. The most common methods of pathogen and disease transmission are through:

* Direct contact: This includes skin-to-skin contact, kissing, and sexual intercourse.
* Indirect contact: Transmission through inanimate objects, such as a doorknob or faucet handle.

* Aerosol or droplets: This includes coughing or sneezing.
* Vector: This includes transmission by a living organism, such as a flea, tick, or mosquito.

In the health care setting, the primary method of disease transmission is through direct contact, especially with the hands. Hands make contact with thousands of different surfaces, objects, and people every day. Thus special attention needs to be paid to the handwashing technique.

Hand Washing

There is no question that the most important thing you can do to prevent the transmission of disease is to wash your hands frequently and properly. Poor hand hygiene practice may endanger your own health, as well as that of your patients. Therefore you must establish routine handwashing procedures right now while you are training and follow them throughout your career.

Much of the effectiveness of hand washing depends on the *frequency* and *timing* with which you wash your hands. First, you should recognize that your hands will accumulate dirt and germs over time, even if you have not had exposure to pathogens through contact with a contaminated dressing or during the collection of a urine specimen. Almost every surface or object you touch, whether a sink faucet or a computer keyboard, will transfer germs to your hands. Box 13.7 lists common places in the workplace where germs lurk. Develop the habit of washing your hands every hour or two at least, regardless of the type of work you are doing.

There are also many occasions when you *must* wash your hands—sometimes *before* an activity, such

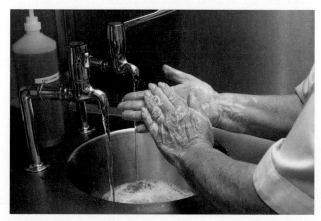

Thorough hand washing helps workers maintain a safe, sanitary health care environment.

as changing a dressing, and sometimes *after*, such as working with laboratory specimens or bodily fluids (Box 13.8). Your workplace may even have specific rules about when to wash your hands. Ultimately, however, effective hand washing depends on your good judgment, persistence, and personal commitment to the best possible sanitation you can bring to your work.

The best hand washing method is with soap and warm water. Avoid using hot water because it may cause skin irritation and may make the skin more vulnerable to scratches and scrapes. Before hand washing, remove rings and bracelets; plain wedding bands are permissible. The length of time when scrubbing your hands is important. Scrub your hands for at least 20 seconds. As a timer, recite "Happy Birthday" twice. Box 13.9 outlines the steps for properly washing your hands.

BOX 13.7

Common Sites for Germs in the Health Care Setting

- Floors and floor drains
- Cooling coils and cooling ducts
- Medical equipment
- Trash and medical waste receptacles
- Sinks, spigots, and handles
- Computer equipment, especially keyboards
- Examination tables and chairs

BOX 13.8

When to Wash Your Hands

Before
- Touching a patient
- Examining a patient
- Putting on new gloves
- Preparing food
- Consuming food
- Cleaning equipment and preparation surfaces

After
- Visiting the restroom
- Touching any bare human body part, including skin, ears, nose, hair, or eyes
- Handling garbage, trash, or hazardous medical waste
- Smoking or doing other activities that soil your hands

BOX 13.9

Proper Handwashing Steps

1. Wet hands with warm water.
2. Apply enough soap to cover the front and back of your hands and in between your fingers.
3. Rub hands together and scrub the front and back of your hands and in between your fingers.
4. Wash the front and back of your hands, in between your fingers, and under your nails.
5. Rinse your hands with clean water.
6. Dry hands completely using a clean towel or single-use towel or air dry.

(Source: Centers for Disease Control and Prevent, https://www.cdc.gov/ncird/index.html.)

Hand Sanitizers

There may be times that soap and water may not be readily available, such as if you are located at the front desk. In these cases, use an alcohol-based hand sanitizer. Alcohol-based hand sanitizers are now standard equipment at most health care facilities, sometimes with stations placed outside every patient or examination room. Alcohol-based hand sanitizers that contain at least 60% alcohol should be used and are effective at killing germs.

When using alcohol-based hand rub or sanitizer, apply the product to the palm of one hand and rub the product all over the surfaces of your hands until your hands are dry. Read the label of the hand sanitizer to learn the correct amount of product to rub.

Alcohol-based hand sanitizers, however, do not eliminate all types of germs and are not effective on hands that are very greasy or heavily soiled. In addition, hand sanitizers may not remove harmful chemicals, like pesticides and heavy metals, from the hands. Thus washing with soap and water whenever possible is recommended, especially in these circumstances.

Gloves

Gloves play an important part in protecting hands from infectious agents and chemicals in the health care setting. They are the most common type of protective equipment for health care professionals. There are many types of gloves, and they should be selected depending on the purpose. For example, in most patient care situations, gloves made of nitrile or vinyl are appropriate. Due to concerns about allergic reactions, most health care organizations have eliminated or limited the availability of latex gloves.

Gloves should fit your hands comfortably and should not be too loose or too tight. They also should not tear or damage easily. Gloves are sometimes worn for several hours and thus need to stand up to the task. In general, nitrile gloves are preferred over vinyl because some vinyl gloves do not fit snuggly over the hand. Furthermore, vinyl gloves should not be used if extensive use is required.

Gloves may also be sterile and nonsterile. When surgical procedures are needed to be performed, sterile surgical gloves must be used. Sterile surgical gloves are worn by surgeons, surgical technicians, sterile process technicians, and other health care professionals who perform invasive procedures on patients or need to ensure what they are doing is performed under sterile procedures. Unlike nonsterile gloves that are usually packaged as 100 to 200 gloves in a box, sterile gloves are individually packaged. To use sterile gloves, proper techniques must be performed to maintain sterility when donning or putting on the gloves.

Gloves protect you against contact with infectious materials. However, once contaminated, gloves can become a means for spreading infectious materials to yourself, other patients, or surfaces. Thus, it is important to change gloves when they become torn or heavily soiled. Gloves must be changed after every patient encounter. Generally, gloves can be disposed of in the trash in the health care facility or medical office. However, if the gloves are heavily soiled, such as with blood, they need to be disposed of in the biohazard container.

Disposable gloves become dirty, just like hands. Change your gloves every time you wash your hands, and wash your hands every time you change your gloves. However, using gloves properly and consistently helps establish a safe, sanitary environment for you and your patients. You should know how to don, remove, and dispose of gloves in a safe, effective manner. It is important to remember that gloves do not replace proper hand washing.

Skin Wounds and Hand Sanitation

Working in health care, you will inevitably fall prey to cuts and burns on your hands. Every little incident, from a paper cut to a scrape against a rough surface, opens a new pathway to pathogens. A finger cot, a waterproof bandage, or gloving can minimize the risk of cuts and open sores. You should treat even the most minor abrasion as having the potential to result in an infection.

A common incident in the health care setting is an accidental needlestick injury, which is any wound caused by a needle that accidentally punctures the skin. Needlestick injuries are a hazard for health care professionals who work with hypodermic syringes and other needle equipment when using, disassembling, or disposing of needles. To prevent needlestick injuries, almost all health care organizations and medical offices should use sharps containers and needles with "safety-engineered devices," which include safety winged butterfly steel needles and self-retracting syringes.

CASE STUDY 13.3
Twenty-One Days a Habit Breaks

During her last year in high school, Elena enrolled in the licensed vocational nursing (LVN) program at the adjoining Vocational-Technical campus. She was good at science, and she had a natural warm and caring nature.

Elena passed her NCLEX-PN Examination on her first try and got a good job at a medical clinic. She was happy with her first job, where she got to triage patients, provide vaccinations, and manage medical records. She was a good writer, and she was assigned to various writing jobs, including revising procedures manuals and creating the monthly internal newsletter.

One day she was working with Alberta, the community liaison manager, on a brochure on diabetes screening and management to be distributed at area work sites and migrant camps. During one of their meetings, Alberta said, "What are you doing to your nails, girl? It looks like a wild animal has been chewing on your fingernails."

Elena was surprised and looked down at her nails. Her fingernails were all chewed down at different degrees. Her fingertips and cuticles were red and some of the tips looked infected. She felt embarrassed and quickly put her hands underneath the table.

"Well, I bite my nails occasionally."

"Occasionally? Your fingers look like you do it all the time, and I've noticed that you bite your nails, especially when you're concentrating."

"Okay, I bite my fingernails a lot. A lot of people do. What's the big deal?" Elena replied, feeling more uncomfortable with the conversation.

Alberta replied, "Well, the big deal is that you work closely with patients, and a lot of patients. What do you think your patients think when they see your fingernails? They don't see what a competent nurse you are. They see someone with gross nails that they don't want near them."

Elena had to agree and remembered what she learned in the LVN program about good hygiene and having clean and trimmed fingernails.

"You're right. But I've had this habit since I was 10 years old. I don't know how to stop it."

"Well, I'm going to help you by breaking that habit in 21 days."

"21 days? I've been biting my fingernails for more than 21 years." Elena laughed nervously.

"I read a self-help book that taught me how to break habits by forming new habits in just 21 days." Alberta went on to explain that it takes 21 days to form a new habit. "But you have to do the new habit every single day—no exceptions. It doesn't always work, but do you want to try?" she said.

Elena looked very interested and said, "Okay, it's worth a shot."

"And, if you can make it to 21 days straight with no exception, I'm going to take you out to get a manicure." They both laughed.

QUESTIONS FOR THOUGHT AND REFLECTION

1. Why did Alberta think Elena's bitten fingernails would be such a problem for her as a nurse?

2. Look at your hands. What do you think patients or clients would think of your fingernails?

3. Have you ever had to tell a friend or co-worker about their poor hygiene? How did that conversation go?

? WHAT IF?

What if you saw a colleague biting their fingernails? How would you explain and illustrate the dangers of this habit?

← JOURNALING 13.7

Explain the importance of personal cleanliness to health care professionals in a health care facility. Include your thoughts on why this skill is named *Displaying Good Grooming and Personal Hygiene*.

A Different Path

THE HISTORY OF TYPHOID MARY

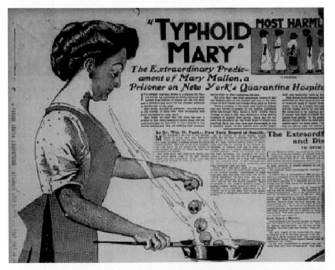

(Filio Marineli, Gregory Tsoucalas, Marianna Karamanou, George Androutsos, Mary Mallon (1869–1938) and the history of typhoid fever. *Annals of Gastroenterology*. 2013;26(2):132–134.)

Mary Mallon was born in Ireland in 1869 and immigrated to the United States when she was 15 years old. She settled in New York City. Like many Irish Americans at the time, Mary found work as a domestic servant for wealthy families, until eventually settling into a career as a cook.

In the summer of 1906, a wealthy New York banker, Charles Henry Warren, rented a house in Oyster Bay, Long Island, for a family vacation. He hired Mary as a cook. Within 3 weeks, 6 of the 11 members of Mr. Warren's family became ill with typhoid, a serious bacterial infection spread by contaminated food and water. Symptoms of typhoid include high fevers, weakness, abdominal pains, headaches, and loss of appetite. Although typhoid was fairly common among poor people around the 1900s, especially those living in unsanitary living conditions, it was a rare disease among the wealthy.

The owner of the summer rental, George Thompson, feared that he would never be able to rent his house again unless the cause of the outbreak was found, so he hired an investigator, George Soper, a sanitary engineer, to determine the cause of the illness. Soper eventually discovered that, between 1900 and 1906, Mary had worked as a cook for seven different families with 22 of the family members contracting typhoid after her hiring. Soper thought this was more than a coincidence, and he wanted to obtain stool and urine samples from Mary.

However, Mary refused to provide any samples for testing to Soper. She told him she never had any of the symptoms from typhoid and felt healthy, so it could not be her. However, more and more families were becoming ill from Mary, and there was a growing suspicion that she was the culprit. News spread about her contagiousness, as well as her refusal to be tested, so the newspapers began calling her "Typhoid Mary."

Soper brought his suspicions and evidence to the officials of the New York City Health Department, who agreed with his conclusion and requested samples from Mary, but were met with the same refusal. Eventually, the health department contacted the police, who took her into custody and restrained her in order to obtain stool and urine samples, which confirmed she carried the bacteria for typhoid, *Salmonella typhi*.

Mary admitted that she did not understand the purpose of hand washing because she did not have any of the symptoms, and thus she did not think she posed a risk. The courts remanded Mary to a hospital on an island in the East River, where she remained in isolation for 3 years. In 1909, Mary sued the health department for her release, but the New York Supreme Court denied her petition.

It was not until 1910, when the new commissioner for the New York State Board of Public Health decided that carriers of diseases should not be kept in isolation and that Mary could be freed, as long as she agreed to stop working as a cook and take reasonable steps to prevent disease transmission, such as frequent hand washing.

Unfortunately, Mary failed to keep her promise and returned to working as a cook at Manhattan's Sloane Maternity Hospital. She used the name Mary Brown in order to be hired and to avoid being identified as Mary Mallon or "Typhoid Mary." Unsurprisingly, during her 3 months as a cook at the hospital, she infected at least 25 people, including physicians, nurses, and other staff members. Two of them died.

From Leavitt, Judith Walzer. *Typhoid Mary*: *Captive to the public's health*, Boston, 1996, Beacon Press, p. 180.

QUESTIONS FOR THOUGHT AND REFLECTION

1. How fair was it for Mary to be forced to submit stool and urine samples and then remanded to a hospital? How would Mary Mallon's case be different if it occurred today?
2. Why did Mary not understand the purpose of hand washing?
3. How did George Soper determine Mary was the cause of typhoid?
4. Why is typhoid fever so much less of a health problem today than it was just 100 years ago?

⭐ EXPERIENTIAL EXERCISES

1. Identify a habit you would like to start or break, create a 21-day chart, and record the successful completion of the habit.
2. Use sticky notes to label places in your classroom or workplace where pathogens are likely to lurk.
3. What are the regulations in your workplace regarding smoking? Hand washing? Grooming and cleanliness?

☯ CROSS CURRENTS WITH OTHER SOFT SKILLS

DRESSING FOR SUCCESS: So much of what you wear to work and at work has a direct bearing on your grooming, hygiene, and cleanliness (Chapter 12).
READING AND SPEAKING BODY LANGUAGE: Your personal hygiene is part of your body language. Poor personal hygiene *screams* in body language (Chapter 4).
FOLLOWING RULES AND REGULATIONS: Some aspects of your grooming and cleanliness are non-negotiable. Whether they are universal precautions established by the CDC or rules in force at your workplace, your commitment must be to follow them without exception (Chapter 14).

Planning for Career Success

- Explain the Importance of Rules and Regulations in the Health Care
- Discuss the Patient's Bill of Rights
- Understand Your Responsibilities under HIPAA and in Maintaining Patient Confidentiality
- List Federal and State Agencies That Oversee Regulations and Compliance in Health Care
- Identify Ethical and Illegal Actions That Would Warrant Disciplinary Actions
- Discuss Compliance Plans and the Role of the Compliance Officer

Following Rules and Regulations

It's not wise to violate rules until you know how to observe them.

—T.S. Eliot

LEARNING OBJECTIVE 1:
FOLLOWING RULES AND REGULATIONS

- Identify specific standards and regulations in health care.
- List the different rights in the Patient Bill of Rights.
- Explain what fraud and abuse are in health care.
- Understand the importance of establishing and following rules and when exceptions are needed.
- Understand the importance of a compliance plan and types of disciplinary actions.

Since health care deals with the lives and health of people, it is understandably one of the most regulated industries in the United States. There are many laws and regulations to protect that set privacy and usage standards for patient information, ensure quality patient care, prevent fraud, and protect health care staff. Health care regulations and standards are necessary to ensure compliance and to provide safe health care to every individual who accesses the system. The health care regulatory agencies in turn monitor health care providers and facilities, provide information about industry changes, promote safety, and ensure legal compliance and quality services.

Patient Bill of Rights

An important aspect of patient care is defining the rights and responsibilities for both the patient and health care provider. For patients, the American

Hospital Association (AHA) created the original Patient Bill of Rights in 1973, which provides guidelines for ensuring the protection and safety of patients. Although the Patient Bill of Rights was originally intended for the hospital setting, most medical practices, hospitals, insurance companies, and even governments have adopted some form of the Patient Bill of Rights.

The purpose of the Patient Bill of Rights is to help patients feel more confident in the health care system in the United States, to strengthen the relationship between patients and their health care provider by defining their rights and responsibilities and those of their health care provider, and to emphasize the role patients play in their health. With that, the Patient's Bill of Rights outlines 15 guarantees for all patients seeking medical care in a health care organization and basic rights and responsibilities for effective patient care. A summary of these guarantees is as follows:

1. You have the right to be treated fairly and respectfully.
2. You have the right to get information you can understand about your diagnosis, treatment, and prognosis from your health care provider.
3. You have the right to discuss and ask for information about specific procedures and treatments, their risks, and the time you will spend recovering. You also have the right to discuss other care options.
4. You have the right to know the identities of all your health care providers, including students, residents, and other trainees.
5. You have the right to know how much care may cost at the time of treatment and long term.
6. You have the right to make decisions about your care before and during treatment and the right to refuse care. The hospital must inform you of the medical consequences of refusing treatment. You also have the right to other treatments provided by the hospital and the right to transfer to another hospital.
7. You have the right to have an advance directive, such as a living will or a power of attorney for health care. A hospital has the right to ask for your advance directive, put it in your file, and honor its intent.
8. You have the right to privacy in medical exams, case discussions, consultations, and treatments.
9. You have the right to expect that your communication and records are treated as confidential by the hospital, except as the law permits and requires in cases of suspected abuse or public health hazards. If the hospital releases your information to another medical facility, you have the right to expect the hospital to ask the medical facility to keep your records confidential.
10. You have the right to review your medical records and to have them explained or interpreted, except when restricted by law.
11. You have the right to expect that a hospital will respond reasonably to your requests for care and services or transfer you to another facility that has accepted a transfer request. You should also expect information and explanation about the risks, benefits, and alternatives to a transfer.
12. You have the right to ask and be informed of any business relationships between the hospital and educational institutions, other health care providers, or payers that may influence your care and treatment.
13. You have the right to consent to or decline to participate in research studies and to have the studies fully explained before you give your consent. If you decide not to participate in research, you are still entitled to the most effective care that the hospital can provide.
    You have the right to expect reasonable continuity of care and to be informed of other care options when hospital care is no longer appropriate.
14. You have the right to be informed of hospital policies and practices related to patient care, treatment, and responsibilities.
15. You also have the right to know who you can contact to resolve disputes, grievances, and conflicts. And you have the right to know what the hospital will charge for services and their payment methods.

Rules and Regulations in Health Care

Health care is among the most highly regulated of all industries. Rules govern how health care is delivered, how patients and employees are treated, and how health care is paid for. Much of your education has involved learning the rules associated with your health care profession, such as following universal and standard precautions, completing insurance forms, performing sterilization techniques, and administering medications.

There are several federal, state, and local regulatory agencies that establish rules and regulations for the health care industry to ensure compliance and to provide safe health care to every person who accesses the system. Box 14.1 lists the most common laws and regulations that affect medical practices and patient care.

BOX 14.1

Common Health Care Laws and Regulations

- Patient Protection and Affordable Care Act: Commonly called the Affordable Care Act (ACA) or "Obamacare," named after former President Barack Obama, who signed it into law in 2010, this federal statute was a major step in health care reform by expanding access to more affordable, quality health insurance; increasing consumer insurance protection; emphasizing prevention and wellness; and curbing rising health care costs.
- Health Insurance Portability and Accountability Act of 1996 (HIPAA): HIPAA gives patients rights over their health information and sets rules and limits on who can look at and receive patients' private information. HIPAA applies to protected health information (PHI), whether electronic, written, or oral.
- Health Information Technology for Economic and Clinical Health Act (HITECH): The HITECH Act expanded on HIPAA and includes provisions that allow for increased enforcement of the privacy and security of electronic transmission of patient information, such as prohibiting the sale of PHI, making business associates and vendors liable for compliance with HIPAA, and creating a penalty and violation system.
- Occupational Safety and Health (OSH) Act: The OSH Act is overseen by the Occupational Safety and Health Administration (OSHA) and states that employers are accountable for providing a safe and healthful workplace for employees by setting and enforcing standards and by providing training, outreach, education, and assistance.
- Controlled Substances Act (CSA): CSA is a federal policy that regulates the manufacture and distribution of controlled substances. Controlled substances can include narcotics, depressants, and stimulants. The CSA classifies medications into five schedules, or classifications, based on the likelihood for abuse and if there are any medical benefits provided by the substance.
- The Emergency Medical Treatment and Active Labor Act (EMTALA) of 1986 requires any hospital emergency department that receives payments from federal health care programs, such as Medicare and Medicaid, to provide an appropriate medical screening to any patient seeking treatment. This was enacted to eliminate "patient dumping" where a facility would transfer a patient based on a potentially high-cost diagnosis or refuse to treat a patient based on their ability to pay. This legislation requires the emergency department to determine whether a condition is emergent or not and to provide stabilizing treatment in the case of an emergency medical condition. It does not require that treatment be given for nonemergency conditions. Furthermore, outpatient clinics are not medically equipped to handle emergencies and therefore are not bound by the EMTALA.
- The Clinical Laboratory Improvement Act (CLIA) of 1988 is a group of laws that regulate all laboratory facilities for safety and handling of specimens. The objective of CLIA is to regulate the accuracy and timeliness of testing regardless of where the test is performed. The Food and Drug Administration (FDA) is the federal agency that authorizes and implements the CLIA laws and determines the test complexity categories.
- Title VII of Civil Rights Act of 1964: The Civil Rights Act prohibits an employer with 15 or more employees from discriminating on the basis of race, national origin, gender, or religion. The Civil Rights Act has also been amended several times to protect other groups. For example, the Pregnancy Discrimination Act of 1978 amended the Civil Rights Act and prohibited discrimination based on pregnancy and other related medical conditions. Sexual harassment is a form of sex discrimination that also violates the Civil Rights A.
- Americans With Disabilities Act of 1990 (ADA): ADA forbids discrimination against any applicant or employee who could perform a job regardless of a disability. ADA also requires an employer to provide "reasonable accommodations" that are necessary to help the employee perform a job successfully, unless these accommodations are unduly burdensome.

Policies and Procedures

Every health care facility and medical office has some form of a policy and procedures manual. These detailed manuals cover every aspect of the employer's policy to ensure smooth, correct, and legal operation of the company. Large health care organizations likely have an institutional approach to policies and procedures, with established committees and even employees dedicated to creating policies and procedures, disseminating them to all employees, and developing the training solutions necessary to implement and enforce them.

The implementation of policies and regulations requires training. New employees must be trained in all types of rules, ranging from procedures to safety and ethics issues. New regulations demand company-wide training, and refresher training should be routinely conducted. Policies and procedures are constantly being evaluated and improved to strengthen best practices and reflect any changes to the company and the environment it works in.

These policies should provide answers to questions such as who gets seen first in the emergency room. What obligations are satisfied by the patient discharge process? How can infectious diseases be better controlled? What dental materials should be used? What happens when a patient misses an appointment? What is the protocol for creating an incident report when there is an employee injury at work? For health care professionals, following the rules of policies is an important duty and critical to the success of their job (Figure 14.1).

Fraud and Abuse in Health Care

Fraud and abuse in health care are national problems that cost consumers, insurance companies, and governments billions of dollars a year. Fraud is the

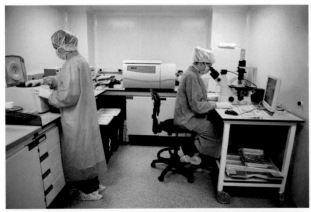

Figure 14.1 Laboratory workers follow strict safety and sanitation procedures to ensure accurate results. (Copyright © istock.com.)

intentional act to misrepresent facts or mislead for financial gain. Fraud in health care is an intentional misrepresentation, deception, or act of deceit for the purpose of receiving greater reimbursement. It is a criminal offense that can lead to, for example, health care professionals and medical billing and coding personnel incurring fines, loss of license, and even imprisonment. Examples of fraud include billing for services not provided or up-coding services to gain larger reimbursement for services provided. It is important to note that it is the attempt at deceit that is fraud, regardless of whether it is successful. Abuse in health care is a reckless disregard or conduct that goes against acceptable business and/or medical practices resulting in greater reimbursement.

Fraud and abuse can bring big financial penalties to a physician or medical practice. As an employee in any health care organization, it is important to understand that the penalties outlined earlier in the text are levied not just on the physician but may also be levied on the employer. Coding and billing personnel can also be subject to fines and imprisonment if they take part in a fraudulent activity, even if they were only following the employer's direction.

As a result, a number of laws and guidelines, especially by the federal government, are in place to prevent, identify, and penalize acts of fraud and abuse in health care. Federal health care fraud statute prohibits "knowingly and willfully executing, or attempting to execute, a scheme or artifice in connection with the delivery of or payment for health care benefits, items, or services to either:

* Defraud any health care benefit program
* Obtain (by means of false or fraudulent pretenses, representations, or promises) any of the money or property owned by, or under the control of, any health care benefit program."
* Violations of key federal fraud and abuse laws can be either civil or criminal offenses.

JOURNALING 14.1

Think of situations you have been in when you broke the rule or thought you should have. What was the rule and what were the circumstances that made you feel that the rule should have been broken?

Best Practices

If there are no established rules or guidelines, people often follow best practice, which is a generally accepted method of doing something that has been established through research or experience. Best practice often occurs in the health care setting and, most likely, will occur in your health care profession. Examples of best practices may be making sure the patient is only kept waiting in the waiting room or patient room for less than 15 minutes or making sure the patient is seen by the same medical assistant at each visit (Figure 14.2).

Similar to best practice is the scientific method, which is a process or procedure that uses observation, measurement, and experimentation to support or contradict a theory. How we practice medicine is often based on the scientific method because it establishes the way we deliver health care, along with the standards and guidelines in health care.

 EXPERIENTIAL EXERCISES

1. Think of a clinical skill you have learned. List how many different ways you can perform that skill.
2. On your next major decision, weigh the risks and outcomes of possible solutions. Which one did you decide on and why?

Compliance Plans

In most situations, people want to know what the rules are in order to know what to do and to be compliant. New employees are especially eager to learn the rules, both written and unwritten, so they can make sure they are compliant and have a sense of knowing what they are doing and how best to do it. Following rules and standards is important to ensuring that you and your employer avoid legal issues and negligent behavior, including malpractice. Most importantly, rules and guidelines in the health care setting help keep patients safe and ensure they get quality care.

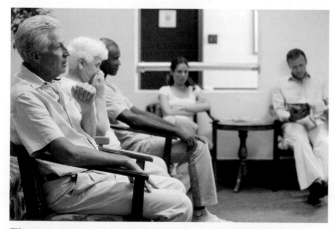

Figure 14.2 Many medical offices use the best practice of limiting patients' wait time. (iStock.com/ monkeybusinessimages/95838760.)

Rules should establish order and prevent chaos but still allow people to be able to comply with them. Workplaces that are too strict may find that employees are unable to comply with the rules, and multiple violations may occur. However, workplaces without rules feel chaotic and unsafe.

To ensure compliance with all health care laws and regulations, almost all health care organizations create a compliance plan. A compliance plan is a written set of policies and procedures that describe how an organization will operate and conduct itself in an ethical and compliant manner. It also includes guidelines and regulations and protocols for addressing infractions when discovered.

The Office of the Inspector General (OIG) is the department that fights waste, fraud, and abuse; improves the efficiency of federal programs; and offers guidelines on how to create and implement a compliance program for individual and small group physician practices, as well as larger health care organizations. The goal of the OIG's compliance program is to detect erroneous claims or prevent the engagement of unlawful conduct, especially involving any federal health care programs, such as Medicare and Medicaid. The OIG's compliance program includes seven key components:

* Conduct internal monitoring and auditing.
* Develop written standards and procedures, such as a compliance plan.
* Designate a compliance officer.
* Conduct appropriate training and education.
* Respond to detected offenses and develop a corrective action plan.
* Develop open lines of communication.
* Enforce disciplinary standards.

An important component of a compliance program and plan is the designation or hire of a specific individual to act as a compliance officer to ensure that these policies and procedures are being followed and that any violations are being appropriately addressed. The position of the compliance officer may be a dedicated full-time position, or it may be included in the duties of an existing supervisor or manager in any given area or department. The role of the compliance officer is to ensure that the compliance plan is followed by all employees and to provide training on the policy and procedures.

Ongoing monitoring is crucial to determine whether a compliance plan is working and to keep up with ever-changing standards and rules. Education and training should be tailored to a specific practice specialty.

Enforcement and Disciplinary Actions

There are a number of different disciplinary actions that a health care professional may receive from one of the regulating agencies, including sanctions, monetary fines, and even imprisonment. State and federal regulations focus on violations in the areas of fraud, substance abuse, illegal activities, practicing without a license or practicing outside the scope of practice, and malpractice.

Illegal and unethical acts can be penalized by law, licensing, and/or ethics boards, certification boards, and employers, with consequences varying depending on the severity of the act or lack of action. In the case of a minor infraction, the consequences may include a performance improvement plan or corrective action plan by an employer or a temporary loss of license or small fine/penalty to an accrediting agency. In the case of a more serious infraction or violation, the health care professional may incur a permanent loss of license, heavy fines and penalties, and imprisonment.

For example, if a physician is found to be guilty of illegal billing practices, the state licensing board may revoke the physician's license and ability to practice medicine.

In the health care field, violations can range from the unethical treatment or negligence of care of a patient to a violation of privacy, fraud, or other illegal actions. In addition to the legal consequences of breaking a law, employers and agencies may also impose sanctions that extend beyond these. Although committing an illegal act may lead to fines and possible imprisonment, professional and workplace sanctions depend on professional codes of conduct and may include corrective actions, termination of employment, or loss of license.

JOURNALING 14.2

Think about your career as a health care professional. Record what inspired you to pursue this goal. What action steps did you take to pursue your goal? Would you have done anything differently in the way you went about achieving this goal?

CASE STUDY 14.1
43 Folders

Sue Yang had been a medical assistant at the pediatrics practice for more than a year, and she started to see the same serious issues crop up repeatedly. There were missing immunization records. Forms for schools were frequently late, causing a last-minute rush that interrupted the patient workflow. Appointments were missed or, in some cases, never even scheduled. Sue thought that all these problems had one thing in common: poor planning and follow-up.

Sue discussed her concerns with the managing partner, Dr. Richardson. She agreed with Sue. "I tell you what, Sue. You're very efficient, organized, and have a good understanding of the workflow in the office. I would really appreciate it if you developed some possible solutions."

Sue was excited by the opportunity because this could help her advance in the clinic, but she soon realized that it was a difficult assignment. One evening while doing research, Sue came across a website called "43 Folders," which described a method to track documents for the 31 days of the month and the 12 months of the year. Sue felt that this could be a great solution.

Over the weekend, Sue collected and labeled 43 folders. On Monday, she put the folders in her personal file cabinet and started using the system. When a health care provider ordered a laboratory test, she put a note in the folder for the day that the results were due. If a booster shot was needed for a baby, she put a note in the file for the month it should take place. By the end of the week, her files were filling up. She began each day by reviewing that day's file and scheduling its tasks. Then, she scheduled any follow-up appointments and addressed any unfinished tasks. At the end of the day, she moved that day's file to the back, so the next day would be in front when she arrived in the morning.

Sue also added files for the next few years for more long-term reminders. She could see that the August file was filling up with school-related activities, forms, and requirements.

Sue made an appointment with Dr. Richardson to share her solution.

Sue explained the 43 folders system and how she had been implementing it in the clinic. Dr. Richardson loved the idea. "It's a simple idea, but that's what makes it so brilliant," she said.

Over the next few weeks, Sue continued to pilot the system she had proposed. She wrote a short manual describing the system and how to use it. She identified all the kinds of documents that would go into the 43 folders. She designed a simple form that could be used to record a task or reminder. Finally, Dr. Richardson asked Sue to make a presentation to the staff explaining the system, provide any needed training, and implement it.

By the end of the month, the system was fully implemented, and all the medical assistants were using it. Patients and staff both noticed significant improvements.

One day, Dr. Richardson invited Sue into her office. "Sue, we'd like to make you the training supervisor for all the new medical assistants. We've hired quite a few new staff recently, and we are confident that you can train them on the new system, as well as on the policy and procedures of the clinic. There's a promotion and a raise involved, if you're interested."

Sue beamed with the knowledge that she had earned her employer's trust. "I am interested, and I will do a good job, Dr. Richardson."

"Sue, you already have!"

QUESTIONS FOR THOUGHT AND REFLECTION

1. What made Sue want to propose a solution to Dr. Richardson?
2. Why did Sue try out the idea herself before proposing it to Dr. Richardson?
3. How would you describe Sue's personality and attitude as an employee?

A Different Path

Linda was a bright student who was a natural leader in class, easy to get along with, and helpful to her classmates. Linda was always dressed appropriately in clean, pressed scrubs.

After she graduated, she found a job in a family medicine clinic working for Dr. Short. It was a hectic and busy practice, with a large staff of physicians and medical assistants. She had worked there for 3 years and generally performed well. But she was getting frustrated with not being promoted.

Last month, Sherita, who was also a medical assistant and was hired a year after her, was promoted to a lead medical assistant. Linda noticed that Sherita was good with both patients and staff. She often went out of her way to help patients and even helped train new medical assistants without being asked.

But Linda felt she was good at her job as well and that should have been enough. She often did not volunteer for extra duties because she did not think she should do them without being paid more. However, when one of the new medical assistants asked her a question, she would answer and would help them if she was not too busy. She decided to schedule a meeting with Dr. Short about being promoted.

"Dr. Short, I've been at the clinic for 3 years and I think I do a good job. I just don't know why I'm not being promoted like Sherita."

"I do think you do a good job, Linda. But the lead medical assistant is truly a lead position and that person must have leadership and management skills. I just have not seen you step up and take initiative," Dr. Short replied.

"Well, I will take on more responsibility once I get promoted," Linda said. "I'm just not sure why I would do it now without being paid more."

"To be honest, that's not a good attitude to have as a professional, especially if you want to be promoted."

Linda left the meeting feeling even more frustrated and deflated about her advancement opportunities. She still did not understand why she should work for free. The more she thought about it, the more frustrated she became.

"I think I'm going to have to find a job somewhere else. Somewhere where they will appreciate me," Linda thought to herself.

QUESTIONS FOR THOUGHT AND REFLECTION

1. What made Linda think she should be promoted?
2. What made Dr. Short promote Sherita over Linda?
3. If you were Dr. Short, how else would you advise Linda?
4. If Linda quits, do you think she will be promoted at her new clinic?

◀ JOURNALING 14.3

Identify a problem that you have noticed at school, at work, or at home. Develop a plan to resolve this problem. Where would you go to find a solution?

⭐ EXPERIENTIAL EXERCISES

1. Find out what written rules you should be aware of at work.
2. Determine how policies and procedures are maintained and updated at your place of employment.
3. Review a recent journal in your profession. Are there new "rules" for best practices being reported?

 CROSS CURRENTS WITH OTHER SOFT SKILLS

ACHIEVING HONESTY AND INTEGRITY: Following rules leads to a positive reputation (Chapter 1).
BUILDING TRUST: People who follow rules can be trusted to work more independently (Chapter 5).
CONTRIBUTING AS A MEMBER OF THE TEAM: Health care is a team activity, and teamwork requires adherence to the rules (Chapter 13).

Professional Code of Ethics

Health care professionals are accountable to a health care provider or a hospital, but this does not exclude them from personal responsibility. Understanding the laws, standards of practice, and ethical principles that govern you and your profession will help you make legal and sound decisions when confronted with an ethical situation or dilemma.

Ethics are the rules, standards, and moral principles that govern a person's behavior and on which the person bases decisions. Ethics are concerned with questions of how individuals in a society should act by defining right and wrong and appropriate conduct to serve the greater good. Ethics encompasses several different facets. One aspect is morals, which describes the goodness or badness or right or wrong of actions. Similarly, values, or an individual's ethics, refer to one person's moral principles or what an individual believes is right or wrong. Values govern a person's decisions, with a goal of maintaining one's integrity or conscience. An individual's values may be influenced by concepts of honesty, fidelity, equality, compassion, responsibility, humility, and respect for life.

There are many types and fields of ethics, including personal, common, and professional. Personal ethics determines what an individual believes about morality and right and wrong. It includes one's personal values and moral qualities and is influenced by family, friends, culture, religion, education, and many other factors. Personal ethics have an impact on areas of life such as family, finances, and relationships and may change during one's life. An example of one's personal ethics may be for a person to believe in the death penalty but support a woman's right to an abortion.

Common ethics, also called group ethics, is a system of principles and rules of conduct accepted by a group based on ethnicity, political affiliation, or cultural identity. An example of common ethics is for a person who is religious to believe all abortion and the death penalty is bad and all life should be preserved.

Professional ethics is a type of ethics that aims to define, clarify, and critique professional work and its typical values. Professional ethics sets the standards for practicing one's profession and can be learned only through education, training, or on the job. It involves attributes such as commitment, competence, confidence, and contract. Professional ethics is often used to impose rules and standards on employees in an organization or members of a profession. Examples of professional ethics are in employee handbooks, the code of ethics, and the Hippocratic Oath taken by physicians.

A branch of ethics is medical ethics, which is the morals, moral principles, and moral judgments that health care professionals use to determine whether an action should be allowed based on "right and wrong." In addition to examining facts, medical ethics uses moral analysis to assess the obligations and responsibilities of health care professionals on various issues and challenges related to health care and medicine. It specifically addresses how to handle ethical issues arising from the care of patients and focuses on the health care professional's duty to the patient.

Informed and Implied Consent

Consent is a critical aspect of patient autonomy, in protecting the legal rights of patients, and guides the ethical practice of health care. Consent's literal meaning is the "permission or agreement for something to happen." Consent is an act of reason. The person giving consent must be of sufficient mental capacity and be in possession of all essential information to give valid consent. Consent must be free of force or fraud. There are many distinct types of consent. It is important for all health care professionals to be aware of them to protect themselves and their employers against cases of malpractice.

General consent is an individual's permission to be touched. General consent can be explicit or implied. Explicit consent, also known as express or direct consent, means that an individual is clearly presented with an option to agree or disagree or to express a preference or choice, often verbally or in writing. Explicit consent is usually required when clear, documentable consent is required, and the purpose for which it is being provided is sensitive, such as the collection, use, or disclosure of personal information.

Conversely, implied consent is not expressly granted by a person, but rather inferred from a person's actions and the facts and circumstances of a particular situation. There are many situations when health care professionals routinely obtain implied consent when treating a patient. For example, a medical assistant may ask a patient to roll up their sleeve while they are holding a syringe. If the patient rolls up their sleeve, this is implied consent for the patient to receive the shot.

Implied consent may also be given in emergency situations. The situation must be life threatening or pose a risk of significant physical injury to the patient if the procedure or action is not performed. Only those procedures that are necessary are authorized, and explicit consent should be obtained as soon as possible. Furthermore, only a health care provider, such as a physician, can make the determination that a true emergency exists that necessitates proceeding without explicit or informed consent. All states have statutes that specify when consent is implied. Medical assistants must be aware of their individual state laws and ensure they are following them in order to protect patients' rights and to prevent any occurrence of malpractice and negligence.

In the health care setting, one of the most important types of consent is informed consent, which is a clear and voluntary indication of preference or choice, usually oral or written, and freely given in circumstances where the available options and their consequences have been made clear. Informed consent involves shared decision-making between the patient and the health care provider. The health care provider must disclose appropriate information to a competent patient so that the patient may make a voluntary choice to accept or refuse treatment. The health care provider must detail all possible risks and potential prognoses for having a treatment or procedure performed and the available alternatives. Failure to obtain informed

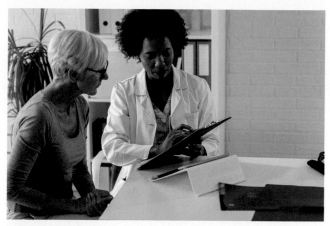

Figure 14.3 All patients should be provided informed consent before any procedures. (iStock.com/Lordn/1211390857.)

consent may lead to a case of medical negligence and malpractice. Unless it is an emergency, health care professionals should not proceed with any procedure without the consent of the patient (Figure 14.3).

Maintaining Confidentiality and Discretion

Patients are far more willing to share the intimate details of their private lives when they have confidence that their doctors will not post those details on Facebook.

—Jacob Appel

LEARNING OBJECTIVE 2:
MAINTAINING CONFIDENTIALITY AND DISCRETION

- Understand the importance of confidentiality.
- Explain the significance of HIPAA.
- State the rights that HIPAA bestows on patients.
- State your obligations as a health professional under HIPAA.
- Discuss what is prohibited and not prohibited under HIPAA.

Confidentiality in medicine and health care has never been more important than it is today. Maintaining the confidentiality of patient medical information has always been a matter of ethics and professionalism. However, with the passage of the Health Information Portability and Accountability Act (HIPAA), patient medical information is now protected by federal law. For example, gossip is never professional. But gossip that involves confidential medical information is a violation of federal law and, most likely, the policy and procedures at your workplace.

The Health Information Portability and Accountability Act

One of the most important laws is HIPAA, which outlines patient privacy and confidentiality and how patient information is managed. HIPAA gives patients rights over their health care information. They have the right to get a copy of their information, ensure the medical record is correct, and know who has had access to the record.

HIPAA, like many laws, can seem complicated and extremely detailed at first. However, regulations and other efforts have been made to simplify its laws and guidelines for easier understanding so that everyone who works in the health care field can be compliant. Every health care professional must understand the HIPAA law and implement it in their daily practice. In fact, regardless of the type or size, every health care facility is required to designate a privacy officer who monitors and ensures the protection of patient medical information, provides staff training, and oversees the implementation and enforcement of the HIPAA law. At your job, you should know who your privacy officer is and use that person as a resource in your efforts to comply with HIPAA.

Patient Rights Under HIPAA

You may already be familiar with the practice of providing patients with the health care facility's policy on protecting personal medical information. All health care facilities must obtain the patient's signed acknowledgment of the policy to further protect the facility (Figure 14.4).

Under HIPAA, patients have rights regarding their protected medical information. For instance, patients may elect to protect their privacy by asking that you communicate confidential information to them in a specific way, such as using a post office box or calling a specific phone number. A health care facility is prohibited from providing and releasing a patient's medical information to anyone without the patient's permission. Thus, a patient can release medical information to an attorney or another health care provider and can even request that parts of the medical information not be disclosed, such as mental health treatment or medication use. These patient rights regarding medical information are further summarized in Box 14.2.

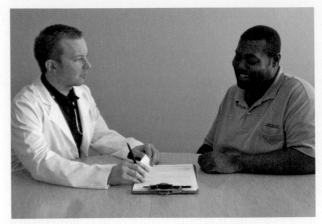

Figure 14.4 Health professional explaining a HIPAA form to a patient.

BOX 14.2

Patient Rights Under HIPAA

- Right to receive a copy of your facility's privacy policy
- Right to determine how they receive confidential information
- Right to restrict parts or uses of medical information, except those required by law
- Right to review your own private medical information
- Right to request that errors in your private medical information be corrected
- Right to know how and to whom your private medical information was disclosed

When patients exercise any of their rights related to how their medical information is handled, the request should be documented in their medical chart. Always review this information for special requests whenever you access a patient's chart to avoid any mistakes or accidental disclosure of patient information.

It is important for you to understand that although your facility owns the patient's medical record, the patient is now entitled to see it. This right was not always honored before the implementation of HIPAA. There should be no question about the patient's right to see their medical information and, if it is incorrect, to have it corrected.

If medical information ever becomes the subject of a lawsuit or legal dispute, you will usually not be involved if you have protected confidential information and observed patients' rights. However, that is why it is important for you to understand and observe these rights.

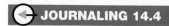

Think about yourself as a patient. What information would you not want to be disclosed to unauthorized people? Who would you want to have access to your medical information? Why?

Your Responsibilities Under HIPAA

Many of your responsibilities are covered in the privacy policy disclosure your health care facility distributes to patients. However, the most important aspects of your responsibilities are listed in Box 14.3.

If you receive a patient request regarding their medical information and you are not sure what is required or permissible, you should check with your privacy officer. Not taking the proper steps to ensure compliance with HIPAA laws will make you and your health care facility vulnerable to violations and lawsuits.

Monitoring Your Activities Under HIPAA

The purpose of HIPAA is primarily to put into law what was best practice for most health care facilities. However, the establishment of the HIPAA law also has helped enforce confidentiality by preventing past abuses in how patient medical information was handled.

Before 1996, it was not uncommon for insurance companies to use private and confidential medical information to deny health insurance to Americans with preexisting conditions. There were also incidences of employers denying employment to applicants based on their medical history. Further, there were no penalties to prevent health care professionals from sharing and disclosing health information about

BOX 14.3

Duties of Health Care Professionals Under HIPAA

- Inform all patients of their privacy rights under HIPAA.
- Be able to explain the proper use of medical records.
- Protect medical records from everyone not involved in the care of the patient.
- Keep medical charts and records secure.
- Follow the privacy policies created by your facility.
- Know who your privacy officer is and complete any mandated training.

patients, especially those they may know from other areas of their lives such as church, school, or neighborhood organizations.

However, HIPAA is not intended to restrict normal communication necessary to provide patient care. While reasonable precautions and efforts should be observed, the law favors the well-intentioned provision of quality care. Box 14.4 includes examples of HIPAA-compliant situations in the health care setting.

? WHAT IF?

What if you receive a call from a patient's spouse asking for a condition update on a patient in your clinic? What would you do?

General Confidentiality

Anything you learn about a patient in your capacity as a health care professional should be considered confidential (Figure 14.5). If the patient discloses personal information, even in a friendly conversation, you are

BOX 14.4

Examples of HIPAA-Compliant Situations in the Health Care Setting

- A physician talks to a patient in a semiprivate hospital room, within earshot of the patient in the other bed.
- A patient is not immediately informed of their HIPAA rights in an emergency.
- First responders do not inform disaster victims of their HIPAA rights when they arrive on the scene of a public health emergency.
- A doctor talks to a pharmacist about a patient's medication within earshot of other patients.
- A medical assistant addresses a patient by name in the presence of other patients.
- Patients sign into an office and see other patients' names.
- One patient has an incidental view of another patient's chart or prescription.
- A patient sees other records come up while the dentist is searching for the patient's record.
- A nursing assistant overhears a nurse talking to a patient on the other side of a screen.
- Nurses speak about patient care issues in a nursing station.

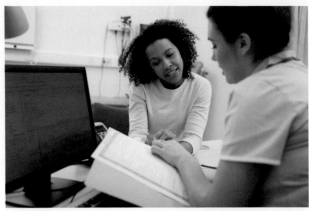

Figure 14.5 A health care professional discusses records with a patient. (Copyright © istock.com).

prohibited from repeating that information to anyone. Information you overhear at work is confidential.

It is not appropriate to discuss any patient information in idle conversation; during break time; and in elevators, hallways, lobbies, or any other place inside or outside the health care facility. You should avoid mentioning a patient's name, as well as any other information that could identify the patient. This is especially important when you have patients who may be known to the public or of interest to the media. In this age of social media and instant communication, you have a special obligation to protect all confidential information.

CASE STUDY **14.2**
St. Nowhere

Al Berks was extremely concerned about his long-time business partner, Jeffrey Galloway. They were great friends, but their medical supply business had not been doing well, and Al could see that Jeffrey was becoming depressed. He had not been himself for the last several months. He spent long days sequestered in his office, and Al had no idea what he was doing in there. Then Jeffrey started showing up only 2 or 3 days a week. Now, Al had not seen Jeffrey in more than a week. Jeffrey was divorced, and his children were grown. So there was no one he knew of that could check on him.

Al decided to drop by Jeffrey's house, but there was no answer to his knock, no car in the driveway, and no evidence that anyone was at home.

Al became very concerned. He continued his search and knocked on a neighbor's door. An older man answered the door and said, "He's in St. Nowhere," which was slang for the state psychiatric facility.

Al went back to his office and called the state psychiatric facility. A staff member told him that she could not "confirm or deny" that information and that she was not allowed to disclose patient information.

He tried a different approach. He called the hospital's general number and asked for the "depression clinic."

"We don't have a clinic specifically for depression but let me forward you to our nurse manager for this floor."

"This is Maria. How can I help you?"

"Oh, hi, Maria. My name is Al Berks and my friend, Jeffrey Galloway, is a patient there. I need to talk to him."

"I'm sorry Mr. Berks, but I can't disclose any patient information without consent from the patient."

"Oh, I know. I don't want to put you in an awkward position, but please hear me out. Jeffrey doesn't have any family nearby. I've known him for a long time, and I may be the only family he has right now. I know he's been having a hard time. I just want to make sure he's okay and that he's not missing somewhere."

"I'm really sorry, Mr. Berks. I wish I could help you but it's against policy for me to disclose any patient information, including if a patient has been admitted or not."

"I know, I know. But can you have him call me? I just haven't seen him in a week. Wouldn't you be worried if your friend was acting depressed and you hadn't seen him in a week?" Al asked, exasperated.

"I understand your concern, sir. But, again, I am not at liberty to disclose any information without patient consent. Have a good day." Maria hung up the phone.

Al slammed the phone down. What kind of rules are these, he thought to himself. I just needed to know if he was there or not.

QUESTIONS FOR THOUGHT AND REFLECTION

1. If you were friends with Al and heard his frustration with the medical staff, what would you tell him to better explain the situation to him?
2. Did Maria handle Al's call correctly?
3. Why was merely confirming if Jeffrey was a patient there a violation of patient confidentiality?

Carlene was scanning laboratory results into patients' electronic medical records when she came across a laboratory report for her friend Leslie, who had married Carlene's cousin, Bob, 2 years ago. She and Bob were very close, and she thought they had an ideal marriage. Leslie's laboratory results showed that Leslie was pregnant. Carlene was thrilled for them.

Carlene continued her scanning and uploaded Leslie's laboratory results to her chart. But she was so excited to learn that Leslie was pregnant. She wanted to congratulate her but had to be mindful of not disclosing Leslie's medical information. She needed to wait until the physician had a chance to give Leslie her results. She checked the appointment book and confirmed that Leslie had an appointment with Dr. Darby on Friday.

Carlene worked in the back office on Friday afternoon. She did not want to see Leslie in case her expression would tip off Leslie as to the results. She did not want to spoil the surprise.

She was proud of herself for keeping such wonderful news to herself. She did not even tell her mother. Anyway, she would see Bob and Leslie at the bowling league on Monday night.

When Carlene got to the bowling alley, Bob said Leslie could not come because she was not feeling well. She was hoping they would both be there to announce the good news. Without Leslie there, it was unlikely that Bob would share the news, but she was hoping he would somehow let it slip.

All evening, well into their third game, Carlene kept an eye on Bob. But he acted like this was just another night at the lanes.

By the end of the night, she decided to say something because she was his cousin, after all. While they were returning their shoes, Carlene says, "So how does it feel, Pops?"

"Pops? What does that mean?"

"The baby, silly."

He just looked at her with a confused look on his face.

"Look, Bob. I work at the clinic. I saw Leslie's pregnancy test. You don't have to pretend around me."

Bob darkened. "She's not pregnant," he said. "How could she be? I had a vasectomy 5 years ago."

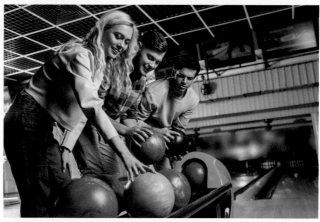

iStock.com/LightFieldStudios/1208330009

QUESTIONS FOR THOUGHT AND REFLECTION

1. Where did Carlene act appropriately and inappropriately?
2. Did it matter that Carlene disclosed Leslie's laboratory results outside of the clinic?
3. Are there ever times or situations when a health care professional is permitted to disclose patient medical information without their consent?
4. What do you think the repercussions will be if Leslie informs Dr. Darby about the disclosure?

EXPERIENTIAL EXERCISES

1. Review your facility's protected patient information policy. Read the fine print.
2. Find out where special confidentiality requests are entered into patients' charts.
3. Describe the qualifications of being a privacy officer.
4. Visit http://www.hhs.gov/ocr/privacy/hipaa/understanding/index.html to learn more about HIPAA.

CROSS CURRENTS WITH OTHER SOFT SKILLS

ACHIEVING HONESTY AND INTEGRITY: Protecting confidential information always comes down to your personal integrity (Chapter 1).

BUILDING TRUST: Confidentiality only works if, like trust, it is observed 100% of the time (Chapter 5 and 6).

PROFESSIONAL PHONE TECHNIQUE: Confidentiality is especially challenging when you are on the phone and may not be sure with whom you are speaking (Chapter 4).

COMMITTING TO YOUR PROFESSION: Professions are identified, in part, with codes of ethics, which include confidentiality (Chapter 13).

Documentation and Medical Records

The shortest pencil is longer than the longest memory.

—Mark Batterson

LEARNING OBJECTIVE 3: DOCUMENTATION AND MEDICAL RECORDS

- Explain the purpose of documentation and medical records.
- Know the different types of records and the medical charting formats.
- Describe the principles and best practices of medical documentation.

Documentation and medical records play an important role in health care by recording the care given to a patient, including who provided the care, what type of care, and when it was delivered. Medical records help health care providers and other health care professionals evaluate and plan the patient's treatment and monitor the patient's health over time.

Medical records also serve multiple functions for billing, legal, and research purposes. Insurers may require accurate and detailed documentation on the medical services provided to make sure the service was covered under the patient's policy and to ensure the medical necessity of the service before providing reimbursements.

Medical records serve as legal documents to protect the patient and health care provider in cases of negligence and malpractice. A medical record can be used as evidence in court to support the patient's case against the health care provider or help defend the health care provider's actions. Additionally, patient data from medical records are collected for health care statistics for research and public health purposes. Being able to monitor and track health data, such as birth and death rates and the incidence and prevalence of different diseases, allows federal, state, and local health departments to plan and implement best practice standards and allocate funding to address specific diseases or communities.

Purposes of Medical Records

Medical records have many purposes, including planning, coordinating, and delivering quality patient care. As you document, keep in mind all the users that will be accessing the medical records, as well as its many purposes.

Continuity of Care

The primary users of the medical records you create are your co-workers and other members of the health care team who will be managing the patients' care, now and in the future. Physicians, dentists, laboratory and imaging technicians, medical billers and coders, and a series of other health care professionals need to obtain accurate information quickly and easily from the medical records. This information is available to them only if you put it there. There is a very common saying in health care: "If it wasn't documented, it didn't happen." Thus, it is critical for you to document any relevant patient information to help in the diagnosing and treatment of the patient.

Every patient is a puzzle, both from a diagnostic and treatment point of view. Just as soon as a patient enters the medical office, the medical documentation process begins. All the compiled, relevant information about the patient creates a holistic picture of the patient's health status. Whether the patient's condition is accurately diagnosed depends on the knowledge and clinical skill of the health care provider. But it is also largely dependent on the information that has been documented in the medical record.

CASE STUDY 14.3
A Thought Bubble

Sara was a night shift nurse at the local hospital and nearing the end of a long night on the floor. Her feet were aching. As she was finishing her rounds and entering her last patient's room, all that was on her mind was a hot bubble bath. The patient's wife began speaking as soon as she entered the room.

"Please … my husband … his color is so bad … the last nurse said it was the narcotic and not to worry, but …" said Mrs. Walsh.

Sara pulled up Mr. Walsh's chart on the monitor and read the last entry, then assessed the patient. She was alarmed at the bluish tinge around the patient's mouth and nail beds. She also had difficulty in rousing him but was able to give him oxygen.

She decided to read his medical records and progress notes to see if there was information that could help her figure out what was going on with Mr. Walsh. According to his medical records, he was recovering from surgery. The previous nurse wrote that she felt the wife was "a bit of a worry wart." Otherwise, she did not find anything in his history to indicate a breathing problem, although he was on a strong narcotic for his pain, and that could cause drowsiness.

Sara decided to alert the physician on call but was afraid the physician would ridicule her for waking him up and

mistaking narcotic suppression for a pulmonary problem. She also knew she would not be leaving on time today.

The physician arrived in 15 minutes, and Mr. Walsh was found to be suffering from an embolism that required immediate treatment. The physician gave Sara high praise for her observation and critical thinking skills, and Mrs. Walsh gave Sara a great big hug. Mr. Walsh sent a gratitude card after leaving the hospital when his wife described Sara's diligence and fast action.

QUESTIONS FOR THOUGHT AND REFLECTION

1. Why do you think Sara was more successful at assessing Mr. Walsh than the nurse before her?
2. What are the factors that were against her decision to call the physician? What factored into supporting her decision to call the physician?
3. What were the critical thinking steps you would take to assess this situation?

⟳ CROSS CURRENTS WITH OTHER SOFT SKILLS

ADOPTING A POSITIVE MENTAL ATTITUDE: Your attitude can cloud your thinking and affect your ability to think critically (Chapter 2).

READING AND SPEAKING BODY LANGUAGE: Your inferences and observations are based in large part on the body language of others. Note that in health care, body language is often substituted for spoken word to keep out of the patient's earshot (Chapter 6).

FOLLOWING RULES AND REGULATIONS: Any critical thinking decision should be made with the rules and regulations of the facility in the forefront (Chapter 9).

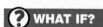

Figure 14.6 Medical records are legal documents that can be subpoenaed in a trial or civil case. (iStock.com/gorodenkoff/1346156637.)

Legal Considerations

Medical records are considered legal documents. They can be subpoenaed and used as evidence in a trial or civil case, such as a malpractice lawsuit. If the medical records are comprehensive, accurate, and objective, they will most likely protect you and your employer in court. However, if they are inaccurate, incomplete, or judgmental, the information in the medical record can harm you or your employer and expose you to legal action (Figure 14.6).

More important, poor or sloppy documentation can harm a patient because it contributes to poor decision-making and treatment. Thus, nothing strengthens patient care and protects your employer from liability more than ensuring complete and accurate medical record documentation.

❓ WHAT IF?

What if you notice someone's documentation in a patient's chart that is judgmental, prejudicial, or derogatory? What actions should you take? How can such a record be properly corrected?

Medical Insurance and Reimbursement

Insurers use medical records to reimburse health care providers for the patient care they provide. Without accurate, properly documented information, insurance claims can be denied. When claims are denied, it means that either your employer does not get paid or reimbursed for the care they have provided or the costs they have incurred, or the patient is obligated to pay for the entire cost of care.

Health insurers are businesses that have structured their premiums in a way that allows them to pay fair claims for providing patient care. Insurers need to verify the legitimacy, accuracy, and medical necessity of the claims before they pay the health care provider. Thus, it is your job to ensure that the documentation you create is clear, complete, and recorded in the proper format, so that financial and reimbursement issues can be properly managed and promptly paid. The care and quality of your medical record keeping can ensure that financial concerns do not harm your employer or add stress to your patient.

Types of Medical Charting and Record Keeping

In the past, the majority of medical records were written by hand and maintained on paper. However, in the last few decades, electronic record keeping has become more common and standard practice. Electronic records increase accuracy and legibility, and they save precious time. They are easy to use and can be quickly transmitted to other health care professionals and health care facilities as needed. If it is easy to electronically record notes and measurements at the time they are observed or taken, the medical record will be more accurate and immediately accessible. However, it is not always possible or practical to record every important piece of information electronically, so you must also be effective and efficient in recording information by hand. Figure 14.7 shows how properly maintained medical records can provide fast access to information when it is needed.

One of the main purposes of a good medical record system is to impose logic and order on the patient care process. Medical practices typically use problem-oriented charting that is organized based on the patient's problem or problems. Some of the most common problem-oriented charting methods are SOAP notes, CHEDDAR, and ADPIE (Figure 14.8).

SOAP notes stand for:
* **Subjective**
* **Objective**
* **Assessment**
* **Plan**.

The charting method using the CHEDDAR format is:
* **Chief Complaint**
* **History**
* **Examination**
* **Details of Complaints**
* **Drugs and Dosage**
* **Assessment**
* **Return Visit**.

The charting method, ADPIE, is more commonly used by nurses and stands for:
* **Assessment**
* **Diagnosis**
* **Planning**
* **Intervention**
* **Evaluation**.

Other charting method systems may be used in your facility, and it is a good idea to become familiar with the most common ones in case you will need to learn and use them in the future.

Regardless of which system you use, all charting methods require that you document patient information in an accurate, organized, and logical manner to allow other health care professionals or providers to easily read and understand what you have documented. In addition to these basic charting approaches, there are many other kinds of patient information that must be recorded, including vital signs, progress notes, and drug administration records.

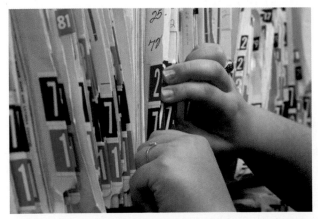

Figure 14.7 Medical charts. (From Proctor DB, Adams AP: *Kinn's the medical assistant: an applied learning approach*, ed 12, St. Louis, 2014, Elsevier.)

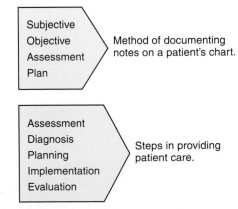

Subjective
Objective
Assessment
Plan

Method of documenting notes on a patient's chart.

Assessment
Diagnosis
Planning
Implementation
Evaluation

Steps in providing patient care.

Figure 14.8 Acronyms SOAP and ADPIE.

Accuracy and Consistency of Medical Records

It is important to understand and practice the proper and correct procedures for recording medical information. For example, every patient encounter should have a date and time to establish the order or chronology of a patient's history, diagnosis, and treatment. Your observations and measurements should be recorded objectively in the medical records, such as vital signs and weight and height. But an important part of the medical chart is also documenting your subjective impressions—as long as they are not judgmental—that can provide clues for accurate diagnosis and treatment. You might document a change in the patient's skin tone or note that they are having difficulty in breathing. You can even document that the patient "appears agitated and is combative." However, you should avoid judgmental or overly personal comments, such as the patient "did not know how to act and started calling me names like a silly child."

Use accurate words and appropriate terminology. You should ask yourself the questions that the reader will ask and record as much information as precisely as you can. Box 14.5 provides best practices for medical charting.

BOX 14.5

Best Practices for Medical Charting

- Think about your audience: Who are they, and what do they need to know?
- Anticipate your audience's questions and record accordingly.
- Record only what you did or observed yourself.
- Never make judgmental statements.
- Focus especially on changes in the patient's condition.
- Spell correctly and use only approved or common abbreviations.
- If writing, use legible handwriting.
- Use descriptive words accurately.
- Reread your notes and make any necessary corrections or clarifications.
- Follow policy in making corrections.
- Chart after providing care only.
- Use the patient's own words when significant; identify them with quotation marks.
- Always sign your entries in the medical record.
- Follow all policies in place to standardize charting.

JOURNALING 14.5

Think about the last time you went to the clinic. What was the reason you went to the clinic, and what kinds of questions were you asked? Using the SOAP note method discussed earlier, complete each category based on your medical visit.

❓ WHAT IF?

What if you forget to document important medical information? What can you do about it? How do you make corrections in a paper medical chart? Or in an electronic medical chart? What can you do to ensure that it never happens again?

Date	Time	Nursing Margin	Other Depts Margin		
7/8	1700			750 mL tap water enema given with the resident in the L side-lying position.	
				The resident was asked to retain the enema for at least 15 minutes. Bed in low	
				position. Signal light within reach. No resident complaints at this time. Resident	
				informed that I would check on her in 5 minutes or when the signal light was used.	
				Angie Martinez, CNA ———————————	
	1715			Assisted resident to the bedside commode. Privacy curtain pulled. Signal light and	
				toilet tissue within reach. Resident reminded to signal when finished expelling the	
				enema or if she needs assistance. Angie Martinez, CNA ———————————	

Charting sample. (From Kostelnick C: *Mosby's textbook for long-term care nursing assistants*, ed 7, St. Louis, 2015, Elsevier.)

CASE STUDY 14.4
Heightened Vigilance

Ken McGuire, a patient admitted to an outpatient psychiatric hospital, seemed to be going downhill fast. The staff was commenting on his mental deterioration and increasing depression. The nursing staff discussed restricting his activities and adding video monitoring of his room.

Gary, a psychiatric technician, was about to start his shift and said, "Let me keep an eye on him. I told Ken I would escort him to the drugstore in the Square. Why don't I do that as an assessment and I'll let you know if he does anything alarming."

"Do you think that's safe?" asked Kathy, the nurse manager.

"He'll be safe with me," said Gary.

On their way to the Square, Gary was getting uncomfortable with Ken's condition. Ken walked slowly, as if each step required great effort. He said very little, barely acknowledging Gary's efforts at conversation. At one point, he just stopped, suddenly crying, unable to say why. Although Gary suggested turning back, Ken insisted he was able to go on because he wanted to buy a birthday card for his daughter.

Gary kept a close eye on Ken the rest of the way. When they reached the bottom of the hill and prepared to cross the street, Ken said, "What if I ran in front of a car? You couldn't stop me."

"Ken, unless you want me to turn you around right now, you are going to have to convince me that you won't do that."

Ken hesitated but then said, "Okay, I won't."

"Do you know how I would feel if you did that, Ken?"

"I won't," said Ken. "It was nice of you to take me. You didn't have to. I won't do anything."

In the store, Ken quickly picked out a card. He then filled a basket with candy. "For the others," he told Gary. "It's the least I can do while I'm here."

They returned to the unit without further incident, but Gary was relieved to be back. He documented the trip in Ken's medical record.

He discussed his concerns with Kathy. "I think we need to put him on 5-minute checks just to be on the safe side," Kathy said.

In the morning, Gary was back for the second half of his back-to-back shift.

"Everybody to Ken's room," shouted a nurse, followed by two shifts of people.

One of the night workers was physically restraining Ken. "Found him in the closet tying his shoelaces to one of the hooks," said the worker. The team went into action to place Ken in a safe seclusion room, and the night nurse called the physician on call for the necessary order.

The next day, Gary was stopped by Dr. Andersen, the psychiatrist in charge of Ken. "That was good work, Gary. Your documentation was really thorough and it really helped alert everyone to Ken's state of mind. Because of that, we were able to closely monitor him and that saved Ken's life."

QUESTIONS FOR THOUGHT AND REFLECTION

1. How did Gary's documentation save Ken's life?
2. Do you think Gary quoted Ken's exact words about running in front of a car? Why, and does it matter?
3. What would you have told Ken when he threatened to jump in front of a car?

A Different Path

Dr. Raj was angry. He was a physician at a long-term care center, and he was reviewing the medical record of a patient, Ms. Gillespie, which was full of gaps. He was trying to monitor her blood glucose levels in order to adjust her medication. Her diabetes had not been well controlled, resulting in several episodes of hyperglycemia.

As a result, Dr. Raj ordered routine blood sugar draws and asked Ms. Gillespie to keep a food diary to record what she ate on a daily basis. However, her medical records showed inconsistent patterns of blood draws, and what the patient was served during meals was recorded but not what she ate. He could not adjust her medication without more accurate medical information.

Dr. Raj decided to meet with Ramona Hernandez, the nurse manager, about his concerns. Ramona was aware of the issues her staff was having with charting. Some of

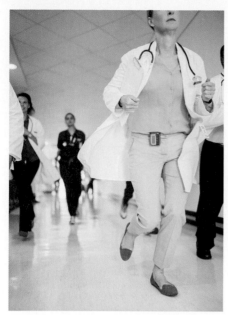

her nurses and nursing assistants needed more training on proper documentation. Others were not documenting in a timely manner and were forgetting to include important information in the patient's medical record.

During Dr. Raj's and Ramona's meeting, one of the nurses burst into the nursing station. "We have an emergency in Room 14A! Emily Gillespie. She's unresponsive, and her breathing is shallow."

QUESTIONS FOR THOUGHT AND REFLECTION

1. Who was affected by poor charting?
2. How do medical records play a role in Dr. Raj's treatment of Ms. Gillespie?
3. If you were in charge of retraining the nursing staff on documentation, what steps would you take?

CROSS CURRENTS WITH OTHER SOFT SKILLS

THINKING CRITICALLY: Record keeping should be an occasion to think analytically about the data you have collected and its implications (Chapter 9).

WRITING, GRAMMAR, AND SPELLING: Your record keeping should reflect correctness and professionalism (Chapter 4).

TAKING ACCOUNTABILITY: In the end, no one can document your observations and care except you, and your patients and colleagues depend on you to do it consistently and accurately (Chapter 5).

References

For additional information on the OIG's compliance programs, visit the OIG website at: https://oig.hhs.gov/compliance/101/index.asp.

Advancing in Your Career

- Set Goals and Make Their Achievement a Reality
- List Ways You Can Maximize Your Role on Your Teams
- Learn How to Develop Personal Skills to Make You a More Valuable Employee
- Learn How to Form a Positive Relationship With Your Supervisor
- Explain the Difference Between Gross and Net Income and the Types of Deductions That Affect Gross Income
- Understand Fiscal Responsibility by Establishing a Personal Budget
- Explain the Benefits of Joining a Professional Organization
- Define and Plan for Your Career Success

Setting Goals and Planning Actions

Goals are dreams with deadlines.

—Napoleon Hill

**LEARNING OBJECTIVE 1:
SETTING GOALS AND PLANNING ACTIONS**

- Create and design achievable goals using the SMART format.
- Identify obstacles and ways to overcome them.
- Learn how to visualize your goals to achieve them.
- Create actionable steps toward your goals.
- Understand the need to continually review and reevaluate goals.

There is no shortcut to anywhere worth going.

—Beverly Sills

To advance in your career and profession, it will take more than a desire to do so. It will take hard work, your skills and knowledge, and your personal attributes. Fortunately, there are actions you can take to help advance your career. In this chapter, we address the importance of developing personal skills, creating a positive working relationship with your supervisor and your co-workers, and making yourself more competitive in your profession. You can start by establishing a record of personal accomplishments and by taking personal accountability not only for your work but also for your success. Expand this notion by thinking not just in terms of your own accomplishments but in terms of those of the entire team. Health care is a team sport, and you want to distinguish yourself as a contributing member of every team you are part of. Finally, to excel in your career, you need to play an active role in your profession.

Importance of Goal-Setting

If you don't know where you're going, any road will get you there.

—George Harrison

Imagine getting in your car and driving to a destination, but you do not have an address. It sounds rather pointless and maybe even ridiculous. But that is what is happening when you do not think about what you want to achieve in your life. This is important to do in both your personal and professional lives. For example, in your personal life, consider what you want to achieve in 1 month, 1 year, 5 years, or even 20 years. This can include buying your first home or paying off all your student loans. In your career planning, you may want to be hired on at your first job as a dental technician or to be a clinical manager one day. If you can achieve goals that are related to your health, finances, personal growth, family, social life, and spiritual life, they will also enhance the success of your career goals.

Goal-setting is something we must do as a part of a health care team. The goal of your health care team or employer is to improve the health of the patient by operating as a business. Whether you are directly providing care or supporting a co-worker who is providing direct care, you are part of a team working toward the same goal. If you are doing something unrelated to the mission of the team, you are pulling the team away from its goal. For example, if you are rude to patients and not providing excellent customer service to them, your clinic may lose patients and money, potentially jeopardizing the operation of the clinic and patient care.

When you lack goals, you will not achieve as much because you do not have a direction or a destination. Goals give you purpose; they clarify your values and give you a sense of meaning.

Goals can be set at many different levels and timelines. Goals can be daily, short term, or long term. However, all your daily or short-term goals should support your long-term goals in one way or another. If you had a long-term goal, for instance, of getting promoted at work, you would want some short-term goals to get you there. These might include obtaining specialized certifications, volunteering for additional

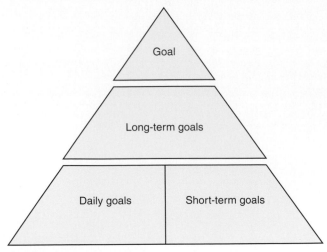

Figure 15.1 Goal levels.

responsibilities, helping your co-workers, and contributing to problem-solving at work.

In this way, your daily or short-term goals contribute not only to your ultimate professional goal but also to your health care team's mission. A complete hierarchy of your goal system, therefore, includes daily, short-term, and long-term goals that are all internally consistent and support one another (Figure 15.1).

How to Set Goals

When setting goals, think about what you ultimately want to achieve. Create a picture of where you want to be in the next 10 or 20 years and then plan steps going back to what you can do right now, next month, or next year. Make a routine schedule—daily, weekly, or monthly—to monitor your progress. After each schedule, review your goals and adjust them as needed.

JOURNALING 15.1

Consider a time when you accomplished a goal. What was the goal, and how did you achieve it? Did you write it down or keep it in your head? When you achieved it, how did it make you feel?

Creating Your Goals

In a previous chapter, we discussed visualizing as an effective tool. Once you have settled on a goal, your chances of achieving it are vastly improved by how vividly you can "see and feel" the results and outcome. If you can imagine reaching your goal, you have taken the first step toward fully realizing it. You will know where you want to go and what it feels like when you get there. For example, you are a health information technologist in charge of assisting a surgical practice's move from paper to electronic record keeping. You currently work with more than 4,000 patient records, which are taking up a massive amount of storage space. First, visualize the entire cabinet space cleared and the cabinets removed. Now, you can feel how freeing it is to have more space and to have the ability to access records at the touch of a finger. Once you feel how great it is to have a paperless office, you will be ready to tackle the next step to accomplish this task. If the outcome feels positive and looks achievable, the steps will follow with greater ease.

When thinking about your goals, be ambitious and dream big. However, the goal must be realistic. If it is not realistic and is unachievable, you may find it demoralizing, resulting in your more realistic goals not even being achieved. Create realistic goals and then visualize achieving them; this will help make them a reality (Figure 15.2).

Once you have a positive and specific goal in mind, enhance this visualization by writing out what the overall goal looks like once it is accomplished in the present tense. The physical act of writing down your goals makes them feel real and achievable. Further, if you write them down, you are less likely to forget about them.

Motivational speaker and author Hilary Hinton "Zig" Ziglar said that people should strive to be a "meaningful specific" rather than a "wandering generality." Writing down goals encourages you to state them with great specificity and detail. For example, write down "I will be employee of the month" if that is a goal for you.

Then, imagine how encouraging and amazing this will be for you as a recognition of your hard work and commitment. Avoid making negative goals, such as not getting into an argument at work or not being terminated. Negative goals will inevitably influence how you feel at home and at work and most likely will make it more difficult for you to focus on achieving them. Thus, reframe any negative goals into positive sounding ones.

Be cautious about setting too many goals. It is, of course, a good thing to have lots of goals and aspirations. However, if you list too many, you may find that you are stretched too thin and do not have the time or energy for all of them, resulting in potentially no goal being achieved. To prevent this, your goals must be prioritized, which will be discussed in the next section.

Prioritizing Your Goals

It is likely that you will have multiple goals. How do you prioritize and decide what to do first? In order to prioritize, you must decide what is most important to you right now. Although that may appear simple, it can be challenging for some people and in some situations. If it is hard for you to determine this because you have so many goals and they all seem important, one effective method is to rate your goals on a scale from 1 to 10, with 1 being the least important and 10 being the most important to you right now. Write down all your goals and rate them. As you go through your list of goals, you may notice that you will start making comparisons of your goals. What you once thought was a priority may not be as high of a priority compared to your other goals. For example, if you have a priority of buying a new car, it now may not be as important as making payments to pay off your student loan.

Another method of prioritizing is based on time. With your list of goals, write down next to each one how long it most likely will take to accomplish that goal—1 week, 6 months, 5 years, 10 years, or more, and so on. Consider which goal needs to be accomplished first. Or a particular goal may take more time to complete and needs to be started right now.

Creating a Plan

Once you have determined what your goals are, what should you do next? Although there are different methods, one of the common methods of goal-setting is using the SMART goal method, which stands for

* S—Specific
* M—Measurable
* A—Attainable or achievable
* R—Relevant
* T—Time-bound

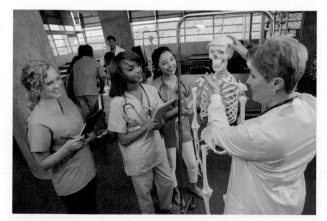

Figure 15.2 Create realistic goals and then visualize achieving them; this will help make them a reality. (Copyright © istock.com.)

Specific. What exactly do I want to accomplish? Your goal should be clear and specific. What do I want to accomplish? Why is this goal important to me?

Measurable. It is important to be able to track and monitor your progress on your goals in order to stay motivated. Try to create milestones to assess your progress. How will you know when it is accomplished?

Attainable. As mentioned earlier, your goals need to be realistic and attainable. How can I accomplish this goal? Can I accomplish this goal based on constraints, such as finances and time?

Relevant. Set goals that are important to you and lead to what you want in your life and career. If they are not meaningful to you, it is likely that you will not focus on them, and you will waste your time trying to complete them. Does this seem worthwhile? Does this align with the other goals in my life?

Time-bound. To successfully complete goals, you must give them a deadline. When there is a deadline, you have a sense of urgency and will work toward it. Having goals that are time-bound will also prevent your goals from being pushed aside by everyday tasks.

Since SMART goals are designed to be achievable, you can better stay motivated when pursuing them. Also, it will help you develop your self-discipline and focus on the task ahead.

Overcoming Obstacles

Obstacles are those frightful things you see when you take your eyes off your goal.

—Henry Ford

Once you have set and prioritized your goals and visualized them, think about all the obstacles you will need to overcome. Do not get discouraged by the presence of obstacles. There will always be obstacles and they can be overcome. First, you must know what they are. Some of the most common obstacles are controllable and controlled by you. For example, procrastination, or the habit of delaying doing or completing tasks, is a common obstacle to achieving a goal. There are many reasons why procrastination occurs, usually due to fear or anxiety about the things you need to perform and complete to achieve a goal. As a result of this fear and anxiety, you may avoid pursuing your goal.

One good method of confronting obstacles is to evaluate your goals. Are they realistic? Have you given yourself enough time to accomplish them? It is important to set yourself up for success and to create a positive, motivating environment.

Other methods may be to perform the tasks or goals in pieces. Can you break that goal into smaller tasks that are more manageable? Also, put those tasks and goals on your calendar as a reminder to set time for it.

Successful people aren't people without problems. They are people who deal with their problems successfully.

—Dr. Scott Peck

Review and Reevaluate

As a final phase, you must review your goals at regular intervals to sustain them. Planning is not a one-time event; it is an ongoing process.

Every week, maybe on a Sunday night, review your current goals. Are they still what you want? Are you making progress? Do you see a clear path of achievement through the next actions you have selected? Are the next actions on your calendar for the coming week? If you see that you are close to achieving them, you are more likely to push forward to complete them.

In some cases, a few of your goals may lose their appeal or they are no longer relevant to you. There may be new goals you want to add to your goal-setting. For example, your goal was to become a clinic supervisor. But, after working in the field for several years, you decide managing people is not something you want to do. Instead, you want to return to school and advance your education to become a respiratory therapist.

It is important to periodically reevaluate your goals to ensure they are still aligned with what you want to do with your life. The most successful people are always reevaluating and reimagining new futures. Be careful that you are not discarding a goal because you are just discouraged. Box 15.1 lists tips for achieving a goal.

The key to goal achievement is to make it a persistent, methodical pursuit. The smartest way to stay on track in pursuing your goals is to keep a written

BOX 15.1

Tips for Achieving Goals

- Write down the goal.
- State it positively and specifically.
- See and feel what the goal will look like when it is accomplished.
- Set reasonable deadlines for the goal or task.
- Ensure that the goal is tied to a purpose or a mission.
- Anticipate and overcome obstacles.
- Review your plans to ensure that the goal makes progress.

record of where you have been, what you have done, and what you want to do next. Studies show that only 3% of Americans have written goals. So, logging your goals and the steps you will take to achieve them will put you far ahead of the game.

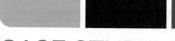
WHAT IF?

What if you were suddenly making twice as much money? How would that change your goals?

What if you had two more children? How would that change your goals?

The only thing that has to be finished by next Tuesday is next Monday.

—Jennifer Yane

⭐ **EXPERIENTIAL EXERCISES**

1. Watch the movie *Groundhog Day*. Determine how the main character played by Bill Murray manages to improve his daily life through goal-setting.
2. Interview your parents or other respected people about their goal-setting methods.
3. Pick a goal to achieve this week or month.

CASE STUDY 15.1
Looking for a Lift

Joe started out as a firefighter and eventually became certified as an EMT. When he was 43, he retired from the St. Louis Fire Department and took a full-time job as an EMT with the Green Ambulance Service. He did that for a few years until he was injured. Joe was out of work for almost 6 months on short-term disability, causing him to become unmotivated personally and professionally.

One day he attended a motivational workshop because his sister bought him a ticket for his birthday. To his surprise, what the speaker was saying really resonated with Joe. The speaker said that anybody could live a fulfilling, challenging life and that goal-setting and achievement were the way to get it. Joe went home and wrote down his positive and specific goals. He included everything he could think of that he wanted to accomplish in his life. He came up with 85 goals spread across six aspects of his life. He wrote each goal on an index card and put them in a recipe box.

Next, Joe created a to-do list. It was a modest list that allowed for all the unexpected calls he would get in the ambulance service. One of the goals for the day was to get all his work done, and he made a separate list for that. Another goal involved gaining his paramedic certification. He had done some work toward his intermediate EMS certification, but he always quit before he completed the program.

Joe liked this goal-setting method. Pursuing goals gave him direction and energy. Once he returned to work, even his supervisor noticed his sudden enthusiasm for his job.

Several months later, Joe completed his paramedic certification. With that being completed, he reevaluated his goals and thought of pursuing a leadership position. Joe

knew he could be the kind of leader the other EMTs could look up to, so he brainstormed a list of new goals and what he needed to do to achieve them. "There is nothing I can't do," he thought to himself.

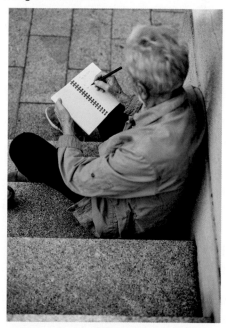
iStock.com/millann/1387005211

QUESTIONS FOR THOUGHT AND REFLECTION

1. How was Joe able to change his life?
2. What methodology did Joe pursue in reaching his goals?
3. What gave Joe enthusiasm and confidence?

Ivana stopped attending her career college where she had enrolled to become a medical assistant. Her program director called her many times and tried to help her with her attendance and missing assignments and exams, but she stopped taking the calls just before the phone company canceled her service.

Ivana had lots of problems. First, she was working nights at a nursing home to cover her living expenses and pay for school. She worked the late shift and would often sleep through her first class. She had also hoped that the job would help improve her English because Russian was her native language. Unfortunately, there were few opportunities for interactions with the sleeping residents or the busy staff. Finally, she hoped her 1990 Oldsmobile would last a little longer, but it eventually broke down. Without transportation, she could not get to work or school.

QUESTIONS FOR THOUGHT AND REFLECTION

1. What advice would you give Ivana in her difficult situation?
2. How would you help Ivana with her goal-setting?

 CROSS CURRENTS WITH OTHER SOFT SKILLS

MANAGING YOUR TIME AND ORGANIZING YOUR LIFE: Planning goals and actions provides meaning and structure to your time and your life (Chapter 1).

THINKING CRITICALLY: Planning is an excellent application of critical thinking (Chapter 8).

COMMITTING TO YOUR PROFESSION: This should be reflected as a major element of your goal-setting (Chapter 13).

Contributing as a Team Member

I am a member of a team, and I rely on the team, I defer to it and sacrifice for it, because the team, not the individual, is the ultimate champion.

—Mia Hamm

LEARNING OBJECTIVE 2: CONTRIBUTING AS A MEMBER OF THE TEAM

- Define what makes a good team.
- Understand the roles of team members.
- Describe the benefits of teamwork in a health care setting.
- Know what it means to be a team player.
- Describe five problems that teams could encounter.
- Observe the purpose of meetings.

The effective delivery of patient care requires teamwork. Not one health care professional or provider can do it alone. It calls for the expertise of multiple professionals, who must work together toward a common goal and mission. Teams are built on trust, and each team member must feel confident that every member of the team will do their part. Everyone needs to do their best because the team depends on them. Thus, to advance and be successful in your new profession, you must know how to be an effective member of a team.

Purpose of a Team

Teams are a group of people with special characteristics, having a unified purpose and common goals, and with an internal structure and specific expectations for each member. The purpose of a team is to accomplish specific tasks and goals. You will likely be a member of one or more permanent teams at work. You may be on the team that supports a physician. You may be on a team that performs a specific function, like providing emergency care, dispensing medication, providing diagnostic images, or providing rehabilitation services. You may also be on a team with the other members of your health profession. As a dental assistant, you and your fellow dental assistants may jointly manage the reception area, the supply room, or cover shifts for each other. As a physical therapist, you may join your fellow physical therapists in planning or reviewing care for a specific patient, evaluating and purchasing equipment, or assisting and consulting one another. These are the kinds of permanent teams that function every day at work. Few health professionals operate in solitude or isolation.

Other teams you may serve on may be temporary and have a specific short-term goal. Once the goal has been achieved, the team dissolves. Often, these are called committees or ad hoc teams. Such teams could include recruitment groups for new employees, planning teams for accreditation visits, teams to review the hospital formulary, or teams that plan the holiday party. In every case, though, the team has been formed for a specific purpose, and the purpose is achieved by meeting criteria everyone approves and agrees with.

For any team to be successful, the goals of the team must be clear to everyone. Moreover, everyone needs to agree when the goals have been achieved. What are the desired outcomes? Providing effective patient care? Maintaining smooth operations? Creating an employee policy manual? Planning a successful event?

In some cases, a team gets a specific reward, like a bonus, a plaque, or public recognition. More often, however, the reward is a job well done. Your contributions as a member of a team can be meaningful and lead to promotions, increases in pay, and career success. But, more importantly, they show your employer and co-workers that you can work effectively as a team member.

? WHAT IF?

What if you are asked to join a team? What information will you want before deciding? What questions will you ask?

Team Structure, Leadership, and Size

Research shows that teams function best when they are made up of between 5 and 12 people. Fewer than 5 members makes it impossible to spread the work effectively. Having more than 12 members makes communication difficult and slow and may minimize the idea of ownership and accountability because too many people are responsible for too few things.

Teams do not function effectively without some organization or leadership. Every team has to have a leader in some form. The leader is often the supervisor; other times, an employee may be assigned or volunteer as the leader. The leader's role is to combine, organize, and leverage all the members' special skills and expertise to accomplish a task or goal.

To ensure progress is being made toward the goal, the leader will schedule regular team meetings. During these meetings, records of what is discussed, policies, and a list of action items may be created. Some examples of these documents appear in Box 15.2.

BOX 15.2

Documents Used in Team Meetings

- Mission statement
- Member list
- Timelines
- Task list
- Milestones
- Notes
- Templates
- Project charts
- Flowcharts
- Mind maps

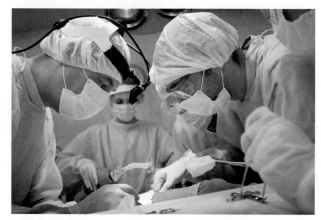

Figure 15.3 Teamwork is essential in health care. Members of the surgical team rely on each other during procedures, just as teams of technicians, aides, and others work together to provide before and after care. (Copyright © istock.com.)

A team is ideally structured so that the members' varying talents can be optimally combined to accomplish specific goals. Therefore, it is important to understand and define the expected contributions of each team member. As an individual, are you there to lead, take notes, do research, write a report, or contribute ideas? To succeed as a team member, you must know exactly why you were picked for this team and what you are expected to contribute (Figure 15.3).

Benefits of Teams

Establishing teams is an efficient and effective way to manage a demanding workload because teams allow for specialization. For example, when providing patient care, one member of the team checks them in and starts to collect data for the patient registration, including insurance verification and patient demographics. Another member of the team will perform the clinical examination, which will include the medical history and vital signs. Other members of the team may include specialists in imaging, laboratory work, or other diagnostic tests; nurses; and physicians. As you can tell, health care is too complex to be delivered by any one person.

Expertise

There are more than 100 different health care professions and providers, each with their own skill set, body of knowledge, and role and function in the health care setting. Remember how long it took and how difficult it was for you to master the skills and knowledge of your own profession. In general, health care professionals are experts in one aspect of patient care. Your expertise is needed, and you and your patients need the expertise of your co-workers.

Because of the varying types of expertise represented on a team, there must be a clear role for each team member, with each member contributing. This is one reason that working in a team often can be a pleasure and produce positive feelings about work. An often-overlooked benefit of teams is the social connection they offer to their members. Trust and a sense of responsibility to the team prompt team members to go to extra lengths to perform and not let their team members down.

> **JOURNALING 15.2**
>
> Consider a team you are part of. What is the expertise you bring to this team? Record your expertise in the form of skills and knowledge. Be as broad and specific as you can be.

None of us is as smart as all of us.

—Ken Blanchard

Problems Experienced by Teams

Teams can and will experience problems from time to time. Conflict is not necessarily a problem or as detrimental as it may appear for teams. Conflict and constructive disagreement, if managed correctly, may lead to discussion and a better understanding for the team to ultimately improve outcomes. When working together on a team, people must agree to put their differences aside and work together to achieve the team's goals. Use some of the conflict resolution and communication skills you have mastered from earlier chapters to resolve these problems.

When someone on the team has proven to be untrustworthy, the work of the team can be severely compromised. Often, the work of one team member depends on the work of another team member. Of course, even the most committed individuals may make mistakes or fail to complete a task. At other times, however, you might have a team member who does not really want to be there or who is not committed to the team's mission. When that happens, their poor performance and lack of participation and contribution are noticeable and will negatively affect the team. In severe cases, sabotage and bad team behavior may manifest in communication. A team member may omit key data, falsify data, or offer misleading information. Such behavior, if deliberate, can be dangerous to your patients, and the team member should be immediately released from the team. The best way to prevent this from happening when setting up a team is to ensure that everyone supports the mission and goals. In some cases, a supervisor or manager may need to replace those who cannot or will not support the team's goals.

Even if you have everyone's commitment from the start, teams and their goals often need to change. Many of us are able to adjust to change, due to our initial commitment to the team and its mission. Sometimes, however, a team member may be unable or unwilling to adapt to the change. Just one person resistant to change can sabotage the team's mission. It is sometimes necessary to replace someone who is resistant with someone who can support the new goals and be a team player.

All team members must uphold their responsibilities and contributions to the team. Anyone not holding up their end will soon be apparent to everyone else. If you ever find yourself lacking commitment to your team, failing to take accountability, or not caring about the outcomes, take time to assess. Are you overcommitted? Or do you feel like you may not have enough to contribute to the team? If you are unable to resolve this issue, it may be better for you to recuse yourself from the team than for you to continue in it. Speak to the team's leader to discuss your concerns.

The name on the front of the shirt is more important than the name on the back.

—Herb Brooks

CASE STUDY 15.2
The Wine Tasting

Rachel was honored to be chosen to lead an ad hoc team to select a new electronic health records (EHR) system for the hospital. She had been involved with a similar effort at her previous employer, and her experience with EHR systems was one of the reasons she was hired.

Her manager, Saul Bremer, gave her the authority to run the task force, giving her the goal of evaluating and recommending a new EHR software system by the end of November. The EHR system should be purchased and implemented early in the new fiscal year. He assigned members to the task force from different departments in the hospital, so there would be a broad range of recommendations. He asked Rachel to give him weekly status reports by email, so he would have a record of the team's progress. But he said he would also meet with her each Friday to discuss the team's progress in more detail.

Because Rachel was new and the team members did not all know each other, she planned a social event for their first meeting. She was also concerned about the challenges of having a large, 12-person team. She wanted to make sure everyone felt comfortable participating in the team. She had a small team-building budget, and she thought a wine tasting would be fun. She had a lot of knowledge about wines and thought her wine expertise might translate to the leadership style she wanted to establish.

Rachel rented a banquet room at the Bella Vina restaurant, which she knew had a good wine list. She met with the wine steward there ahead of time to plan the event. She thought it would be fun to set up tastings of three different vintage years for three different wines, so the team members could appreciate the differences in grape qualities from previous years.

The event included appetizers and took place on a Friday evening from 5:00 to 7:00 p.m. Rachel arrived before her team, so she could greet and introduce herself to everyone individually. Once everyone arrived, she asked everyone to stand up and introduce themselves. During the introductions, one man from the IT department, Chet, explained that he was good at "stress-testing" software. Rachel made a mental note that she would put him in charge of that and would pair him with two clinicians to tap their knowledge and educate them about stress-testing. A woman from medical records, Velma, had been with the hospital for several decades, and she was skeptical about the changes a new EHR system would bring compared with the existing one. Rachel needed to remember this to prepare for any concerns or resistance from Velma.

After a couple of rounds of appetizers, the three wine stations were mixing up the group and everyone was getting along well.

However, Rachel noticed that one team member, Sue, was off by herself, so Rachel approached her. Rachel learned that Sue did not know too many people on the team. "I'm good at data processing," Sue volunteered.

"That's great, Sue. We're lucky to have your talent on the team," said Rachel.

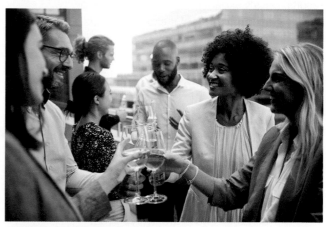

iStock.com/monkeybusinessimages/1146473379

QUESTIONS FOR REVIEW AND REFLECTION

1. What steps did Rachel take to make sure her social event was successful? How will this success translate to her effectiveness as a leader of the team?
2. What did Rachel learn about her team at the wine tasting?
3. How was Rachel able to effectively establish her leadership of the team?
4. Why was it important for Rachel to notice Sue standing alone?

Gary from the accounting department was rotating into the leadership role of the team responsible for keeping the policy manual updated. The team had representation from all different departments. Each member served for 3 months as the leader before leaving the team and being replaced by a new member, just to keep things fresh and provide everyone with a leadership opportunity. Gary called the team's next meeting for a Monday morning at 8:00.

"Oh, boy," said Della to her co-worker Evelyn, who was also on the committee. "Can you believe he called a meeting for 8:00 a.m.?! I'm still listening to my alarm at that hour." Evelyn laughed. She represented the nursing staff on the team, and Della was the administrative medical assistant for one of the orthopedic surgery units.

Della made it to the meeting on time, but she was not happy about it.

Gary passed out the agenda. "You received this by email, but I made hard copies for everyone. Let's get started." The first thing on the agenda was reporting and filing laboratory results. Della's expertise would come in handy.

"I hope everyone's had a chance to review this already. Della, do you have any thoughts on the proposed procedure?" Gary asked her.

"Uhm, not really. But let me look at it right now."

Gary took a deep breath and waited patiently, with the rest of the team, while Della read over the procedure.

"Well, it looks okay, except our current EHR software doesn't have that capability," she responded.

"That's true. That's why we're discussing the option of either meeting with the vendor to add that application or choosing new software. Didn't you read the meeting announcement?" Gary asked.

"The one that said we're meeting at 8:00? I'm here, aren't I?"

"Yes, and thank you for being here. But we don't have much time and we really need everyone working together to make sure this project is successful," said Gary.

Della crossed her arms. She had had just about enough from this guy.

QUESTIONS FOR THOUGHT AND REFLECTION

1. Did Della understand the goal of her team?
2. Did the time of the meeting or Gary's personality have anything to do with the team's work?
3. Is Della living up to her commitment to the team and sharing her expertise?
4. What is Della's role on the team? How is she functioning in that role?
5. How do you think Della will manage once it is her turn to lead the team?

⭐ EXPERIENTIAL EXERCISES

1. List all the teams you are a part of. Consider both your personal and professional lives.
2. If you wanted to create a positive working relationship with your co-workers, what kind of event would you organize?
3. Think of a team you are a member of, whether it is a bowling group, a PTA, a church group, or a book club. Who leads these teams? Describe their leadership qualities.

🔄 CROSS CURRENTS WITH OTHER SOFT SKILLS

BEING DEPENDABLE: Your team members count on you, and you on them (Chapter 1).

BUILDING TRUST: Trust is the basis for team function (Chapter 5).

DEALING WITH DIFFICULT PEOPLE: Unfortunately, being a member of a team forces you to confront difficult people, because you must work effectively with everyone on your team (Chapter 7).

READING AND SPEAKING BODY LANGUAGE: Team settings require you to transmit and receive a full range of communication to get the team's work done (Chapter 6).

Managing Your Manager

LEARNING OBJECTIVE 3: MANAGING YOUR MANAGER

- Have a strategy for developing a positive relationship with your supervisor.
- Learn how to manage difficult interactions with your supervisor.
- Learn to develop solutions to problems.
- Use your supervisor as an advisor and source of feedback.
- Manage the performance evaluation process.

One of the most important tasks on your first day at work is to begin building a positive relationship with your supervisors. Your supervisors play an important role in your success at work, as you do in theirs. Only your knowledge, competence, hard work, and attitude are more important. As you manage your workload, your effectiveness and your ability to do your job well will reflect positively on them. In turn, gaining experience on a successful team makes *you* look good and will help you advance in your career.

Managing Up

Many new employees are intimidated by anybody who is in a position higher than theirs. They are shy, insecure, or fearful around their supervisors, and they seek to avoid rather than engage their supervisors. This is a mistake that can set their careers back. Your supervisors are just people with responsibilities and pressures, just like you. Your supervisors want to quickly feel they can depend on you and trust you to do your job well.

However, conflicts and tensions between employees and supervisors are unfortunately common. If there are conflicts between you and your supervisors, they often can be resolved through open communication. Thus, it is important to prioritize creating a good relationship with your supervisors to manage stressful situations and to develop a sense of trust. This is often called "managing up" or creating a smooth and productive relationship with your supervisors. Sometimes, people may interpret this as a political maneuver or "brown-nosing"; however, you and your supervisors both have jobs to perform and are mutually dependent on one another. Your supervisors need you to perform your job well for them to do their jobs well. You also need your supervisors to support and guide you while you are doing your job.

Consciously overcome any fears and plan to have frequent positive interactions with your supervisors. It is important to understand your supervisors, not just when you first start your job but throughout your working relationship. Try to have some insight into yourself and your supervisors, specifically each of your strengths, weaknesses, work styles, and goals. One of the most important things is to try to view things from your supervisors' perspective. For example, there may be times when you do not understand why you are being asked to do something and may be

resistant. Remind yourself that you are paid to perform a job in the way your employer wishes it to be done. Further, your supervisors also have supervisors, and they may have directives that they need to execute.

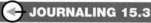

JOURNALING 15.3

Describe your ideal supervisor. Consider how you would want to use them as an asset. Include their role and influence in your organization, communication style, and how they could motivate you to give your highest performance.

Your Supervisor's Duties to You

Your supervisor is there to offer you training, guidance, feedback, and encouragement. Rather than waiting for your supervisor's feedback, try to be proactive and ask for feedback and guidance from them instead (Figure 15.4).

Supervisors differ in their personalities and work styles. Some are highly focused on work, and your relationship with this supervisor will be based solely on work-related issues. Many other supervisors are more relationship oriented. They feel that the best way to work is to motivate their team and do this by developing relationships with the people on their team. Others are creative types who are always seeking new, better, and more innovative ways to work. Supervisors who are "process" types are sticklers for detail and seek smooth operations. Your response to

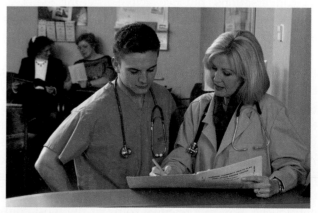

Figure 15.4 A medical assistant interacting with his supervisor. (From Proctor DB, Adams AP: *Kinn's the medical assistant: an applied learning approach*, ed 12, St. Louis, 2014, Elsevier.)

and interactions with your supervisor depend a lot on the supervisors' personality and work style. Work to develop compatibility with your supervisors, so you can feel more comfortable approaching them.

In addition, try to determine your supervisors' communication styles and preferences. Do they prefer verbal communication, emails, or both? How should you use emails to communicate with your supervisors, and what issues should you copy them on? Some supervisors want highly detailed emails, so they have a written record and documentation to refer to later. If you are uncertain about your supervisors' communication preferences, ask them.

You should also be mindful of when are the best times to approach your supervisor with your ideas and suggestions. When will they be the most receptive? Are they more formal and prefer meetings and appointments to discuss issues? Or are they more informal and receptive to hallway conversations?

Conversations With Your Supervisor

Your supervisors' time is valuable, but you and your ability to do your work well are important as well. Plan to speak with your boss when you need guidance, when you have something important to communicate, when your needs are not being met, or when you have ideas and solutions to problems. Think about your conversations before you have them. Visualize and anticipate them. Imagine what could go right or go wrong. When you plan for a successful outcome to a conversation, you are more likely to get one.

Proper body language helps people bond and treat each other as professionals engaged in a professional discussion. Smile if it is appropriate. Make small talk at the beginning but keep it short. Get to the point and clearly state the purpose of your conversation. As in all conversations, practice active listening skills, as you learned in previous chapters. By allowing your supervisor to speak, the more you will learn, and the better the questions you can ask.

Be appreciative of your supervisor's time but be sure you clearly understand any directions you receive or commitments you make. Ask questions to be sure you understand. If necessary, summarize your understanding verbally or in a follow-up email. Always inform your supervisor of actions you took in response to your conversation. Clarity and follow-up are two qualities all supervisors prize in their employees. Box 15.3 reviews some of the most common mistakes people make when communicating with supervisors.

BOX 15.3

Behavior to Avoid When Talking to Your Supervisor

- Being offensive to others in any way: inappropriate dress, coarse language, poor hygiene, immaturity, holding grudges, refusing to apologize or accept apologies, being sarcastic or cynical
- Treating your peers disrespectfully
- Wasting time and goofing off; making personal calls; texting; surfing the Internet; checking Facebook; listening to music with headphones
- Being discourteous to anyone
- Being late
- Not listening, writing things down, or following directions
- Acting bored or unenthusiastic
- Lying or demonstrating a lack of integrity
- Failing to learn on the job; making the same mistakes over and over
- Failing to control your emotions by shouting, crying, or sulking
- Inability or unwillingness to solve problems
- Refusing to go beyond your job description
- Being messy, disorganized, or disheveled
- Not being a team player; skipping company events; not contributing
- Undermining change or managerial initiatives

Problem-Solving With Your Supervisor

Pretend you are a supervisor. Two employees knock on your door at the same time and want to talk about the same issue. Which one are you more eager to listen to? Employee A or Employee B?

Employee A: "We have a big problem. It's going to cause a lot of issues next month."

Employee B: "I noticed a problem and I think I see a way we can avoid facing a big mess next month."

We would probably agree on Employee B. When bringing a problem to your supervisor, try to use your critical thinking skills first to come up with solutions to the problem, if possible. Consider the following questions when you encounter a problem at work: Is this a problem you can solve yourself? Do you have enough knowledge to solve this problem? Are there co-workers who you can ask for help?

You might not always have a solution. But your ability to show critical thinking and problem-solving skills will demonstrate your value as an employee. When presenting a problem, use the following tactics:

* Bring the problem to your supervisor's attention as soon as you become aware of it. Problems are more easily dealt with the sooner they are known.
* Gather as many facts and details about the problem as you can. If you are unclear on the facts, investigate and confirm their accuracy before you inform your supervisor. Revising the facts later can be difficult and damaging when a solution built on false information must be reversed.
* Be objective, not emotional.
* By being thoughtful and creative, your supervisor can rely on you as a valuable employee and depend on you to solve workplace problems.

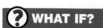

What if you received a directive from your supervisor and you think there is a better way to do it? What would you do?

Feedback From Your Supervisor

How would you react if your supervisor said one of the following statements to you?

* "I noticed that you're spending a lot of time talking to your co-workers when there are patients waiting to be seen by you."
* "I asked you to add that medication to Mrs. Sambora's medical record and you forgot. Now, she's upset because she wasn't able to refill her prescription."
* "You seem to be a little rushed during the patient interview. I would like you to pay more attention to the details."

Nobody likes to be criticized, but it is important to try to take these comments as constructive. Feedback from supervisors is actually meant to help you perform better in your role. Providing constructive criticism and feedback on your performance is part of your supervisor's job and can be the most important gift your supervisor can give you.

Although it may not always be easy, try to receive this feedback as constructive. No one is perfect, and none of us can see ourselves with the clarity with which others see us. If your supervisors have taken time to make you aware of some of these problems, they are helping you by giving you an opportunity to correct any problems that would otherwise negatively affect your performance and career. Box 15.4 lists six steps to receive constructive criticism.

BOX 15.4

Six Steps to Receiving Constructive Criticism

- Stop your first reaction
- Remind yourself of the benefit of receiving feedback
- Listen for understanding
- Say "thank you"
- Ask questions to deconstruct the feedback
- Request time to follow up

? WHAT IF?

What if your supervisor was angry with you and told you that you were a poor communicator because you should have disclosed a problem to them that has now blindsided them and created an even more difficult problem? What would be your response? Would your reaction be different if they said it but were not angry?

Performance Evaluations

Most organizations require that a regular performance evaluation be conducted on all employees. Performance evaluations can be quarterly or annually. For new employees, there may be a 30- or 90-day performance review. The performance evaluation should cover the entire period since the last evaluation, and it becomes part of your employee file for the Human Resources Department to manage.

The performance evaluation is a major opportunity for you and your supervisor to agree on your strengths and areas for improvements and decide what developmental and learning goals you will work on in the coming review period. You may also want to discuss any goals and share your professional development and career growth opportunities during this time. The performance evaluation is often used to determine merit increases and promotions.

Of course, this periodic evaluation is not the only time you should solicit feedback from your supervisors. Between reviews, refer to your practice's performance evaluation form as a reminder of growth opportunities. Figure 15.5 shows a sample evaluation.

You can help yourself in this process by preparing your own evaluation. First, start a file of your accomplishments, including dates and details, and keep track of aspects or skills you would like to improve. Then, a week or two before performance evaluations are due, and before your supervisor has a chance to

Employee Performance Evaluation Form

Employee name: _____ Date: _____

Position: _____ Hire date: _____

Description of responsibilities:

_____

_____

_____

_____

Performance on a scale of 1 to 10, with 10 being outstanding/exceptional
performance and 1 being poor/below expectations.

Professional performance	Self-appraisal rating	Manager rating
1. Knowledge of office procedures		
2. Patient awareness and communication		
3. Adhering to office policies		
4. Judgment and ability to recognize/solve problems		
5. Administrative/organization/working within system		
6. Quality of work		
7. Productivity/results		
8. Willingness to learn/grasp of instruction		

Figure 15.5 A performance evaluation form.

write yours, compose a "self-evaluation" and send it to your supervisor. Your supervisor might have forgotten events or duties that you performed that happened months ago. Your supervisor will most likely be impressed when you remind them in your detailed self-evaluation.

Be as objective as you can be in your self-evaluation. Your honest self-evaluation is certainly an opportunity to cast yourself in a positive light and show initiative. But if it is too glowing and lacks objectivity, your supervisor may not put too much weight on it.

The objective of the performance evaluation is to receive regular feedback from your supervisor on your performance (Figure 15.6). Use the performance evaluation to identify areas for improvements and to learn how you can do even better in your job.

Challenging Supervisors

Supervisors are not perfect. They are human. At best, they are supportive, understanding, and patient. At worse, you could have a supervisor that is rude, unappreciative, and intimidating. You rarely get to pick your supervisor and, thus, hope for a good one. If you

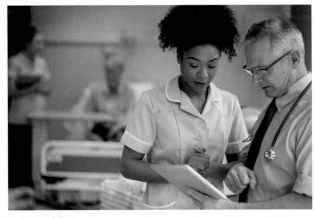

Figure 15.6 A nurse receives feedback. (Copyright © istock.com.)

have a difficult supervisor, there are tactics you can take to manage your situation.

Approaches to Dealing With a Difficult Supervisor

Some supervisors may not be equipped to be in a leadership role. They may have done their previous job well but may not have the skills or personality to be in a management position. Other supervisors may have gotten promoted through their connections, who may or may not be aware of their performance as a leader. Few of them, however, will see themselves as bad managers. Regardless, it is unlikely that you will be able to remove your supervisor from a position, and you should not try to.

Avoid complaining and "bad-mouthing" your supervisor to your co-workers. This does not improve the situation, and if your supervisor found out, it could worsen your working relationship. Instead, there are several strategies you can pursue to manage the situation. First, ask yourself some of the following objective questions:

* What is driving my supervisor's behavior? Why are they acting like that?
* Is this a temporary behavior or a personality problem?
* Am I a target, or is everyone treated this way?
* Am I doing anything to contribute to my supervisor's behavior?
* What can I do to improve the situation?

Second, whatever you do, maintain the quality of your work and a positive attitude. Both are under your control. Acting sullen, unproductive, insubordinate, uncooperative, and argumentative only makes a bad situation worse. These reactive strategies are totally unproductive and may result in disciplinary action. Control these impulses and try to choose more productive strategies. Never embarrass, publicly confront, or threaten a supervisor you are having difficulty with.

If all else fails, you may need to accommodate and adjust to your supervisor's behavior and management style. Do a good job, and let your boss know what you have accomplished. Other strategies for dealing with challenging supervisors appear in Box 15.5.

The higher a monkey gets up the tree, the more rear end he's got showing.

—Louis Harris

If your boss demands unreasonable performance, explain what you will have to prioritize to complete this goal. This sometimes may mean stopping some of the tasks and projects you are currently working on. However, refuse to do anything you feel is unethical. Doing so will seldom cost you your job. Above all, stay calm, especially when your supervisor is being emotional. If you are the target of abuse, you may need to contact your Human Resources Department to submit a complaint.

BOX 15.5

Tips for Dealing Positively With a Demanding or Difficult Supervisor

- As always, first seek to understand the supervisor's difficult behavior.
- Be politely assertive, not attacking or threatening. Acting intimidated will invite more of the same bad treatment.
- In private, provide your boss with feedback following this structure: "When you _____, it makes me feel _____."
- When being criticized, ask for details. Explain that you want the details, so you can improve next time. Details require the supervisor to be more thoughtful.
- Control your emotions and choose your response carefully.
- To protect yourself and preserve details, document any instance in which your boss engages in any dishonest, unethical, or abusive behavior.
- Refuse to do anything dishonest, unethical, or abusive.
- Don't do anything rash that could jeopardize your career, no matter what the provocation.
- If all else fails, consult with your Human Resources Department, which exists in part to help employees deal with difficult bosses. However, you should exhaust all other remedies before taking the matter to Human Resources.

Coping With Change and Stress

Keep in mind that a supervisor's negative behavior may be a reflection of how that person behaves when stressed. Recognize that your supervisor is under a great deal of stress, and some supervisors are better at dealing with stress than others. One of the best ways you can support your supervisors is to help them manage change.

If change is difficult for you and your co-workers, it may even be harder for your supervisor. You may have co-workers with negative mindsets who want to resist or sabotage the change. Do not be one of these employees. Many times, your supervisors did not choose the change; they are responsible for helping to implement it.

CASE STUDY 15.3
Dr. Jekyll and Mr. Hyde

Everybody who worked in Dr. Ray Brazos's pediatric practice marveled at how he could be the beloved, kindly, gentle physician his patients loved while treating his employees so disrespectfully.

"Look at this *Newsweek*. It's from last summer. Do you think patients want to read last summer's news?" Dr. Brazos said, while slamming the magazine down on the table. Just then, Brenda, one of the medical assistants, arrived. "Nice of you to join us today, Miss Flores," he said. "You're visiting Starbucks on my time," he said, pointing at her coffee.

"Actually, I'm on time, Dr. Brazos" she said, annoyed with herself for sounding defensive.

"Well, get to work then," said Dr. Brazos, stalking down the hallway to his office.

Brenda followed him. "I need to speak to you," she said.

"Make an appointment," he said brusquely.

"I did make an appointment, and it's on your calendar."

"Okay. What's on your mind then?"

"I've only been here 2 months, but you have a lot more no-shows than other offices where I've worked."

"What's your point?" Dr. Brazos asked impatiently.

"Well, there are ways you can reduce the number of no-shows."

"Don't you call patients the day before?"

"Yes, but we can also call them the morning of the appointment to remind them again. Many say they forget."

"They do?!"

"Yes. If you call them again in the morning, and they can't come, at least they can tell us, and we can book somebody else when they call. There are a lot of patients that call in, and they would be happy for a same-day visit. Instead, we're having patients come in as walk-ins, and they have to wait until you have a break or when we have a last-minute cancellation."

"Hmm, that's interesting. That's a good idea, Brenda. Please share it with the rest of the staff and let's begin implementing it immediately."

QUESTIONS FOR THOUGHT AND REFLECTION

1. How was Brenda able to successfully look past Dr. Brazos's behavior?
2. Why did Dr. Brazos's attitude change toward Brenda?
3. Did the relationship between Dr. Brazos and Brenda Flores change today?

A Different Path

Saul, the health service administrator, could see Sue, the medical office specialist, circling outside of his office again. "Did you want to talk to me, Sue?" he called to her.

"If you have a minute. I just wanted to let you know that I'm way ahead of schedule," she said with a big smile, although Saul did not know what she meant by that since the waiting room was full of patients.

She sat down in the chair in front of Saul's desk. "I don't know if you know or not," she said, "but our medical records committee is making great progress. We have already identified the five market-leading software systems, and we're putting together a pilot and a sample of the data to run through each system."

"Yes, I'm aware," said Saul. "That's great. I get regular updates from Rachel, who is overseeing the electronic health records implementation."

"I wouldn't be surprised. She's great for reports. But it took me 4 hours to compile the test data, the information we're using for the pilots, to test the software. The vendors gave us samples."

"Right. I am aware of that. That's great work, Sue."

"The samples limit the number of records we can enter, but I compiled the maximum number. I just wanted to be sure you were up to date, because the software samples expire at the end of the month, and we really need to get going."

"So, you think we're behind schedule?" said Saul.

"Oh no, ahead of schedule," said Sue. "I've already got the data entered and everything."

"Well, that's great."

"I do what I can. I try to contribute."

"OK," said Saul with a wan smile. "I appreciate your letting me know, but you should probably get back to work now."

At lunch, Sue sat with some of her co-workers. "This Rachel is driving me nuts," she said as she sat down. "Just because she's in charge of this electronic health records adoption committee, she hasn't given me an ounce of credit, even though I'm doing almost all of the work. If this place ever gets electronic medical records, they'll have me to thank for it."

"Why don't you talk to her about it?" said Alex, a co-worker, said.

"Like she talks to me? No way. I don't have a speaking relationship with one single medical assistant here, and that's fine with me. They all drive me nuts. I swear, Saul does the worst job in the world of hiring these people. He's clueless. If I didn't keep him informed, he wouldn't know half of what's going on."

Back in the unit, Sue ran into Rachel in the hallway and put on a big smile. "I got that data all compiled now," she told Rachel.

"Thanks! You told me that yesterday. I appreciate your help," said Rachel.

Sue lost the smile and headed toward Saul's office again, peeking through the glass. He waved her in.

"Did you need to talk to me again, Sue?" he asked.

"Well, I'm just a little bit concerned," she said. "I just ran into Rachel, and I'm not sure she understands the importance of compiling the test data. I mean, did she mention me in her report?"

"I don't really remember, Sue."

"I didn't think so. Saul, without that test data, this project is going nowhere. Are you sure Rachel is the right one for this job?"

"I'm confident in Rachel's ability," said Saul.

"Well, I wouldn't want to doubt your confidence in her, Saul, but I would keep a close eye on her if I were you."

QUESTIONS FOR THOUGHT AND REFLECTION

1. What do you think Sue's objectives are? Do you think she is going about it the correct way?
2. What kind of a working relationship does Sue have with her peers?
3. How would you describe Saul's opinion of Sue?
4. If you were Saul, how would you manage Sue?

⭐ EXPERIENTIAL EXERCISES

1. Think about the best and worst teachers you have had. What were the three best and three worst qualities they had?
2. Create a self-evaluation. Include all your accomplishments and achievements and the goals you hope to achieve for the next year.
3. Ask someone you know who is in a supervisory position to describe their ideal employee.

CROSS CURRENTS WITH OTHER SOFT SKILLS

THINKING CRITICALLY: Thinking skills are what managers are paid to have. You can interact with your supervisor more effectively by thinking critically, too (Chapter 8).

SPEAKING PROFESSIONALLY IN YOUR WORKPLACE: How you speak matters as much as what you say (Chapter 6).

LISTENING ACTIVELY: In your communications with your manager, listening is paramount (Chapter 4).

READING AND SPEAKING BODY LANGUAGE: You put yourself and your boss at ease by mirroring their body language (Chapter 4).

Financial Literacy

Managing Your Money

The safest way to double your money is to fold it over and put it in your pocket.

—Kin Hubbard

> ### LEARNING OBJECTIVE 4: MANAGING YOUR MONEY

- Establish a personal budget.
- Explain the difference between gross and net income.
- Plan for your retirement.
- Describe ways to build a good credit record and explain how your credit record is used.
- Discuss differences in types of student loans.
- Explain the process for making a loan decision.
- Develop a plan for getting out of debt.

How Do You Manage Your Money?

In your health care training program, you gained a great deal of knowledge and learned many different skills to prepare you for your new profession. However, most training programs do not teach you how to manage your personal finances. Being able to effectively manage your finances by budgeting and saving will help you achieve many of the goals you may have set for yourself, such as buying a new car, buying your first home, or paying off your student loans.

The way you manage your money is heavily influenced by how you grew up. We get many of our financial habits from our families and observing them manage their financial situations. For example, parents who provide good examples of frugality and saving money for the future are more likely to have children who are also good with money. Conversely, parents who live paycheck-to-paycheck and have a lavish lifestyle that exceeds their means are more likely to have children who are financially unstable.

Other factors that influence your financial decision-making are your personality and emotions. Some people are naturally good savers whereas others enjoy spending money and may find it difficult to control their money. You might have heard some people refer to themselves as "emotional spenders." These are people who shop or spend money when they are happy, sad, and even bored. As a result, it is easier for some people to make good financial decisions. Gaining financial knowledge by understanding your own budget, including how much you earn and how much you spend; learning about investments, loans, and debt; and setting clear financial goals will help you keep more of the money you have earned.

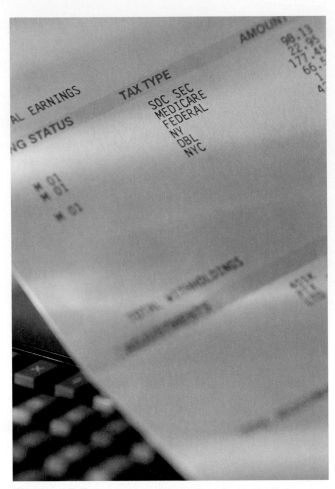

Figure 15.7 Itemization of deductions from a typical paycheck. (Copyright © thinkstock.com.)

← JOURNALING 15.4

- Who or what do you think has been the greatest influence on how you manage money? How would you describe their financial decision-making?
- Describe how you make financial decisions about your money. When do you like to shop? Are you able to save any money at the end of the month, or do you live paycheck-to-paycheck?

Your Paycheck

To begin to talk about money management, you need to understand what is included and taken out of your paycheck. When you got your first paycheck, you might have been surprised that it was not as much as you expected.

What you expected to make is called your *gross* salary, which is before any deductions are taken out. Your net salary is what you receive after deductions, which includes any employee benefits, Federal

Insurance Contributions Act (FICA) taxes, state and federal taxes, and a retirement savings plan, if applicable (Figure 15.7).

Taxes

Federal taxes are calculated as a percentage of your income. How much you pay is dependent on how many people you claim on your W-4 form, also called the Employee's Withholding Allowance Certificate. When you first get hired, you will be asked to complete this form, which will help determine how much federal income tax should be withheld from your pay.

The amount of your federal taxes may change, for example, based on the number of people you claim. For example, if you have children and you claim them when you filled out your W-4 form, less money will be taken from each paycheck. However, it is incorrect to think that the more claims you have, the more you will get to keep. Although you will be able to keep more per paycheck, you will most likely receive less tax refund at the end of the year when you complete your taxes, and you may even end up owing money for federal taxes. The same logic goes for withholding money from your paycheck. You will get less each pay period, but you will most likely receive a larger refund at the end of the year.

Some states collect income tax in addition to federal income tax. Some local governments may also impose an income tax, which is calculated based on state income tax.

Employee Benefits

One of the most valuable things that your employer can offer you, besides your salary, is employee benefits. When you are choosing a job or company, weighing employee benefits against net income is an important factor when deciding on different job offers. Benefits may differ widely from one company to the next. For example, smaller organizations and businesses may not be able to afford and provide fewer benefits.

When you receive a copy of the employee benefits package, read it carefully so you know what you are being offered. Typical employee benefits include:
* Paid vacation days
* Personal days (either paid or unpaid, sometimes called sick leave)
* Maternity/paternity leave (paid or unpaid)
* Education or training reimbursement
* Health insurance
* Retirement plan

In some cases, you may have a choice of several insurance plans. Often, the lower the premium, which is the amount you pay each month for the insurance policy, the higher the deductible, which is the amount you must pay for covered medical services before your insurance plan starts to contribute.

JOURNALING 15.5

■ At what age would you like to retire? Using the online retirement planning tools, how much money should you have saved by then? How much money would you have at retirement if you invested 6% of your income into a 4019(k) or IRA?
■ When you think about saving for retirement, what kind of lifestyle do you imagine is realistic after you stop working?

Establish a Personal Budget

Once you have a job and receive a regular paycheck, it is easy for someone to tell you, "Just save your money." But that may be difficult to do without an organized plan or proper tools. A few simple strategies are all you need to start taking control of your personal finances.

Step 1: Track and Monitor

The first step to financial responsibility is simply becoming aware of where your money goes. Start keeping track. Carry a small notebook with you and write down how you spend your money over the course of each day. Do not judge or second-guess yourself—just keep track. At this stage, avoid thinking of any spending as right or wrong. You want to be able to review your spending to identify what you spend your money on and what you see as valuable.

Make sure you include rent, food, utilities, medical costs, gas or bus money, clothing, childcare, and student loan payments. This may seem like a time-consuming exercise, but it is important to do it as accurately as possible.

Step 2: Review and Evaluate

At the end of documenting your expenditures each day for 1–2 weeks, you are ready to make your first assessment. Are you seeing a pattern of where you spend your money?

Most Americans spend an average of 25%–30% of their income on housing and 8%–12% on utilities. Food bills run 10%–15% of expenditures, and transportation or gas money is roughly 15%–20%. Health care and health insurance usually comprise 7%–10%. Entertainment for most Americans runs around 5% of overall income.

After the first week or two of tracking your spending, how does your spending compare with some of the general figures given above? Which category did you spend more on?

Step 3: Create a 1-Month Balance Sheet

In the next step of budget planning, you can start establishing your budget. There are many systems for doing this, including good software packages.

Using your most current paycheck that does not include any unpaid days, draw four columns on a sheet of paper. Title the first column "Date," the second "Money Available," the third "Expenses," and the fourth "Balance."

Include only the money you want as part of your monthly budget. Do not account for any money that you want to reserve for savings or an emergency fund. In general, after determining how much your expenditures are in Step 1, you should start saving 6–9 months of living expenses for emergencies. You should also calculate how long this will take you and how much money you should be deducting from your paycheck for this emergency fund.

Step 4: Do the Math

At the end of the first month, add up all the numbers under "Expenses" (third column) and subtract the total from the "Money Available" column (second column). This is your balance (fourth column), which is what you have left after 1 month's spending.

Step 5: Analyze Your Spending Patterns

How did you do? Hopefully, the balance in the fourth column at the end of the month is a positive number, suggesting that you make more than you spend. This is the position you want to be in, and you can put the excess money toward your emergency fund, savings, or retirement plan. However, if your balance is negative, this means you spend more than you make, and you will need to make some decisions about your spending.

When analyzing your spending, make sure you allocate money to cover the following in this order (Figure 15.8):

1. necessities—food, housing, utilities, health care, and transportation
2. emergency fund—6–9 months of living expenses
3. entertainment and incidentals—clothing, home repairs, etc.
4. savings

You might think that savings should come before entertainment and incidentals, but this is rarely practical. Everyone needs to relax and have a little fun on a regular basis. Your budget needs to be realistic and something that you will be able to do each month. If it is too rigorous, it is likely that you will abandon it.

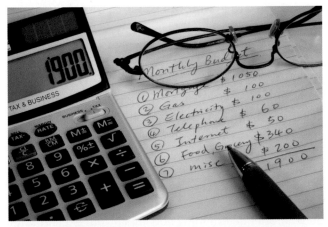

Figure 15.8 Estimate what you need to cover monthly expenses, then subtract that from your net salary for the month. Make saving for emergencies, retirement, entertainment, and incidental expenses your priorities for the balance. (Copyright © thinkstock.com.)

Step 6: Make Good Financial Choices

If you are tempted to overspend, stop and make choices. Most of the time if you have a reasonable income, even if it is not very high, you can manage to do *something* for fun. Would you rather buy this book or that CD? Do you want the mocha latte with your best friend, or would you rather chip in on the pizza party later? Often, you really can do any *one* thing you like. You just cannot afford to do them all!

Learn to separate wants from needs. Do you really need the expensive, name-brand shampoo, or is there a less expensive, plain-label product that is just as good? Have you tried the store-brand milk instead of the brand-name one you grew up with? Do you need the multicolored note pens for class, or will the cheap multipack do? Slowing down to make choices not only saves you money but also gives you the feeling of being in control (Figure 15.9).

Step 7: Set Your Financial Goals

Financial goal-setting—for the short term and long term—cannot be started soon enough. In the short term, write down your more immediate money goals. Do you need to save for books for next semester? For a prescription refill? Or can you afford to start setting money aside for a new smartphone? Set your priorities.

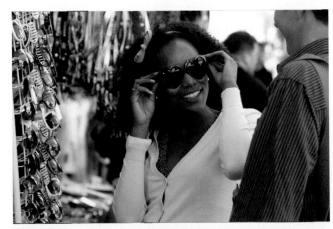

Figure 15.9 Slowing down to make choices not only saves you money but also gives you the feeling of being in control. (Copyright © thinkstock.com.)

In the long term, you will want to start building an emergency fund, something you can fall back on if you lose your job or have an accident. It is important to add money to your emergency fund every month until you have 6–9 months of living expenses. On average, it takes approximately 8 months for a person to find a new job.

Step 8: Open an Account and Follow Your Game Plan

Open a checking or savings account as soon as you can. Many banks have free accounts, but some accounts have nominal fees or require a minimum balance. This is a smart, easy, inexpensive way to keep track of your income and spending.

Bank accounts are helpful in many ways. They are like electronic piggy banks where you deposit money to save for the future. Keep in mind that a checking account is not the same as a savings account. A savings account offers interest earnings to inspire you to *keep* your money *in* the account.

What Is Credit and Do You Need It?

Neither a borrower nor a lender be.

—**William Shakespeare**

Credit is money that is borrowed now to purchase goods or services and is paid back later. The amount to be paid back may or may not include interest, depending on when you pay back the full amount of the borrowed money. How much credit you have depends on your credit score and credit history. The better or higher both are, the more trustworthy you are as a borrower and the more money you likely can borrow. However, a poor credit report and score can affect your ability to get a loan, rent an apartment, or even qualify for a job.

Credit Reporting and Score

Your credit report is created and kept by a company called a credit bureau, which studies patterns in your borrowing history to produce a profile of your performance and generates a credit score. Your credit report shows your bill payment history, current debt, and other financial information.

Your credit score is then calculated by your credit report, which is a number from 300 to 850. The higher the number, the better your credit. This means that if you have a credit score of 750, you may be able to qualify for a loan or be offered a credit card with a lower interest rate.

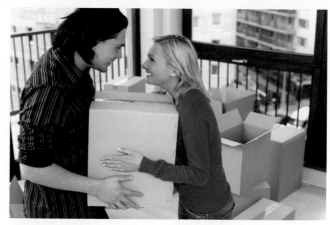

Figure 15.10 Good credit is often required for approval for employment or for leasing an apartment. (Copyright © thinkstock.com.)

It is difficult to make large purchases, such as a car or home, without credit. Thus, it will be important to carefully monitor your credit score and history and manage any loans and debts you have. The most important factors in establishing good credit are having a good payment history, specifically making payments on time; your debt-to-income ratio; and having a long history of credit. Try to pay the full amount on your credit card bill each month. This will require careful monitoring of what you charge. More debt on your credit card will negatively affect your credit score.

Banks and lenders are not the only agencies looking at your credit score. Insurance companies now assess your credit before deciding whether to insure you and when determining your rate. Good credit may also be necessary for approval for employment, leasing an apartment, or buying a car or house (Figure 15.10).

JOURNALING 15.6

- Calculate how much credit card debt you have. Based on your monthly balance, how long would it take you to pay off all your credit card balances?
- What are your credit card interest rates or annual percentage rates (APR)? If you have a balance on your credit cards, calculate how much interest you will accrue if you only pay the minimum balance.
- Do you know what your credit score is? Identify two ways you can improve your credit score.

? WHAT IF?

What if you had just one credit card that you only used for emergencies or purchases larger than $250? Would that change the way you spend money?

Never spend your money before you have it.

—Thomas Jefferson

Personal Loans

Depending on where you are in your life, you may already have taken out several loans for large purchases, such as your education, a car, or a home. Loans may be a necessity; however, they can create a lot of stress in your life. But, if you are selective in the loans you take out and prepare for them, you are more likely to manage them.

Student Loans

Many students must take out student loans to pay for their education. Depending on your situation, there are several kinds of educational loans available to you as a student. Thus, it is important to understand the differences in student loans to ensure the best rates and terms.

Federal student loans. The terms of these loans are subject to change and include limits on the amount you may borrow. They tend to be low-interest loans for people who can demonstrate significant financial need. Some federal student loans offer a *deferment*, which is the postponement of repayment until you graduate, with no accruing of interest charged to you during that time. In some cases, you may be eligible to apply for a *forbearance*, which is the postponement of repayment, usually due to financial hardship, but interest still accrues. Most federal student loans require complete repayment within 10 years, but there are usually a variety of repayment plans to choose from.

Private student loans. Students who do not qualify for federal education loans or need additional funds to pay for their education may be eligible for private loans. Private student loans often have higher interest rates than federal student loans; thus, they should only be used once options for federal student loans have been exhausted. Additionally, private student loans have some conditions and terms, such as requiring very good credit or a cosigner, that may make them difficult for some students to qualify.

Consolidation loans. These loans may be good, especially if you have credit card debts *and* student loans, because they enable you to combine two or more existing loans to create a new loan with a fixed interest rate, instead of one that may increase over time. Many graduates find consolidating their student loans to be a good option because it often gives a longer period of repayment, often 30 years to pay back the loan.

Student loans are a source of significant individual debt, which is not a good way to start out your professional life. So, when taking out a student loan, consider how much you will really need. It is important to pay student loans back to maintain your credit score. Defaulting on a loan can ruin your credit for decades. Further, student loans cannot be discharged when filing for bankruptcy.

The Five-Step Financial Decision Chain

As a rule, it is wisest not to borrow money unless, or until, you really need to. Before taking on any kind of loan, use the following five steps when making a financial decision. A car loan has been used as an example (Figure 15.11).

1. **Calculate** carefully how much you can afford to pay for a car. Be sure to take into account related expenses such as gas, oil, insurance, maintenance, and parking.

2. **Consider a cash-only purchase of a good used car first**. A used car costs a lot less than a new one, and a new car depreciates rapidly in value the moment you drive it off the lot. Buying a reliable used car saves you from that significant loss (Figure 15.12).

3. **If you decide you do need to take out a loan**, either apply for preapproval at a credit union, which usually offers the lowest interest rates, or see whether your current bank offers discounted loans for existing customers. Once you have this information, compare these rates with the dealer's rates before choosing.

4. **Whether you pay cash or take out a loan**, once you think you have found your car, invest in a

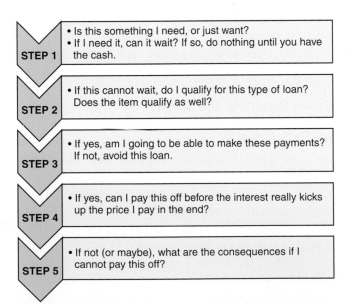

Figure 15.11 The Five-Step Decision Chain.

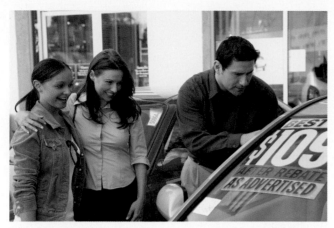

Figure 15.12 Buying a used car rather than a new one may be a good financial decision. (Copyright © thinkstock. com.)

prepurchase inspection by a reputable mechanic to get feedback on the car's condition.

5. **Finally, if you do take out a car loan**, pay it back as soon as possible. However, be careful and check to ensure that there is no penalty for paying back too soon. If there is such a penalty, weigh it against the interest you will be charged on the payment plan.

Managing Debt

What if you are already in debt? Go back to that balance sheet discussed earlier in the chapter. Sit down and make a plan for paying off your debts, 1 month at a time.

* Begin by weighing your income against those necessary expenses, and then look at your balance.
* From that information, assign whatever amount you can to paying back each of your debts. Do not be discouraged if you cannot pay that much at first. Getting out of debt will take time.
* Be sure to talk with your creditors. Explain your situation and express an honest desire to pay them back or try to negotiate a settlement.

Regardless of the payment plan or budget you choose, commit to a plan that you know you can adhere to. Be consistent and eventually you will develop a routine. A big step toward job readiness is understanding key concepts in personal finance. Armed with the skills and tools needed to create and maintain a budget, save money, and build both your savings and your credit record, you will be well equipped to take on the challenges of becoming an independent professional. Financial responsibility is only intimidating if you have never tried it before and do not have a plan. Once you start taking control of your money and planning your financial future, you will feel more empowered and self-confident.

Planning for Retirement

It is important for you to plan early for your retirement. Your employer may be large enough to offer you a retirement savings plan. There are many different types, with the most common ones being 401(k), individual retirement accounts (IRAs), and a pension plan.

A 401(k) plan is a retirement plan sponsored by your employer. It allows you to take a percentage of your paycheck each pay period to invest in a plan that may include different stocks, bonds, and money market investments. A 401(k) plan allows you to delay paying taxes on the amount of money you are deducting from your paycheck to put toward your retirement. This is called a tax deferment. However, once you begin withdrawing funds upon your retirement, you will start paying taxes on the amount you withdraw. Your employer may contribute a percentage toward your retirement in a 401(k) plan. For example, an employer will contribute or match up to 50% of your 6% deduction from your salary. If you contributed 6% of your $30,000 annual salary toward your 401(k), or $1800 for the year, your employer would contribute 50% of this amount, or $900.

Another common retirement plan is an IRA, which is an account set up at a financial institution that allows you to save for retirement. Unlike a 401(k) plan, this is not employer-based, and there is no contribution from your employer. However, it does allow you to deduct money from your income to lower your taxes or defer them until retirement.

A pension plan is a retirement fund sponsored by an employer. Pension plans are managed by the employer and pay out a steady income over the course of the retirement. There are generally two types of pension plans: either your employer contributes a fixed amount of money to your retirement plan each year or your employer bases its contribution to your account on the company's profits for that year. Pension plans are becoming less commonly offered as employee benefits because the cost of running pensions has escalated. Instead, many employers have started replacing them with 401(k)s.

There is a wealth of information when it comes to investing for retirement, and it can be overwhelming. But it is important to start early and learn how to save your money for retirement. Take advantage of the many great online resources for designing your own plan.

CASE STUDY 15.4
Getting Off the Tightrope

Ava does not have enough money to pay for the books for her dental assisting classes next semester. She picked up Chinese food last night before collecting her daughter from the babysitter and now is sitting down at the kitchen table wondering what to do. She calls her friend, Brigitte, to borrow money.

"Again?" Brigitte says. "I'm sorry, Ava, but I barely have enough money for rent this month."

Ava decides to call her brother, Jonah, and asks him to lend her some money.

After a long pause, Jonah sighs. "This time I'm charging you interest if you don't pay me back this month. I can't keep on doing this."

Ava is tired of this, too. She complains to her mother, who says, "That's just the way life is and part of being a grown-up. Your father and I were in the same situation many times and we had five children to raise."

"So, how did you do it, mom?" Ava asked.

"Well, we struggled for many years until we developed a budget. We figured out how much we earned and how much we had to spend each month. The hard part is sticking to it."

"I'm not even sure where to start, mom. Creating a budget sounds already so overwhelming."

Ava's mom helped Ava set up a budget based on how much she makes and all her expenses. Once her monthly balance was calculated, Ava said, "That's depressing. There's barely anything left at the end of the month."

"Well, that's only until you graduate and start to earn more money. But, in the meantime, look at your expenses. Is there anything you can cut out?"

"I don't know," Ava said, glancing over her budget.

"One of the things your father and I did was, we wrote down everything we bought for a week. Try it. I think you'll be surprised at how much you spend that you don't realize."

Over the next few weeks, Ava kept a diary of what she spent each day.

A few months later, Ava invited Brigitte over for lunch at her house. "So, how are things," she asked.

"Things are so much better and I'm less stressed than usual, especially about money."

"That's great! So, what are you doing differently now?" Brigitte asks.

"Well, I tracked how much money I was spending on things, and I was surprised at what I was buying. So, now I make my own coffee instead of buying it at the coffee shop, I pack my own lunches to take to school, and I try not to buy bottled water or sodas at the vending machines."

After a few months, Ava was saving enough that she could not only pay Jonah back but also had a little money left over.

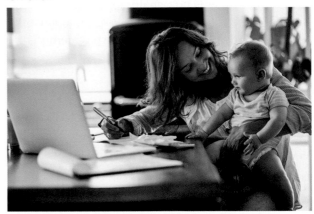

iStock.com/Drazen Zigic/1182823932

QUESTIONS FOR THOUGHT AND REFLECTION

1. What are the main advantages Ava has gained from keeping track of what she spends?
2. What were the root causes of Ava's money management problems?
3. What were some of the expenses Ava could eliminate from her budget?

A Different Path

Sophie was excited. She was about to start her new job as a surgical technologist. Before she starts her job, she is asked to complete several forms for new employees. She asked her older sister, Sara, to help her with completing the forms because she was not sure how to answer some of the questions.

"What's this?" Sophie says pointing at the W-4 form.

"It's a form that lets you control how much income tax is withheld from your paycheck each month," Sara tells her. "For example, you can deduct yourself and Jack as a dependent. You can have your employer take out less from your paycheck for taxes, so you have more money to use every month."

"I like that idea. But what if I keep too much?" Sophie asks.

"In that case, you may have to pay the rest at the end of the year when you do your income taxes."

"Yikes," Sophie says. "Who wants that? But what if I pay too much?"

"Well, you'll just get it back as a refund."

"Now *that's* smart!" Sophie says. "It's like a bonus at the end of the year. Take out the maximum!"

"Well, it's not really a bonus or free money," Sara tried to explain.

"Sign me up!" Sophie says. "Take out the max! Next question!"

Sara shrugs, then continues, "Okay, your employer is offering a 401(k) plan, which is for your retirement, and it looks like they'll match 50% up to 6% of your contribution."

"Retirement?" Sophie laughs. "Are you kidding? I'm only 25! I'm kind of young to start thinking about retirement, especially with a little boy to raise."

"Well, it's never too early to think about your retirement, and you're throwing money away that your employer is contributing," Sara says.

"I'm not thinking about retirement until I'm 50 years old."

QUESTIONS FOR THOUGHT AND REFLECTION

1. What are some of the mistakes Sophie is making in her planning for her taxes and retirement?
2. How would you help Sophie understand that a refund check is not a bonus or "free money"?
3. What potential savings Sophie has lost out on by not contributing to a 401(k) plan this year? Use real numbers as examples of what she's lost. How much money would she retire with if she started contributing at age 25 compared with age 50?

Goal-Setting for Debt

You have already acquired some strategic tools for (1) how to establish good credit, (2) how to save for the future in general, (3) how to get out of debt if you have it, and (4) how to plan for your retirement. The task now is to set your goals. Which of these four aspects of money management is most pertinent to your situation right now? Choose a reasonable, realistic goal that takes your financial needs into account, and then set down your plan of action.

Establishing good credit does more than give you more borrowing power when you need it. Landlords and employers now routinely run credit checks to see how reliable an applicant is. Taking responsibility for your financial obligations and your spending behaviors affects much more than just your financial bottom line.

Advancing in Your Profession

Your work is to discover your work and then with all your heart to give yourself to it.

—Buddha

LEARNING OBJECTIVE 5: ADVANCING IN YOUR PROFESSION

- Know the local, state, and national professional societies for your profession.
- Understand the benefits of society or association membership.
- Develop a networking plan within your profession.
- Access new research being performed and published in your profession.
- Leverage the resources of your profession to improve the quality of your work.

Through your education, you have joined a great profession. You have satisfied the criteria to graduate, may have obtained licensure or certification, and readied yourself to be hired in your chosen profession. You should be aware that your profession has an extensive network to support it, and you can tap into that network by learning more about your profession.

There are a number of professional societies and numerous journals and publications that support your profession. If you are not already aware of what they are, you should learn about as many organizations and publications as you can from your career services departments and co-workers in your field. If there are multiple options, you should determine which best meets your current and future needs. You may even consider joining multiple organizations or subscribing to multiple publications.

Professional Societies and Organizations

Try to join one of your professional societies or organizations. Although there are a few that are free, most require an annual membership fee to join. There are many benefits to joining a professional society or organization. Some of the benefits include discounts on certification examinations and renewals, conferences, free magazines and publications, and continuing education. Additionally, a professional society and organization keep you up to date about what is going on in your profession, emerging trends, specialties, regulations, and job opportunities. Making sure you are current on these issues and trends makes you a more valuable employee at work. A list of typical association membership benefits appears in Box 15.6.

Moreover, national professional societies and associations typically have state and local chapters or affiliates. Sometimes, membership in the state or local chapters comes with the membership fee for the

BOX 15.6

Typical Benefits of Society Membership

- Receive frequent newsletters or magazines updating you on developments in your profession
- Opportunity to attend national or state conventions
- Networking opportunity
- New products and services available for your profession
- Educational events and speeches from important people
- Latest developments in your professions
- Leadership development
- Fun and social events
- Discounts, including products and professional journals
- Job boards
- Certification preparation, examinations, and credentials
- Lobbying services for legislation that would benefit your profession
- Online bookstore
- Research and education grants

national organization; other times, a small additional fee is required. However, most of the benefits of the national organization can be accessed through your local affiliate, including meetings and networking.

JOURNALING 15.7

Based on your current health care profession, research the professional societies and organizations for your profession. How much does it cost to join, and what are the benefits? What is a conference or a meeting you would be interested in attending?

Licensure, Certification, and Continuing Education

One of the main functions of a professional organization is to offer and manage continuing education, licensure, certification, recertification, and specialty certification. Almost every health care profession requires a certain amount of continuing education courses to be completed in a period of time, usually every year or every 3 years, in order to maintain your license or certification.

Additionally, many health care professions require continuing education (CE) courses to maintain your license or certification. Your professional organization usually manages the certification and offers CE, endorses others who offer it, or both. In some cases, a state board or organization will manage a licensure, such as for nursing or massage therapy. But the CE courses may still be taken through the professional organization.

When seeking a renewal of your certification or license, you will be required to submit proof that you completed the required amount of CE units. CE units are usually obtained through the completion of classroom or online courses or attending professional conferences. Requirements vary by profession, so you should make sure you know your profession's requirements and the agencies or associations that manage your certification or licensure.

WHAT IF?

What are the different licensure and certifications offered for your profession? What are the requirements to get them, and what are the renewal requirements?

Professional Networking

One of the most valuable activities any health care professional can pursue is networking. Networking takes the pleasures of socialization and friendship to

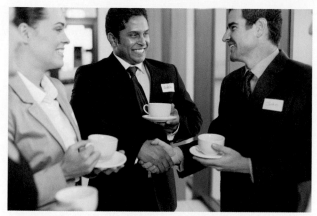

Figure 15.13 Two conference participants greet each other during a networking event. (Copyright © istock.com.)

⊙ JOURNALING 15.8

Create a professional networking plan. Think about the people you currently know and would like to connect with professionally. Locate and connect with them on a professional network website, such as LinkedIn.

❓ WHAT IF?

What if you received an invitation or a friend request on your personal social media site from a co-worker or supervisor? You often post personal comments and photos on your personal site. Would you accept their request? Why or why not?

a broader level. Networking is building on and maintaining relationships with people to help advance your career and professional goals. When you attend professional activities outside of your workplace, whether at a convention or just volunteering at a community center, you have opportunities to meet new colleagues and friends that may help connect you to even more people (Figure 15.13). You already have your instructors, former classmates, and co-workers as professional connections. You should be encouraged to use them, and it will be likely that you will connect with even more people.

Now more than ever, networking is an extremely important part of your professional life. If you have a strong network, you can get answers to and opinions on clinical issues, discuss the important issues in your profession, seek information, and even look for new jobs, consulting engagements, and career specialization paths.

Another common method of networking is establishing a professional presence or "personal brand" on a professional social media site, such as LinkedIn. It is free and easy to do. You simply complete a profile on yourself that includes your educational and work experience. Typically, you can include a photograph of yourself; if you add a photograph, make sure it is professional. Once your profile is online, others can search for you, and you can search for others. The idea is to facilitate networking. For instance, if you are attending a convention in an unfamiliar city, you can locate and contact local professionals there who may be able to recommend restaurants or local attractions. If you are looking for a job, you may be able to leverage your contacts to refer you to others with information about open positions.

Publications and Research

Medical knowledge is always advancing and changing. These changes are often reported in journals and other publications; many of them are specific to your profession, such as *CMA Today* for medical assistants, *Journal of AHIMA* for health information management professionals, and *The Surgical Technologist*. These journals and publications are valuable tools to keep you up to date on new trends and information in your profession.

You may receive a journal as a part of your membership in a professional society organization. Otherwise, you may have to purchase a subscription, which may be costly. However, most university and hospital libraries carry several different professional journals and publications. If you find a journal that you particularly like, you should consider subscribing to it. Many subscriptions usually include electronic access to searchable archives of past issues, making your subscription more valuable. Thousands of scientific and health-related journals are published around the world, almost all of them in English.

Additionally, the Internet offers a wealth of resources. Sites range from government agencies to organizations and foundations to research labs and facilities. You might find additional sources, like blogs or Twitter feeds. Bookmark these sites as you come across them, adding them to a professional folder you keep in your web browser. Then make a schedule to review them occasionally, so you can benefit from the information they offer.

Lifelong learning is the norm in the health care professions. Create a plan and make a commitment to ensure that your learning is continually updated by taking advantage of all the resources covered in this chapter. The more successful you are at maintaining current knowledge of your profession, the more valuable you will be to your employer and to your patients or clients. Moreover, committing yourself to your profession better positions you for advancement, success, and personal satisfaction in your career.

CASE STUDY 15.5
Network Chicago

Rinda Khalif was a speech pathologist in search of a new job. Her husband, Ayman, a pathologist, had just been recruited to a new position in Chicago. They would be moving there at the end of the summer with their two preschool-age children, Randy and Joe. Neither Ayman nor Rinda was familiar with Chicago, and they did not know anybody there. Rinda just knew they would love Chicago, but she was worried about finding a job in a new city.

Rinda subscribed to the *Chicago Tribune* online and registered with the Human Resources Department at the hospital where Ayman would work. She created an attractive resume and started applying for jobs. Despite her efforts, she had yet to find a job and she was getting frustrated. But, instead of giving up, she decided to be more proactive and started using her own professional network.

She wrote emails to her professional contacts, explaining her situation and asking them to keep her in mind if they became aware of any openings. She did not expect this to help much, but she wanted to cast a wide net.

She also remembered that she had three contacts in the Chicago area. She had been introduced to them at separate functions at last year's convention of the American Speech-Language-Hearing Association (ASHA) in Philadelphia. She emailed them all to reintroduce herself and explain what she was looking for. They all agreed to help her and said they would make some inquiries on her behalf. More importantly, they shared information about the area, specifically which neighborhoods and school systems to explore. She sent them her resume electronically.

One of them reminded her of job postings on the ASHA website. When she went to the website, in the searchable job database, she saw seven new positions she could apply for.

Rinda updated her LinkedIn profile and researched her contacts, and she found that five of them were located in Chicago. She decided to send them a message. One of her contacts, Jameel, replied that she knew someone who worked for the Chicago Public Schools Human Resources Department and that she would contact her on Rinda's behalf.

Several weeks later, Rinda got a message through her LinkedIn from a staff member from the Chicago Public Schools Human Resources Department to schedule a time to talk on the phone.

QUESTIONS FOR THOUGHT AND REFLECTION

1. In what ways did Rinda leverage her network to find a job? What else could she have done?
2. What different resources did Rinda use to job search?
3. Do you think health care professionals have better networking and job search opportunities than other professionals?

A Different Path

Caitlyn Day had gotten funding from her new employer to attend a regional meeting of the American Association of Professional Coders (AAPC). It was held nearby in Nashville, and she had been to the Gaylord Opryland Hotel facility many times on family vacations. The registration fee was only $325 for almost 3 days of education and fun events. Specifically, Caitlyn's employer wanted her to learn more about the upcoming ICD-11 implementation and any updates in health care reform. Caitlyn's employer asked her to make a presentation to the coding staff when she got back.

Caitlyn also had some personal goals. She wanted to get an update on what was going on at the AAPC, and she wanted to learn more about specialty certifications. She also wanted to start establishing her professional network.

The first night featured a big networking reception with a sundae buffet. Caitlyn made friends with some young women from Knoxville. When the reception was over, they decided to head down to the bars for country music and dancing. It was after midnight by the time Caitlyn found her room and collapsed into the bed.

The maid's knock on the door woke her up. What time was it? Almost 10:00? She had missed the "State of the AAPC" breakfast session and the ICD-11 update. Caitlyn sobered up quickly, showered, and dressed. She found the next available session on coding for reimbursement for conditions related to childhood obesity, which, much to her relief, was a focus at her practice. She took copious notes. Later sessions bored her though, and she could barely keep awake. At the afternoon break, she ran into the girls from Knoxville again. Even though she knew she should not, she found herself agreeing to meet them at 7:00 for drinks and dancing again.

Before she went out, she checked the following day's events in the program. The Health Care Reform panel was at 9:00 a.m., which she thought would not be too early and she should be able to attend that. There was nothing else that interested her until the exhibit hall opened at noon.

Caitlyn laid out the clothes she would wear the next day. She had hoped to meet more people than just her new Knoxville friends, but she could not think of a way to gracefully excuse herself.

The next day, she overslept again and barely made the exhibit opening at noon. She had no idea what she was going to say about ICD-11 and Health Care Reform because she had missed both sessions. She wondered how she could turn her childhood obesity notes into a respectable presentation. She spent the next hour collecting as many promotional items as she could scrounge from the vendors' booths. She filled up a whole canvas bag. At least she could pass this stuff out when she gave her presentation, whatever that would be.

QUESTIONS FOR THOUGHT AND REFLECTION

1. Did Caitlyn set goals for the regional meeting? Were they the right ones?
2. Where did Caitlyn falter in her planning?
3. How could Caitlyn have fun but still accomplish her goals at the regional meeting?

 EXPERIENTIAL EXERCISES

1. Identify an influential person in your profession and reach out to them via the person's professional online site.
2. Familiarize yourself with all the associations and journals that support your profession.
3. Plan to attend a local professional meeting.
4. Find five sources of continuing education credits for your profession.
5. Bookmark governmental sites related to your professions.

 CROSS CURRENTS WITH OTHER SOFT SKILLS

SETTING GOALS AND PLANNING ACTIONS: Connecting with your profession requires appropriate goals and careful planning (Chapter 13).
EXUDING OPTIMISM, ENTHUSIASM, AND POSITIVITY: Connecting with your profession is a forward-looking, career-developing move (Chapter 8).

Go Forth and Prosper

Not knowing when the dawn will come, I open every door.
—Emily Dickinson

You have learned many skills, so far, to help you build your career and advance in your profession. But how do you know if you are happy or successful in your career? If you do not define what career success means to you, you will never know when you achieve it.

How you define career success is a very personal definition. For some people, it may be having a degree and a title, whereas for others it may be making more money. It is important to define what career success is to you; otherwise, how do you know if you are happy in it and what direction you may need to take it?

When defining your career success, focus on what is important to you, which may change over time. Early in your career, you may define success by being able to build a good relationship with co-workers and supervisors and being proficient and mastering the skills in your profession. Over time, you may want to be promoted and advance in your organization, make more money, to be respected in your profession, or learn more skills and get more education.

You are embarking on a brand-new phase of life. Start the rest of your life right now by using what you have learned in this book to set goals for yourself, make a concrete plan to achieve them, and become the best person and professional you can be. Commit now to setting high standards for yourself at work and in your life. With a solid plan in place, you will meet your targets. Your success and happiness depend on this plan and your commitment to stick to it.

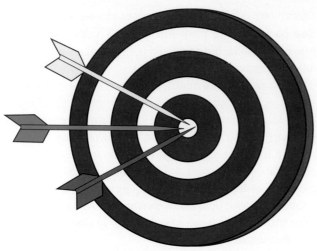

Looking toward your goals by following a plan will help you hit your targets.

Plan for Career Success

Some of the best steps to achieving career success you have already learned in this book. Box 15.7 lists some reminders of best practices that you have learned.

BOX 15.7

Best Practices to Achieve Career Success

- Choose to have a positive attitude.
- Increase your value to your employer.
- Create a professional network.
- Gain the trust of your co-workers and employer.
- Take accountability and ownership in what you do.
- Be your own evaluator.
- Be ready to learn.
- Set goals to achieve.
- When identifying problems, create solutions.

If you integrate these and other positive practices into your work life, and you have good clinical and work skills, you will be a highly valued employee and will enjoy your work. You will be appreciated by your patients and your supervisor, and you will make friends among your co-workers.

 EXPERIENTIAL EXERCISES

1. Define and list what makes you happy and what is important in your life. Prioritize them by ranking them, starting with #1 as the most important. How do your priorities affect your career success? Are they the same or different?
2. List five different career paths that you may be interested in. What are their job responsibilities? What kind of education and advanced training are required for these professions?

CROSS CURRENTS WITH OTHER SOFT SKILLS

ADOPTING A POSITIVE MENTAL ATTITUDE: Adopting a positive attitude will take you far (Chapter 2).

References

Benton DA. *Executive charisma*. New York: McGraw-Hill; 2003:22.

Credit Reports and Scores. USA.gov. https://www.usa.gov/credit-reports.

How the Poor, the Middle Class, and the Rich Spend Their Money. *Money* at NPR.org. http://www.npr.org/sections/money/2012/08/01/157664524/how-the-poor-the-middle-class-and-the-rich-spend-their-money.

Parents Are Likely to Pass Down Good and Bad Financial Habits to Their Kids. T. Rowe Price Group, Inc. at CISION PR Newswire. https://www.prnewswire.com/news-releases/t-rowe-price-parents-are-likely-to-pass-down-good-and-bad-financial-habits-to-their-kids-300428414.html.

INDEX

Page numbers followed by "f" indicate figures, "t" indicate tables, and "b" indicate boxes.

Clarifying, during listening process, 131
Claustrophobia, as anxiety, 57
Cleanliness. *See* Personal hygiene
Clinical Laboratory Improvement Act (CLIA) of 1988, 323*b*
Closed questions, 168*t*
Cloud computing, 174
Cognitive psychology, in anxiety, 58
Collaborating, in conflict situations, 142, 142*b*
Color code writing approach, 87
Combination resume, 245–246, 245*f*, 246*f*
Commitment, to job search, 222–223, 222*b*
Common ethics, 328
Communication, 208
  behavioral interview questions for, 265*t*
  body language. *See* Body language
  conflict, 142–143
  direct, 123, 123*f*
  electronic, 86–87
    blogs, twitter, and digital communication, 87
    emails, 86–87, 87*b*
  in health care, 117–138
  interference with, 168*t*
  listening skills, and conflict resolution, 144
  nonverbal, 79–80, 80*b*, 168*t*
  skills, during job interview, 270–273
  speaking professionally in workplace. *See* Speaking professionally
  with special groups of patients, 129–138, 129*b*, 138*b*
    Alzheimer's disease, dementia, and other organic brain diseases, 135–138, 135*b*
    case study on, 136*b*–137*b*
    co-workers from different generations, 135–138, 136*t*, 138*b*
    elderly patients, 135
    hearing loss, 129–132
    with limited English proficiency, 133–134, 134*b*

Communication (*Continued*)
    patients who are deaf or hard of hearing, 130–131, 130*f*, 131*b*
    small children, 134–135, 134*f*
    speech impairments, 133
    visually impaired, 132
  and trust, 99–100, 100*b*, 100*f*
  verbal, 78–79, 79*b*, 168*t*
  writing skills. *See* Writing
Compact discs (CDs), 174
Compensation, calculation of, 287
Competence
  cultural
    case study, 113*b*–114*b*
    definition of, 108, 108*b*
    examples of influences, 108*b*
    in health care, 112–115, 112*b*, 113*f*
    in United States, 108
    valuing, 108–115, 108*b*, 115*b*
  dressing to reflect, 308
  and trust, 99, 101*f*
Competing, in conflict situations, 141–142
Compliance plan, 325
Compromising
  in conflict situations, 141, 141*b*
  low self-esteem and, 52*b*
Computer-assisted job interviews, 277
Computer literacy, 174–175, 174*b*
Computers, in job interview, 277
Concentration, during observation, 120
Confidence, 54
Confidential calls, 92, 93*f*
Confidentiality, 301, 329–334, 333*b*
  case study on, 332*b*
  externship, 199, 199*b*
  general, 331–334, 332*f*
  Health Information Portability and Accountability Act of 1996, 330–331
  objective for, 329*b*
Conflict, 5, 5*f*
  case study on, 146*b*–147*b*
  and dealing with challenging people, 148–155, 148*b*, 153*b*, 154*b*
  identifying sources of, 142–144, 142*b*

Conflict (*Continued*)
    communication conflict, 142–143
    economic and resource conflict, 143
    power conflict, 144
    relationship conflict, 143–144, 143*f*
    values conflict, 144
  learning from, 145*b*
  managing and resolving, 139–140, 139*b*, 148*b*
    self-awareness, 140
    strategies for, 140
  and problem behaviors
    case study on, 154*b*
    in co-workers, 149, 153*b*, 153*f*
    in patients, 152–153, 153*b*, 153*f*
  strategies for managing. *See* Conflict resolution
  Thomas-Kilmann Conflict Mode Instrument, 140, 141*f*
  at work, sources of, 142*b*
Conflict resolution, 140–142
  act as third-party mediator, 144
  change your response, 144
  checking impulse control, 144
  evidence-based decision making, 145–148
  exchanging ideas, 145
  learning from, 145*b*
  learning how to listen, 144
  personal goals, 144
  recognizing and resolving, 140
  reframing in, 144
  setting positive example, 145, 145*f*
  skills, 144–148
  strategies for, 140
Conscious bias, 111, 111*b*
Consent, 328–329
Consolidation loans, 362
Contact, job interview and, 268, 269*b*
Continuing education (CE), 366
Continuous positive airway pressure (CPAP) device, 70
Control
  lack of, influencing your attitude, 4
  locus of, 63–64, 63*f*

Control (*Continued*)
  of responses to challenging
    people, 149
Controlled Substances Act (CSA),
  323b
Conversations, 123, 123f
  professional behavior and,
    300–301, 301f
Coping skills
  and anxiety. *See* Anxiety
  of manager/supervisor, 355–357
Cornell note-taking system, 161–
    162, 163f
Courtesy
  during interview, 268
  professional behavior and, 303,
    303f
Cover letters in, 250–253, 250b,
    253b
    for advertised position, 251,
      251b, 251f, 253f
    for inquiry, 252–253, 254f
    for unadvertised opening, 251
COVID pandemic, work at home
    due to, 36
Credentials, resume, 241
Credibility
  and dependability. *See*
    Dependability
  and speaking professionally, 78
Credit, 361–362
  checking credit score, 361–362
  establishment of good credit,
    361
Credit score, 361
  checking of, 361, 361f
Critical thinking, 119–120, 119b,
    346b, 357b
  power of observation, 120, 120b
  and problem-solving, 119
  requirement, 119
  skills, 119, 119b
  steps to improve, 120b
Criticism
  accepting, 195
  low self-esteem and, 52b
  and trust, 122
Cultural competence
  benefits of diversity, 108–109
    performance and innovation,
      109
    perspective and experience,
      109

Cultural competence (*Continued*)
    pluralism, 109
  case study, 113b–114b
  definition of, 108, 108b
  examples of influences, 108b
  in health care, 112–115, 112b,
    113f
  skills building for, 113b
  understanding intolerance and
    discrimination, 109–111
    conscious and unconscious
      bias, 111, 111b
    prejudice and bias, 110–111
    stereotyping, 109–110
  in United States, 108
  valuing, 108–115, 108b, 115b
  workplace diversity, 111–112,
    112b
Culture, professional behavior
    and, 300
Customer service skills,
    behavioral interview
    questions for, 265t

D
Daily planner, 14–16
Debt, 363
  goal-setting for, 365
Decision-making, problem solving
    and, 119
Deductions, from gross
    salary, 358
Deep breathing
  controlling anger, 42
  relaxation, 59, 59b
Deferment, of federal student
    loans, 362
Dementia, communicating
    patients with, 135–138, 135b
Dental hygiene, 314–315, 314b
Deodorant, 314
Dependability, 21–25, 21b
  behaviors associated with, 21
  being positive example for
    others, 23–25, 23f
  being trustworthy and reliable,
    22–23
  case study on, 23b–24b, 25b
  definition and importance of,
    21, 22b
  punctuality, 21–22, 22f
  steps to building trust and, 22b
Desensitization, for anxiety, 180

Diagnostic services, 298t
Digital communication, 87
Direct consent, 329
Direct conversations, 123, 123f
Discretion, 329–334, 333b
  case study on, 332b
  general confidentiality, 331–334,
    332f
  Health Information Portability
    and Accountability Act of
    1996, 330–331
  objective for, 329b
Discrimination, in workplace,
    305b
Disposable gowns and gloves,
    as Universal Precautions,
    309–310, 310f
Distraction, listening through, 124
Diversity
  benefits of, 108–109
    performance and innovation,
      109
    perspective and experience,
      109
    pluralism, 109
  in United States, 108
  workplace, 111–112, 112b
Diving board writing approach,
    88–90
Doctor, 296
Doctorate degree, 296
Doctor of Chiropractic (DC), 296,
    297f
Doctor of Osteopathic Medicine
    (DO), 296
Documentation. *See also* Charting;
    Writing
  accurately and timely, 27
  of job search, 223–224
  in teams, 347b
Document, resume and, 248–249
Dress code, 191–192, 191f, 192b,
    310
Dressing, for success, 307–313,
    308b, 310f, 312b–313b
  case study on, 311b–312b
  casual Fridays and, 310, 310f
  everyday professional dress,
    308–313, 308b, 308f
  for first impression, 310–313
  footwear in, 309
  jewelry and body adornments
    in, 309